The Ultimate Guide to Passing Clinical Medicine Finals

MOHAMMED FAYSAL MALIK

BSc (Hons), AICSM, MBBS
CT2 Anaesthetics, London Deanery

ASIYA MAULA

BSc (Hons), MBBS, MRCS(Eng)
Academic GP Registrar, East Midlands Deanery

and

DOMINIC GREENYER

BSc (Hons), MBBS, MRCP(UK)
GP Registrar, East Midlands Deanery

Foreword by
MAURICE A SMITH

Associate Director of Medical Education
Consultant Physician in Geriatric Medicine, Queens Hospital, Romford, Essex
Honorary Senior Clinical Lecturer, Queen Mary's College, University of London

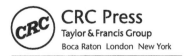

CRC Press
Taylor & Francis Group
Boca Raton London New York

CRC Press is an imprint of the
Taylor & Francis Group, an **informa** business

First published 2012 by Radcliffe Publishing Ltd.

Published 2019 by CRC Press
Taylor & Francis Group
6000 Broken Sound Parkway NW, Suite 300
Boca Raton, FL 33487-2742

© 2012 by Mohammed Faysal Malik, Asiya Maula and Dominic Greenyer
CRC Press is an imprint of Taylor & Francis Group, an Informa business

No claim to original U.S. Government works

ISBN-13: 978-1-84619-524-2 (pbk)

Visit the Taylor & Francis Web site at
http://www.taylorandfrancis.com

and the CRC Press Web site at
http://www.crcpress.com

Mohammed Faysal Malik, Asiya Maula and Dominic Greenyer have asserted their right under the Copyright, Designs and Patents Act 1988 to be identified as the authors of this work.

Every effort has been made to ensure that the information in this book is accurate. This does not diminish the requirement to exercise clinical judgement, and neither the publisher nor the authors can accept any responsibility for its use in practice.

British Library Cataloguing in Publication Data

A catalogue record for this book is available from the British Library.

Typeset by Darkriver Design, Auckland, New Zealand

Printed in the UK by Severn, Gloucester on responsibly sourced paper

 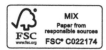

Contents

Foreword

For countless years, generations of medical students have nervously anticipated their final examinations with much understandable trepidation – the culmination of at least five years of intensive academic effort.

Despite the increasing pressure on the typical medical school curriculum and the ever-burgeoning complexity of modern clinical medicine, medical students, as they approach finals, still need to have the ability to convince their examiners that they are proficient in the basic clinical skills and methods. This book, with its relaxed user-friendly style, not only summarises the knowledge base required, but also gives very much more to the student in helping him or her to be confident and well-prepared before facing the final examinations in clinical medicine. Virtually all the underpinning topics of clinical medicine are covered, together with valuable and concise hints and tips on how to convey the unmistakable impression to the examiners that the student knows what he or she is doing. Hopefully, the student will be encouraged to radiate a professional attitude and display a manner consistent with being a safe, reliable and dependable doctor to boot.

In the text there are also frequent and possibly welcome interruptions to the knowledge narrative with 'authors' top tips' and the occasional examiner's comments so that the reader never feels overwhelmed by the myriad of facts necessary to be comprehended and committed to memory. Another thoughtful aspect of the work is the emphasis on examination etiquette, in particular displaying courtesy to all concerned, especially to the patients who give up their time so willingly to help train the doctors of the future.

The authors of this book are three experienced doctors in the latter stages of their postgraduate training who have carefully and wisely pooled their collective knowledge and experience in preparing students for finals in clinical medicine. They have masterfully distilled the essentials for the benefit of their readership. Although principally aimed at final-year students their text will be of interest and benefit to all students from the third year upwards. Furthermore, many Foundation Year 1 doctors will continue to find the medical knowledge contained therein useful as they struggle to cope with the many tasks and impositions on their time once qualified.

The book also includes a thought-provoking chapter on topics such as ethical dilemmas, communication skills with patients and their relatives/carers, factors which are so necessary in these modern times. The book sensibly ends with an important chapter on radiology, clinical procedures and data interpretation which will be both useful for finals and actual clinical practice. Final-year students and other colleagues can consider themselves fortunate to have access to such a well laid out and concise work to assist them. I commend this book to all who read it and hope it will help bring them closer to the success they deserve as they reach this important milestone in their medical careers.

Maurice A Smith
Associate Director of Medical Education
Consultant Physician in Geriatric Medicine, Queens Hospital, Romford, Essex
Honorary Senior Clinical Lecturer, Queen Mary's College, University of London
June 2012

Preface

The key to passing finals is not a secret: adequate preparation and the ability to think logically and speak clearly are all hallmarks of a successful candidate. This book is aimed at teaching final-year students how to tackle the hurdle that is clinical finals. Having organised a successful revision course as well as recently gone through finals ourselves, we have learnt many things as teachers, and this revision guide is the culmination of our efforts. Whilst we do not aim to teach you detailed medical knowledge for written finals, we do hope you will find the advice in this book invaluable to help prepare you for clinical finals, both as a study guide in the final weeks prior to the exam as well as a last-minute revision aid en route to the examination hall.

Objective structured clinical examinations (OSCEs) have now become integrated into medical school finals, so it is important students are well versed in tackling them. Although a degree of luck is required and well appreciated by everyone, there is no substitute for hard work and dedication in the last few weeks. Finals will be a stressful time; however, just remember that once it is over and if hard work is put in for preparation, you will pass and have a sense of achievement. Remember, a well-prepared student takes the initiative to create learning opportunities and propel themselves towards qualification; we find that the better prepared you are, the luckier you become.

Finally, we would like to take this opportunity to wish you all the best for your exams.

MF Malik
A Maula
D Greenyer
June 2012

About the authors

Mohammed Faysal Malik qualified from Imperial College School of Medicine in 2007. Having completed his Foundation Programme training in the North East Thames Deanery, he is currently in core anaesthetic training in London.

Asiya Maula qualified from St Bartholomew's and the Royal London School of Medicine and Dentistry in 2007. Having completed her Foundation Programme training in the North East Thames Deanery, she initially started training in core surgery before moving onto her current training as an academic GP registrar in Nottingham whilst also completing a postgraduate master's in public health.

Dominic Greenyer also qualified from St Bartholomew's and the Royal London School of Medicine and Dentistry in 2007. He completed his Foundation Programme training in the North East Thames Deanery and subsequent core medical training in East Midlands. He is currently working as a GP registrar in East Midlands Deanery.

All three authors have presented at numerous meetings regionally, nationally and internationally, as well as having been published in several peer-reviewed journals. Their teaching record includes competitive selection during their undergraduate years as a mentor for sixth-form students completing exams, the successful organisation and management of a finals revision course, formal training in teaching methodology and theory, as well as teaching statistics and epidemiology to fellow postgraduate registrars. They have also successfully published a companion textbook, *The Ultimate Guide to Surgical Clinical Finals* (Radcliffe Publishing; 2011), a surgical finals revision guide aimed at preparing the student for surgical OSCEs in MBBS finals.

Acknowledgements

The authors would like to acknowledge the invaluable specialist input in reviewing and making suggestions in their respective fields of expertise for this revision guide, from the following individuals:

Dr Javed Ehtisham
Consultant Cardiologist, Kettering General Hospital

Dr Debashish Das MD, MRCP(UK)
Consultant Hepatologist and Gastroenterologist, Trust Lead for Hepatology, Kettering General Hospital

Dr Mike Pierides BSc, MBChB, MRCP
Specialist Registrar Diabetes and Endocrinology, University Hospitals Leicester (UHL)

The authors would like to give special thanks to the following:
- Muzaffar and Uzmah Qureshi, the illustrators, for their excellent line drawings.
- Rownaq and Numann Malik for their patient acting roles in the clinical examination skills photographs.

The medical students whom we have had the pleasure of teaching over the many years since graduating, and our consultant mentors whose guidance, advice and support during our training has been invaluable.

Finally, we would like to thank Radcliffe Publishing for giving us the opportunity to publish this textbook, in particular Gillian Nineham, whose patience and understanding has provided us with the opportunity to complete this manuscript to the fullest of our ability.

List of permissions

The figures from the following books have been reproduced by kind permission of the publisher Churchill Livingstone, ©Elsevier:

Corne J, Carrol M, Brown I, Delany D. *Chest X-Ray Made Easy*. 2nd ed. 1999.
p 22, e; Section 6.4

Jackson SA, Thomas RM. *Cross-Sectional Imaging Made Easy*. 1st ed. 2005.
p 22, Figure 2.4

Chawla HB. *Ophthalmology: a symptom-based approach*. 3rd edition. 1999.
p 67, Figure 8.12
p 69, Figure 9.1
p 76, Figure 9.7
p 168, Figure 23.2
p 169, Figure 23.3
p 170, Figure 23.4

Munro JF, Campbell IW. *Macleod's Clinical Examination*. 10th ed. 2000.
p 58, Figure 2.41

The figures from the following books have been reproduced by kind permission of the publisher PasTest, ©PasTest Ltd:

Wasan R, Grundy A, Beese R. *Radiology Casebook for Medical Students*. 1st ed. 2000.
p 17, Figure 17
p 19, Figure 19

Feather A, Visvanathan R, Lumley JSP. *OSCEs for Medical Undergraduates, Volume 1*. 1st ed. 1999.
p 64, Figure 3Cii
p 70, Figure 3.13d
p 71, Figure 3.13e

Kelly P. *MRCP3 Practice Questions*. 1st ed. 2005.
p 78, figure on page; Ophthalmology Section, Case 4

List of abbreviations

The following abbreviations have been used throughout this book.

A&E	accident and emergency	CK	creatine kinase
AAA	abdominal aortic aneurysm	CKD	chronic kidney disease
ABC	airway breathing circulation	CLL	chronic lymphocytic leukaemia
ABG	arterial blood gas	CML	chronic myeloid leukaemia
ABPI	ankle brachial pressure index	CMV	Cytomegalovirus
ACEi	ACE inhibitor	COPD	chronic obstructive pulmonary
ACL	anterior cruciate ligament		disease
ACTH	adrenocorticotropic hormone	CRH	corticotropin-releasing hormone
AD	autosomal dominant	CRP	C-reactive protein
AF	atrial fibrillation	CSF	cerebrospinal fluid
ALP	alkaline phosphatase	CT	computed tomography
ALS	advanced life support	CVA	cerebrovascular accident
ALT	alanine transaminase	CVP	central venous pressure
ANA	antinuclear antibodies	CX	crossmatch
ANCA	antineutrophil cytoplasmic	CXR	chest X-ray
	antibody	DEXA	dual-energy x-ray absorptiometry
AP	anteroposterior	DIPJ	distal interphalangeal joint
APTT	activate partial thromboplastin	DKA	diabetic ketoacidosis
AR	aortic regurgitation; autosomal	DMARD	disease modifying anti-rheumatic
	recessive		drug
ARB	angiotensin receptor blocker	DoH	Department of Health
ARDS	adult respiratory distress	DRE	digital rectal exam
	syndrome	DSA	digital subtraction angiogram
AS	aortic stenosis	DVLA	Driver and Vehicle Licensing
ASD	atrial septal defect		Agency
ASIS	anterior superior iliac spine	DVT	deep vein thrombosis
AST	aspartate aminotransferase	EBV	Epstein–Barr virus
ATLS	advanced trauma life support	ECF	extracellular fluid
AV	aortic valve; atrioventricular	ECG	electrocardiogram
AvF	arteriovenous fistula	EEG	electroencephalography
BCC	basal cell carcinoma	EMG	electromyogram
BM	Boehringer Mannheim	ENT	ear, nose and throat
BNP	B-type natriuretic peptide	ERCP	endoscopic retrograde
BOO	bladder outflow obstruction		cholangiopancreatogram
BP	blood pressure	ESM	ejection systolic murmur
BPH	benign prostatic hyperplasia	ESR	erythrocyte sedimentation rate
BTS	British Thoracic Society	EUA	examination under anaesthesia
CABG	coronary artery bypass graft	EWTD	European Working Time
CCF	congestive cardiac failure		Directive
CD	Crohn's disease	FAP	familial adenomatous polyposis

FAST	focused assessment sonogram in trauma	KUB	kidneys, ureters, bladder
FBC	full blood count	LAD	left axis deviation
FDP	flexor digitorum profundus	LBBB	left bundle branch block
FEV	forced expiratory volume	LDH	lactate dehydrogenase
FNAC	fine-needle aspiration cytology	LFT	liver function tests
FOB	faecal occult blood	LIF	left iliac fossa
FY1	foundation year 1	LMN	lower motor neuron
G&S	group and save	LOS	lower oesophageal sphincter
GA	general anaesthetic	LRTI	lower respiratory tract infection
GCS	Glasgow Coma Scale	LTOT	long-term oxygen therapy
GFR	glomerular filtration rate	LUTS	lower urinary tract symptoms
GH	growth hormone	LVEF	left ventricular ejection fraction
GGT	gamma glutamyl transpeptidase	LVF	left ventricular failure
GI	gastrointestinal	LVH	left ventricular hypertrophy
GMC	General Medical Council	MC&S	microscopy, culture and sensitivity
GORD	gastro-oesophageal reflux disease	MCPJ	metacarpophalangeal joint
GP	general practitioner	MCV	mean corpuscular volume
GTN	glyceryl trinitrate	MDT	multidisciplinary team
Hb	haemoglobin	MEN	multiple endocrine neoplasia
HCG	human chorionic gonadotropin	MI	myocardial infarction
HDU	high dependency unit	MIBG	metaiodobenzylguanidine scan
HE	hepatic encephalopathy	MR	mitral regurgitation
HIV	human immunodeficiency virus	MRCS	membership of Royal College of Surgeons
HLA	human leukocyte antigen		
HNPP	hereditary non-polyposis colorectal cancer	MRI	magnetic resonance imaging
		MS	mitral stenosis; multiple sclerosis
HOCM	hypertrophic cardiomyopathy	MSU	midstream urine
HONK	hyperosmolar non-ketotic acidosis	MTPJ	metatarsal phalangeal joint
		MTX	methotrexate
HR	heart rate	Na	sodium
HSV	herpes simplex virus	NASH	non-alcoholic steatohepatitis
IBD	inflammatory bowel disease	NBM	nil by mouth
ICP	intracranial pressure	NG	nasogastric
IGF-1	insulin-like growth factor 1	NHS	National Health Service
IGT	impaired glucose tolerance	NICE	National Institute of Clinical Excellence
IHD	ischaemic heart disease		
IJV	internal jugular vein	NIV	non-invasive ventilation
INR	international normalised ratio	NJ	nasojejunal
IPJ	interphalangeal joint	NOF	neck of femur
IV	intravenous	NSAID	non-steroidal anti-inflammatory drug
IVC	inferior vena cava		
IVU	intravenous urogram	OA	osteoarthritis
JVP	jugular venous pressure	OCP	oral contraceptive pill
K	potassium	OGD	oesophagogastroduodenoscopy
KCL	potassium chloride	OGTT	oral glucose tolerance test

ORIF	open reduction internal fixation	SCC	squamous cell carcinoma
OSCE	objective structured clinical examination	SFJ	saphenofemoral junction
		SIRS	systemic inflammatory response syndrome
OT	occupational therapist		
PA	posteroanterior	SLE	systemic lupus erythematosis
PAD	peripheral arterial disease	SOB	shortness of breath
PCA	patient-controlled analgesia	SPJ	saphenopopliteal junction
PCI	percutaneous coronary intervention	STI	sexually transmitted infection
		SUFE	slipped upper femoral epiphysis
PCKD	polycystic kidney disease	SVC	superior vena cava
PCL	posterior cruciate ligament	SVT	supraventricular tachycardia
PCR	polymerase chain reaction	T1DM	type 1 diabetes
PE	pulmonary embolus	T2DM	type 2 diabetes
PEFR	peak expiratory flow rate	TB	tuberculosis
PET	positron emission tomography	TCC	transitional cell carcinoma
PIPJ	proximal interphalangeal joint	TED	thromboembolic deterrents
PMR	polymyalgia rheumatica	TFT	thyroid function tests
PO	by mouth (per os)	TIA	transient ischaemic attack
PPAR	peroxisome proliferators-activated receptor gamma	TKR	total knee replacement
		TPO	thyroid peroxidise
PPM	permanent pacemaker	TR	tricuspid regurgitation
PPI	proton pump inhibitor	TRH	thyrotropin-releasing hormone
PR	per rectal	TSH	thyroid-stimulating hormone
PSA	prostate-specific antigen	TURBT	transurethral resection of bladder tumour
PSIS	posterior superior iliac spine		
PSM	pansystolic murmur	TURP	transurethral resection of prostate
PUJ	pelvi-ureteric junction	U&E	urea and electrolytes
PUVA	psoralen and UVA	UC	ulcerative colitis
RA	rheumatoid arthritis	UMN	upper motor neuron
RAD	right axis deviation	URTI	upper respiratory tract infection
RBBB	right bundle branch block	USS	ultrasound scan
RIF	right iliac fossa	UTI	urinary tract infection
RTA	road traffic accident	UV	ultraviolet
RUQ	right upper quadrant	UVA	ultraviolet A
RVF	right ventricular failure	VUJ	vesico-ureteric junction
SAAG	serum-ascites albumin gradient	WCC	white cell count
SAH	subarachnoid haemorrhage	WHO	World Health Organization
SBE	subacute bacterial endocarditis		

We would like to thank our respective families for all their
patience and continued support throughout this endeavour.

MFM, AM & DG

CHAPTER 1

Introduction to finals, ethics & communication skills

1.1 INTRODUCTION TO CLINICAL FINALS

Clinical medicine finals present a unique challenge to medical students, in that compared to their counterpart, surgical finals, there is an increased emphasis on detailed medical knowledge as well as sound clinical examination skills. However, you must remember that despite what may initially seem to be a hostile environment, the examiners are indeed keen to pass you.

Learning whilst on attachments is ad hoc at best, often with very little time dedicated to teaching you the large number of history-taking, examination and practical skills required. This is primarily because internal medicine is such a busy specialty that teaching students tends to be less of a priority. However, this does not mean you waste your time; a lot of opportunity exists on the wards for you to see patients and examine them. The emphasis being to hone your clinical examination skills, particularly at being apt at picking up clinical signs and presenting your findings. Remember, you must use your time efficiently and effectively by concentrating on what you need to know to pass the exams. It is very obvious to an examiner when a candidate has never performed a respiratory examination.

Often, the candidates who seem to know the most in terms of knowledge, struggle during clinical examinations, whereas their colleagues who may not know as much are doing better. Their successful technique is no secret. The aim of this book is simple: to teach you how to think logically and communicate in a thoughtful but structured manner. This will enable you to not only demonstrate your breadth of knowledge but also your depth of knowledge.

It is necessary to pause here and emphasise this fundamental point to you: it is your breadth of knowledge that the examiner is interested in. There is no point in knowing the pathophysiology of digital clubbing when you cannot name the causes. We aim to teach you the basics and hopefully to enable you to know these well, because it is this that scores you the marks and helps you to pass finals.

Students often ask us what key skills they need to pass finals. While there are many skills that make a good candidate, for purposes of medical finals the most important factor is in knowing your basic core knowledge inside out and being able to communicate this knowledge to the examiner in a methodical manner, as well as being able to collate clinical exam findings into an overall unifying differential diagnosis. The differential diagnosis is a key point, as candidates often tend to commit themselves to a single diagnosis; while this may be the most likely diagnosis, you should still be aware of other possible causes. This is because in internal medicine, as is often the case, the initial presentation may not necessarily be the textbook signs and symptoms we are all well versed in. We emphasise these key skills throughout this revision guide, repeating ourselves as needed because we know it scores you marks and helps you to achieve your aims.

While the majority of topics we cover will be the basics, we will endeavour whenever possible throughout this book to demonstrate to you what constitutes an honours response compared to an average response to a viva question. In cases where we have described this, the honours response is in addition to what the average or good candidate had stated earlier, so you should aim to learn both responses. Further to this, we have highlighted questions or cases that are considered difficult or at honours level. And unless otherwise stated, the answers we provide to such cases will be at honours level. This way, we hope you can identify what is needed to score the top marks in finals.

Wherever possible, we describe to you exactly what you should say in the exam, as if we were in the exam with you. These descriptions are given in italics and take the first-person perspective.

1.1.1 Common reasons for exam failure

For those of you reading this, thinking that there is no way you will make the same mistakes we have highlighted throughout this book and feel that this is all common sense ('Why would anyone do such a thing in their exam?'), take a step back and a moment to think of your predecessors who were in that very same situation and felt the exact same way before their exam. It was they who unknowingly made these same mistakes. That is the paradox here: common sense goes out the window when you are stressed, with the idea reverberating around in your head that 5 years of hard work may be thrown away in one swift afternoon. Fear is powerful, but it can be a powerful motivator too – use it to your advantage. You have an added advantage in that hopefully, with the aid of this revision guide, you will be able to fine-tune yourself to think logically, speak coherently and examine slickly – all key hallmarks of a good candidate. Needless to say, if you prepare for finals with this in mind, you will find that you will be at an advantage and will, we hope, be successful.

EXAMINER'S ANECDOTE

A candidate who performs a good clinical examination will almost certainly pass finals, even if his diagnosis is completely wrong! You can always improve your knowledge set upon qualification; however, once poor examination habits are set, these are very hard to shake.

Finals exams are not easy, so do not, like we once did, listen to your senior colleagues who said they were. They are only speaking in hindsight. While it is true that the purpose of finals is to pass as many of you as possible – as opposed to postgraduate exams, where the purpose is to pass as few as possible – the pressure of passing finals and becoming qualified doctors, coupled with the pressure of being matched to a likeable job, makes finals an all-or-nothing event. Hence the most important piece of advice we will give you is to prepare well, or you may find yourself on the losing end.

Poor communication

When a student is asked a question that they are unfamiliar with, they tend to display what is affectionately known as the 'goldfish' sign. That is, they stand there in front of the examiner with their mouth opening intermittently, trying to speak, but with no words coming out. You cannot score any marks if you say nothing. This is a shame, as most examiners want to pass you and are often urging you to say something, anything that may score you points.

For those who do manage to speak, they often demonstrate what is colloquially known as 'knight's move thinking', where they tend to talk on an unrelated topic and then randomly change to a completely different train of thought, almost as if plucking answers out of the sky. This is the classic case of a student who does not classify or structure their answers.

Likewise, examiners are not psychic and they do not know you have spotted a clinical sign unless you say so, even if to you it appears it must be blindingly obvious to everyone around you. You will only cost yourself marks by assuming this. You must therefore state the obvious.

Single-answer responses do not bode well with an examiner, as this will lead to the examiner and candidate playing what we call 'exam tennis'. This is where the examiner asks for causes of a condition and the candidate answers by giving a single cause, then the examiner asks for another and the candidate replies with another single cause, and so on and so forth. As you can appreciate, this can be frustrating to the examiner, who wishes to go through as many questions as possible. Do not alienate the examiner; if you have them on your side, you will find the exam a more pleasant affair. If you demonstrate a structure to your answers with commonly known classification systems, you can always think of several diagnoses or causes of a certain condition, rather than relying on your memory to bail you out of a stressful viva situation.

Poor examination skills

There is no excuse for a candidate to attend finals having never examined the cardiovascular or cranial nerves before. There are ample opportunities on the wards and clinics. You must be competent in your examination technique and slick in its execution. While there are acceptable variations in technique, a poor clinical examination will lose you many marks.

Behavioural issues

Believe it or not, candidates have in the past and will continue to argue with the examiners. When an examiner says that you are wrong, even if you know that you are right, just accept the examiner's will. It is far better to move onto a new topic and score points than to argue your case. The examiner will almost certainly not accept that you were right and will certainly not admit to you that you are. You do not have the time, and in either situation the only person who will suffer is yourself.

Do not be rude or make haste with an actor; they too are scoring you, and it may well be that their aggregate scores are the decisive ones. Do not hurt or cause pain to the patient under any circumstances. In some medical schools, this results in an automatic fail. Remember that although this is an exam and the patients are likely to be actors, this does not excuse you from such behaviour. You will be a working professional soon, and the examiners want to see that you will be a caring and empathetic doctor. Do what you would do in actual clinical practice. If you know something may hurt the patient, then mention this to them before you do it. Little things like this go a long way to build rapport with a patient and score you many of the communication skills marks that are available; we assure you there are many.

1.1.2 Revision techniques

Clinical examination revision is ideally done in groups of students with not-too-dissimilar levels of ability. We suggest you set up a tutorial group with several of your friends and recruit a registrar to act as your tutor at one of the local teaching hospitals. They can then take you around the wards and show you the sorts of cases you are likely to come across in finals. If you are really lucky, they may even be the one setting the task of recruiting patients for finals and so you have an insider's advantage. If you do not know a registrar, then the next-best place to look is the postgraduate teaching centre, which often keeps a list of doctors who are keen to teach and will help you to contact them.

We find that the best way to learn for finals is to focus your learning objectives and practice. The tutorial group will help facilitate this. Your tutors are ideally placed to assess your examination skills, critique your presentation skills and push your knowledge to the limit in the viva. You are essentially having a mock OSCE with the benefit of receiving immediate feedback. Also, you will learn from the mistakes of your colleagues, and you will pick up on things they did well so you can incorporate this into your routine. Never underestimate the power of group learning. It may be that your percussion technique is inadequate, and only by watching your colleagues would you identify this. Group learning will thus help you to focus your learning needs.

With finals, we sometimes find students locking themselves away in their rooms. This is the wrong approach – there is power in numbers. The tutorial group gives you the opportunity to liaise with your colleagues, who are in the very same situation as you. You may find that your colleagues have been given hints and advice on what is likely to come up in the exam. They can be a useful resource.

We suggest you start early, ideally several months before finals, and decide on the topics you wish to cover with your tutors. Remember they are in full-time employment in a busy specialty, so you need to give them adequate notice. For the more specialist areas like neurology or rheumatology, it is probably best to recruit a registrar from those specialties separately.

We cannot emphasise the benefits of a tutorial group enough; this is how we prepared for finals, and it was invaluable. You have the safety net of being able to examine poorly in front of your tutors and ask silly questions and be corrected, rather than make those same mistakes in finals themselves.

If time does not permit this or you are unable to set up a tutorial group, practise as often as you can, till it is engrained into your mind and becomes second nature. Practise with your friends, family or even by yourself using pillows or having a viva discussion with yourself in the mirror; it doesn't matter so long as you practise. It is all too easy to crumble under the pressure and anxiety of finals, but with repetition and continual practise you will find yourself in autopilot mode and will fly through the actual exam.

1.2　THE EXAM ITSELF

Clinical finals will be unlike any other exam you have ever sat. Most students, however, could probably predict the cases that are likely to appear in the exam; this study guide has already done this for you.

The majority of marks are from inspection alone, so you must say what you see. The examiner will not know that you have noticed the visible pacemaker unless you have said so – do not assume anything.

Do not rush when talking to the examiner. Classify your answers, as we will describe throughout this revision guide, and do not under any circumstances argue with an examiner, make jokes or be rude. This is an exam; treat it as such.

Some medical schools insist you wear your short white coat, whilst others are not so strict on the precise dress code in the exam, as long as it is smart and conservative. The exam is not a fashion show, but definitely do not wear jeans; this is unprofessional and simply not acceptable. For the ladies, in particular, it is important that you do not wear low-cut tops or too short a dress or skirt, as firstly you do not want to be uncomfortable during your exam by constantly having to pull your top up, or your dress down, and secondly it is unprofessional. While you are unlikely to be negatively marked for your attire, first impressions do count for a lot. So keep it simple and professional.

Drug dosages cause anxiety amongst some medical students for fear that they should have memorised the entire British National Formulary (BNF). Rest assured you would not be expected to know drug dosages for the majority of the treatments you offer in the exam. On the whole, if asked for a dose, state that you would check the BNF first before you prescribed any drugs. The only exception to this is during an emergency such that checking a BNF would not be feasible due to comprising patient care. Dosages such as aspirin in an acute coronary syndrome or the dose of adrenaline in anaphylaxis are examples of these. In the medical emergencies chapter, we have covered dosages wherever appropriate (*see* Chapter 11).

Students in the last few weeks leading up to finals tend to get flustered by the many different techniques they see clinicians use to perform the same task; even more so when the clinician says that their method is the best and should be adopted. Remember this key statement for the rest of your careers: everyone examines slightly differently – this is the art of clinical medicine. From the various methods you see, use whatever feels comfortable to you and what works in your already established examination routines. There is no wrong way to do any examination task; there are many acceptable alternative techniques. Remember that in anything you do, under no circumstances cause harm or pain to a patient. Examiners do not look too kindly on candidates who do so, and you will be penalised. If, however, you accidentally do cause pain, apologise immediately and do not repeat the same manoeuvre.

Occasionally you may come across a pushy or hostile examiner. Try not to be intimidated. Unfortunately, despite being a rare breed, they do exist. On the whole, most examiners are very friendly and accommodating. If, however, you do come across a pushy examiner, try and neutralise the situation with your humility and competence. Often the pushy examiner is in fact simply wanting to get through as many questions as possible so as to score you as many marks as possible. Stick to your classification systems and speak clearly and confidently. Remember, do not play 'tennis' with the examiner. Try to hit an ace from the outset!

Sometimes the 'poker face' examiner causes more stress than the talkative ones. This is mainly because candidates are looking for a reaction of approval or disapproval for their answers, and when faced with an examiner who doesn't seem to care, it can be frustrating to not know if you are going along the correct path. It is unlikely an examiner in finals will allow you to take a downward spiral to failure with your irrelevant answers. Often they will gently coax you into re-evaluating your answers or your examination approach.

The cheerful examiner doesn't necessarily mean that you are doing well, either. Many a time have our colleagues come out of an exam saying it was terrible, when in fact they have done superbly well, simply because their examiner was 'poker faced' and vice versa. This is because the atmosphere of the exam, dictated by the examiner, can sway your overall perception of how you performed. We advise that you disregard the examiner's demeanour and approach to you and simply concentrate on answering your questions to the best of your ability. Remember also that there is no harm in saying that you do not know the answer, but follow it up by saying that you would certainly find out before you did anything to the patient or that you would seek advice from your seniors. Do not seek reassurance of your answers from the examiner by stating your answer in the form of a question. The examiner will simply respond by saying, 'Are you asking me, or telling me?' Medical finals examiners tend to be conservative and restrained. Do not take this to mean anything in finals; simply do what you have been practising for months for and you will pass, irrespective of whether or not the examiner smiles at you!

And finally, sometimes it's OK to have no idea what to do, so long as you're confident in your answer and think logically demonstrating your breadth and depth of knowledge, you can convince the examiner that you actually do know. We hope that by the end of this book, this will be the case. Good luck.

1.2.1 Exam talk

In order to communicate effectively in the high-pressure environment of finals, adopting various classification systems will help focus your answers and demonstrate to the examiner your depth and breadth of knowledge. This will probably be the first time you have had to discuss medicine with a medical consultant, and the encounter can be intimidating to say the least. Therefore, having a clear structure in your mind when approaching any question a consultant is likely to ask you will hopefully enable you to remain calm when asked bewildering questions and help you to come out with a logical and intelligent answer, even if you haven't actually answered the question. Even if you do not know the answer, you can give the impression to the examiner that you do know. This will be evident from the way you answer the question, rather then what content you produce. This is one of the reasons why sieves are widely used.

Discussing aetiology

In the stress of the exam, it is easy to try and list as many causes of a condition as quickly as possible. However, this is the wrong approach, as you are only demonstrating your ability to memorise lists; this list you will no doubt soon forget.

AUTHOR'S ANECDOTE

He regurgitated five differentials before I even finished my question! He then sat back and thought he had done enough to pass! I told him I was impressed by his memorisation skills. It is far better for you to classify your answers and state them clearly and confidently than to reel off a list you clearly memorised the night before.

It is far better to classify or structure your answers using well-accepted aetiological sieves. In our experience, we find that surgical sieves you have constructed yourselves are the ones you tend to remember the best. The sieve itself is unimportant; it's the attempt at classifying your answers which will be well appreciated by the examiner. The examiner knows that we simply cannot memorise every single differential diagnosis for every condition we come across, as it is impractical. Classification enables us to access and retain our knowledge.

For example, if you are asked for the causes of chest pain, you might answer:

'The causes of chest pain are myocardial infarction, pneumothorax and pulmonary embolism.'

Average response

In addition to the above:

'There are many causes of chest pain. They can divided into cardiac causes, respiratory causes, gastrointestinal causes and others', before giving details from the following table:

TABLE 1.1 Causes of chest pain

Classification	Pathology
Cardiac	Myocardial infarction (MI), angina, pericarditis
Respiratory	Pneumothorax, pulmonary embolism (PE), pneumonia
Gastrointestinal	Oesophageal spasm, peptic ulcer disease
Others	Rib fractures, costochondritis, anxiety

Good response

Note that this table is not exhaustive.

Another common aetiological sieve is where the causes are classified into their originating physiological system. This can be demonstrated when, for example, you are asked the causes of digital clubbing:

'The causes of clubbing are idiopathic, lung cancer, inflammatory bowel disease and cystic fibrosis'.

Average response

'The most common cause of digital clubbing is idiopathic. However, there are many causes of clubbing and they can be classified into . . .':

TABLE 1.2 Causes of clubbing

Classification	Causes
Gastrointestinal causes	Inflammatory bowel disease, primary biliary cirrhosis, coeliac disease
Respiratory causes	Bronchogenic carcinoma, suppurative lung disease, e.g. bronchiectasis, cystic fibrosis, mesothelioma, fibrosing alveolitis
Cardiac causes	Congenital cyanotic heart disease, endocarditis
Other causes	Familial, idiopathic, Graves' disease

Good response

While the average response is acceptable and will score you some points, the subsequent response demonstrates the breadth of knowledge required to excel in finals.

Discussing investigations

When you discuss investigations, it is helpful to classify them. This helps you not only to order your investigations in a logical manner but also to remember what the next most appropriate investigation is. Remember, always move from simple or non-invasive to invasive, and reserve specialist investigations till the end once all the basic ones have been done.

Investigations can be divided into simple bedside tests, blood tests and imaging.

TABLE 1.3 Investigations

Investigations	Tests
Simple bedside tests	**ECG:** to rule out cardiac ischaemia, rhythm abnormalities or MI
	Urinanalysis: useful to look for blood if you are considering a UTI, protein for renal disease or to perform a pregnancy test in a woman
	BM: to check for the blood sugar level
Blood tests	**Simple tests**
	FBC: to check for a raised WCC in infection or anaemia if GI bleed
	U&E: to look for dehydration, renal failure, raised urea in cases of an acute gastrointestinal bleed, or electrolyte imbalance
	LFTs: if you suspect jaundice or hepatitis, hypoalbuminaemia
	G&S or crossmatch (CX): if you suspect that the patient will require a blood transfusion
	ABG: assessment of respiratory failure can be made. And if your patient is particularly sick, this will help to gauge how unwell the patient is. The lactate and pH are helpful indicators of the level of shock
	Specialist tests: this depends on the diagnosis, e.g. antinuclear antibodies or rheumatoid factor in patients with rheumatoid arthritis, HbA1c to assess glycaemic control in diabetics
Imaging	**Plain films**
	CXR: in cases of respiratory disease or cardiac chest pain, amongst others
	Ultrasound
	USS abdomen/liver: to scan the biliary tree for evidence of gallstones or measure the size of the common bile duct in suspected obstructive jaundice, to assess the bladder and any other gross abnormalities
	CT scans
	CT chest or CT pulmonary angiogram: respiratory disease or suspected pulmonary embolism
	CT abdomen/pelvis: this depends on the case, but useful in patients with suspected intra-abdominal malignancy or liver disease
	CT head: in suspected stroke

You may choose to add additional blood tests or other specialist tests depending on your diagnosis.

Discussing management

Whenever you discuss the management of a condition, the word 'management' here does not solely refer to treatment. It typically covers the entire clinical encounter, starting from the history, the examination, investigations, your list of differentials and finally the treatment options available. So when you structure your answer, ensure you state this. Usually, the examiner will ask you to skip to the treatment options, in which case you should structure your answer as follows.

Treatment options can be conservative, medical or surgical.

TABLE 1.4 Treatment options

Treatment	Options
Conservative	This generally includes anything non-invasive. This may be in the form of IV fluids, physiotherapy, increased monitoring, e.g. continuous ECG monitoring; or a wait-and-watch approach
Medical	This includes any drugs that may be given or drug dosages altered. Remember that oxygen is a drug.
Surgical	This is any surgical procedure performed.

There is a special note on discussing chronic debilitating conditions such as osteoarthritis or cancers. This always takes a multidisciplinary team management approach with input from various disciplines, including occupational therapists, physiotherapists and clinical nurse specialists. Ensure you put this across in your answer.

EXAMINER'S ANECDOTE

When he mentioned an MDT approach to treating arthritis with input from the OT and GP, I almost jumped out of my seat! That was impressive; clearly he knows what happens in actual clinical practice.

1.3   PRINCIPLES OF A CLINICAL ENCOUNTER

As with all clinical encounters, whether it is an examination station or clinical skills, the same general principles apply. There are marks available for beginning and ending a clinical encounter appropriately. Below we describe the key points you will need to remember.

The clinical encounter

Introduction
❑ **Wash your hands**
  ■ There will be alcohol gel available to you at each OSCE station in order for you to wash your hands; this must be done at the beginning and end of every station.
  ■ Almost all medical schools award marks for doing this.
  ■ NICE has also issued guidelines specifically stating that the washing of hands is mandatory.
❑ **Introduce yourself**
  ■ You must introduce yourself using your full name and current medical student status.
  ■ Use the patient's name if offered, or clarify their name at the beginning.
  ■ Always be polite and courteous when addressing a patient and use their surname.

❑ **Explain purpose, gain consent and ask for a chaperone**
- As with any clinical encounter, you must gain consent first by explaining the purpose of the exam and check whether the patient agrees for you to continue.
- This is especially important for intimate examinations, where you must turn to the examiner and specifically ask for a chaperone.

❑ **Expose patient adequately**
- This clearly depends on the situation, but in general you should ask the patient to expose as much as possible whilst maintaining your field of vision and preserving their dignity.
- If you are conducting an intimate exam, you must allow them privacy to change.
- More often then not, the patient is already adequately exposed.

❑ **Position patient appropriately**
- This is particularly important in the clinical examination stations, where correct patient positioning will help make your examination easier and more accurate.
- For example, ask the patient to lie at 45 degrees for cardiovascular examinations.

❑ **Build rapport**
- There are often numerous marks available for building a good rapport with the patient, and so informing them of what you are doing as you go along helps to alleviate their anxieties and reminds you of the routine that you have rehearsed many times before the exam.
- This is of utmost importance when conducting intimate examinations, as there may be intrusive parts to the exam which could be uncomfortable for the patient; by explaining and discussing beforehand with the patient, they will know exactly what to expect, and it will help make them feel more comfortable.
- If you need the patient to do special manoeuvres, use short and succinct instructions as you do not want to confuse them; alternatively, you could demonstrate to them what it is you want them to do.
- Finally, always ask about pain and avoid starting with that part of the body if at all possible. If you know that your examination may exacerbate any underlying pain, take the time to explain to them that your examination may be slightly uncomfortable but should not be painful. Assure them that if you do cause them pain, you will stop.

AUTHOR'S TOP TIP

Remember, most medical schools will fail you if you cause the patient pain, so be gentle and warn the patient beforehand.

Complete the encounter

❑ **Thank the patient**
- Always thank the patient, and if they are undressed ensure that they are comfortable and able to redress.
- If there is a blanket, then offer this to them to cover their modesty.
- If you have just finished an intimate exam, you must again give them privacy to redress.

❑ **Wash your hands** (the second time during the station)
  - You must actually do this; do not simply offer to do this. We emphasise this point, as some medical schools negatively mark you if you do not wash your hands again.
❑ **Further examination**
  - On the whole, use this opportunity for examinations that you feel are necessary but time does not permit.
  - A typical example would be conducting a DRE after examining the gastrointestinal system.
  - You may also choose to state other bedside tests you would like to perform as part of your clinical examination, such as measuring peak flow in your respiratory exam.
❑ **Present your findings**
  - You must turn and face the examiner, and whilst maintaining eye contact as you find comfortable, summarise your findings.

AUTHOR'S TOP TIP

Do not fidget with your hands or look back at the patient; some students like to fold their hands in front or behind them in an attempt to seem professional; do whatever makes you comfortable and be confident in your approach.

1.4 ETHICS & COMMUNICATION SKILLS

There has been a real shift in medical school teaching to encompass communication skills teaching and assessment in preparation for tomorrow's more empathetic doctor. As such, you can almost be certain there will be a communication skills station of some form or other in finals. These should be taken seriously, as often the marks are easy to obtain, so long as you follow the outline given for the cases described below.

Remember, you must at the very least appear to be genuinely concerned for the patient in finals, as you are often given marks for your interactions by the patient themselves, and so it is crucial you build a good rapport and maintain their trust and confidence. Remember your interaction must be jargon-free and patient centred.

The most common cases that tend to crop up are obtaining consent and explaining an investigation, procedure or diagnosis. See our companion text, *The Ultimate Guide to Passing Surgical Clinical Finals*, for these cases. Below, we discuss other commonly occurring cases using examples wherever applicable, bearing in mind that it is the principles that need to be remembered rather than the specific examples, which are purely for illustrative purposes.

Case 1: Breaking bad news

Instructions: This 54-year-old woman admitted with haemoptysis has just been diagnosed with metastatic lung cancer. At an MDT team meeting, it has been decided she is for palliative care, as the disease is not amenable to any intervention. Please discuss this diagnosis with her. Note that she has not been told her diagnosis.

Key features to look out for

❑ **Preparation**

■ **Familiarise yourself with patient's history:** You should read through the patient's notes so you are aware of all test results, patient encounters and any further investigations still awaiting. This may also give you a clue as to how well informed the patient is already of their diagnosis.

■ **Ensure your dedication:** Breaking bad news takes time, so don't be surprised to be still reiterating your initial conversation to family members an hour after you began. This is by its very nature unpredictable. However, it is sensible to set aside at least half an hour where you are free to talk. Mention you will give your bleep to a colleague to hold. Ideally, you should arrange with your consultant a specific time when you can see the patient and family members.

■ **Suitable environment:** Breaking bad news behind a curtain in a four bedded ward bay is not ideal, not to mention the lack of confidentiality. Giving the patient the opportunity to hear news in privacy is a key part of maintaining a positive experience. Therefore, find a suitable room for this. Often, wards have a dedicated patients' family room where such discussions can be held. Also, if the patient is alone, you may ask them if they would like a family member or friend to be present when you talk to them, so as to offer them support or comfort.

– e.g. *'Is there anybody I can call for you to come and be with you while we discuss these important results?'*

■ **Third party:** Ideally, take a senior colleague with you if you can, as the patient and their family may ask questions, many of which you may not know the answer to. Of course, in the exam you will be told that you are the only doctor available. At the very least, take a senior nurse with you, usually the staff nurse looking after the patient, to act as a mediator and to reiterate what you have said to the patient after you have left. This ensures continuity.

❑ **Principles of a clinical encounter:** This is essentially the same with formal introductions and shaking hands, etc., but with some key features to note.

■ **Identify all present:** Identify yourself, with full name, grade and your consultant's name. Confirm the patient's identity; the last thing you want to do is give bad news to the wrong person. Ask if all individuals with the patient can introduce themselves and their relationship to the patient.

AUTHOR'S TOP TIP

In order to ensure confidentiality, you must identify everyone in the room and that the patient is happy for them to stay. In the exam, it is not unheard of to have a lay person in the room, only for you to identify that the patient does not want them to be present for the conversation. You can do this by simply asking the patient at the outset.

■ **Confidentiality:** Ensure you ask the patient if they want these family members to be present, and if so, how much information they should be told in the patient's presence. Ideally, you should ask the patient this when the family are not around, as there may be difficult family dynamics you are unaware of which may be strained if the question is asked in their presence.

- **Explain why you are there:** To discuss the test results or diagnosis.

❑ **Gather information**

- **Ascertain level of current knowledge:** Ask whether they know their diagnosis, what procedure has been planned and why. Ask the patient to go through what initially brought them to hospital and what has happened from their point of view. This allows patients to feel they are in control and enables them perhaps to voice their concerns that they may have been aware they had a serious illness for a long time.

- **Gain consent:** You must ask the patient if they want to know the results of a test or a diagnosis before you tell them. Remember that patients have absolute autonomy, and if they choose not to know their diagnosis then that is their right. You of course should try to explore their reasoning and explain the benefits of knowing, but you must ultimately respect their decision. Take this opportunity to ask that, if they do wish to know, how much information they would wish to receive.
  - e.g. *'Are you the sort of person who wishes to know everything in detail, or just the key facts?'*
  - or *'If your condition is serious, would you like to know, and how much would you like to know about it?'*

- **Pre-emptive warning:** Subtly suggest that the results or next few things you are about to say will be bad news. It is far easier to prepare a patient for this inevitability rather than jumping into conversation with bad news.

- **Non-verbal communication:** The use of long pauses can be a very powerful tool in aiding communication and allows the patient time for the realisation to set in.
  - e.g. *'I have the results of your biopsy . . . [pause] . . . Would you like to know the results of this?'*
  - or some like the cut to the chase: *'I have some bad news . . . Should I continue?'*
  - others like to give the patient the opportunity to guess that it is bad news: *'You had a biopsy done last week because we were concerned about the chest X-ray and the weight loss you've had recently. I remember you said you were concerned about your chest and wondered if there was anything serious going on . . . [pause] . . . What do you think is going on? What are your concerns?'*

- Often, patients already fear the worst and have some idea of the diagnosis already, before you say anything. This method eases the results to the patient, as the patient already 'knows', and all you are doing is confirming their suspicions.

❑ **Set up the bad news**

- **Summarise care given so far:** Give a brief review of the patient's presenting complaint, results so far, management plan and what the patient has told you they know and what they are concerned about.

❑ **Break the news**

'I have looked at the results of the test, and I am sorry to say that you have lung cancer.'

- Do not linger with non-specific terms such as 'growth' or 'suspicious lesion', as this only confuses patients. You must state that it is a cancer, or the patient will not acknowledge the seriousness of your discussion.

- Do not collude with relatives, who may ask you to omit such information in your discussion. Your duty is first and foremost to the patient. You must instead reply to a request for collusion with a question exploring the relatives' reasons for collusion. This may, in fact, be what is being tested in the OSCE.

- Offer apologies/condolences for the news.
- Some may go so far as to be empathetic when breaking bad news. This is particularly helpful when the patient is surprised by the result.
  - e.g. *'I've looked over your results and I was very surprised, so I've checked them again . . . [pause] . . . But I'm very sorry to say . . .'*
- By mirroring the patient's responses, you are demonstrating your empathy.
- Remember to say this statement slowly and offer pauses in between key information to allow the patient to acknowledge the information and appreciate its extent. Speaking too fast and hurriedly only makes you seem impatient, rather than the caring doctor the patient wishes to see.
- It takes time for bad news to sink in; you must therefore be slow and concise. Be prepared to repeat information many times over.

❑ **Offer consolation & address concerns**
- **Demonstrate sympathy:** This may be in the form of lightly patting the shoulder to offer condolences. Holding a patient's hand is discretionary – some candidates are not comfortable with this – but if the patient puts their hand out to you, many of us as junior doctors would find it difficult not to accept. In the OSCE exam, the easiest thing to do is to offer a tissue.
- **Allow time for information sink in:** This is where you can use the pause effectively. Sometimes not saying anything for 15–30 seconds while the patient contemplates their diagnosis is what is needed. Occasionally, this silence can be broken with sensible empathetic comments like:
  - *'I understand this must be a very difficult time for you.'*
- **Offer some reprieve:** If there are treatment options available, then discuss this, although in the exam you are unlikely to know these in detail enough to do so. However, if there are clearly no further treatment options, do not give false hope but reassure the patient that they will have you, the consultant and the hospital staff and services to help them through this difficult time. Being offered a comfortable last few days or weeks to their life and ensuring they are pain-free is what most patients would want.
- **Offer counselling:** This may be in the form of grief counselling or religious counselling via a priest, rabbi or imam if the patient holds a particular religious viewpoint.
- **Expect hostility:** Some patients may react angrily to your diagnosis, even question its validity. This is a normal behavioural response to bad news. Acknowledge this, and explore further with them if you can. Patients all go through these stages of the grief response. However, it is important you do not react to this personally and simply let the patient vent their frustrations and offer your unreserved apologies. Bargaining is a common behavioural response whereby the patient suggests and attempts to convince you that your test may be inaccurate. While this is a possibility, hopefully you would have been fairly certain of your diagnosis before you told the patient, and you can gently reassure the patient that while it is indeed true that not all tests

are 100% accurate, this is the most accurate test available and it is unlikely that it is wrong. It may even be acceptable to offer to repeat the test, but mention that you expect the result to be the same. Often, patients are happy enough to have their request for retesting considered and will accept your initial result as correct.

- **Offer a second opinion:** Occasionally, patients and family are in the denial phase of grief such that they do not believe a word you say and wish to see another physician. Offer this to them if they wish, mentioning that it is unlikely they will disagree. Take this as an opportunity to explore their reasons and try to address this.
- **Prognosis:** Patients commonly ask the infamous question, 'How long have I got, doctor?' To which you should reply that as a junior you cannot say. Unless you are a senior or a consultant and are aware of the published 5-year survival rates, you should not offer any time frames. However, being ambiguous is also not good, as this leaves the patient with uncertainty. It is best in finals to say that this is a difficult question for anyone to answer and that you do not know for sure, but that you will ask your senior for estimates and will come back to the patient with this information. In reality, it is very difficult to quantify as this depends on the TNM classification of the tumour (which you may not know yet due to pending investigations). Sometimes, the easiest answer in finals is *'I honestly don't know. I cannot say for certain, but I can find out.'*

❏ **Conclude the encounter**
- **Summarise discussion**
- **Answer any questions**
- **Arrange follow-up:** Explain what the next steps are, whether this is in the form of a specialist referral to an oncologist, palliative care or hospice referral.
- **Offer availability:** Offer your services to the patient by telling them if they have any other questions later, they can contact you. Inform the nurse of your bleep number.
  - e.g. *'I can understand this may be too much information for you to take on board right now. Why don't you have a think about what we've just said, and if you come up with any questions later, write them all down, and when I come back to see you, we can go through them one by one?'*
- This sentence offers your availability and empathy as well as reassurance that their questions will be answered.

❏ **Documentation**
- This is a crucial part of your clinical encounter.
- Document who was present, what was said by both parties; what the patient understood and the plan agreed by everyone.

Completion

This is a very common OSCE station in finals, and it is therefore crucial you have a good understanding of the underlying principles in dealing with bad news. It is also something you will inevitably come across in your clinical practice, for example, discussing a test result or diagnosis that will negatively impact on a patient, such as telling a patient they have HIV, multiple sclerosis or epilepsy in a taxi driver whose livelihood is affected by your diagnosis. You cannot underestimate the psychosocial impact of such diseases.

Some students may argue that as bad news should ideally be broken by a senior clinician, it is not necessary for students to learn this, as they will not be breaking bad news as a junior doctor. We can assure you that as a junior doctor you may be called upon to discuss bad news with patients and their relatives, often during on-call hours where seniors are not readily available. So we argue that it is an important skill to learn early, as the way you break bad news to a patient and their loved ones can have a profound negative or positive impact on their doctor–patient experience and ultimately affect the way they perceive this news.

Case 2: Dealing with an angry patient (or relative)

Instructions: This lady is about to undergo a gastroscopy after having her procedure cancelled 3 times already: for lack of time, absence of consultant and a priority emergency case from A&E resus. She has expressed anger that she has been made to wait so long for her investigation. Please discuss her concerns.

Key features to look out for

❑ **Gather information**
- Explain that you understand they want to raise some concerns about their management and that you are here to help as much as possible.
- If this is a relative, confirm their relationship to the patient first and ensure confidentiality is maintained.
- Bring a third party with you if you can, usually the ward sister, to help act as a middle person should patients become angry.

❑ **Listen to the patient's concerns**
- Patients often simply want to be heard and have their concerns taken seriously.
- A willingness to listen and help, and an empathetic and caring approach to a patient's concerns may in fact resolve the situation immediately.
- Do not make excuses if at all possible; however, do explain that emergency treatment of other patients will always take priority, and that the other patient must have needed urgent treatment if the elective investigation was cancelled or postponed. Most patients will understand if there was an emergency and priority was given to someone else.

❑ **Acknowledge concerns and state intention to resolve**
- Express sympathy and empathy as required; do not underestimate how expressing empathy can help defuse anger.
- Remain polite and avoid confrontation. It helps if you can find common ground.
- State that you will try and resolve the situation as quickly as possible, for example, by discussing with a senior colleague about rebooking the investigation first thing the next day.

❑ **Outline plan for resolution**
- Offering to put things right and seeking continuous improvement demonstrates to the patient that something is being done about their complaint such that future patients will not suffer the same fate.
- The exact plan will depend on the complaint; however, in the exam it is easier to defer to a more senior colleague for a plan.

❑ **Offer apologies**

- Explicitly apologise for the events, even if you think this is not necessary. Unreserved apologies have been shown to diffuse a volatile situation easily.
- Being patient focused, open and accountable helps resolve issues locally.

❑ **Summarise**

- Summarise the key features of what the patient felt went wrong with their management.
- This demonstrates that you have covered all the important points as well as offered plans to resolve them.
- It also demonstrates that you were listening to the patient, and in some cases that may be all that the patient requires.

❑ **Offer further consultation and contact**

- Offer the patient the ability to speak to the consultant in charge of their care.
- Offer an avenue for formal complaint if needed, even if not requested, such as patient advice and liaison services.
- Offer a follow-up consultation with yourself (to ensure continuity) and a senior, usually the consultant in charge, in the company of a member of their family or friend if required.
- Offer your availability should they wish to discuss things further; usually, your bleep number and name to the nurses so that the patient can request to speak to you again if needed.

❑ **Confirm whether there are any outstanding issues and conclude the encounter**

- Ask if there is anything else the patient would like to say.
- Remind them that their complaint will be dealt with accordingly.

❑ **Documentation**

- Document the encounter clearly in the notes, particularly who was present and what was said by the patient and the doctors.
- Outline any plans of action taken.

Completion

The way you handle the actor in the exam is more important than the details of dealing with a complaint or an angry patient. Empathy goes a long way to defuse a highly tempered situation. In fact, there are guidelines on how to handle complaints drawn up by the Parliamentary and Health Service Ombudsman: *Principles of Good Complaint Handling*. Formal complaints are now handled by a complaints manager at the hospital trust, and timelines are provided whereby complaints are to be resolved to the complainant's satisfaction. Of note, any complaints made by a patient or relative must be made within 12 months of the incident.

Most complaints are about poor communication, and taking the time to communicate with your patients and their relatives helps prevent patient concerns from ever becoming formal complaints.

Case 3: Patient counselling: discuss anticoagulation

Instructions: This 65-year-old woman is about to be started on warfarin therapy. Please discuss this with her.

Key features to look out for
❑ **Gather information**
- Assess patient's current level of understanding: ask if they know anything about anticoagulation treatment already and what they know about warfarin.
- Describe the reason for anticoagulation and the duration of treatment.
- Explain what warfarin is and the reason for taking it, e.g. if the reason for taking it is atrial fibrillation, tell the patient:
    - *'An anticoagulant such as warfarin is a drug which stops your blood from clotting in the blood vessels. This protects you from having an increased chance of clots going to the brain, due to the irregular heartbeat, and causing a stroke.'*
❑ **Demonstrate the yellow anticoagulant therapy record**
- Commonly known as the 'yellow book', this is a helpful pocket-size guide conveying patient information regarding anticoagulation, which is discussed in lay terms using 'dos and don'ts'.
- It also documents the reason, target INR and duration of treatment.
- There is a space at the back for documenting the patient's INR results and current dosage.

Ideally, go though the yellow book with them page by page, if immediately available in the OSCE; if not, then follow the schema below:

TABLE 1.5 Yellow book dos and don'ts

Advice	Description
Dos	● Carry the yellow book with you.
	● Keep your blood-test appointments; this is to check the dose of the tablets you need. If you can't attend, then please arrange another appointment as soon as possible.
	● Inform the doctor of any bleeding or bruising immediately, e.g. nosebleeds, dark urine or black stools, pronged bleeding from cuts, bleeding gums or if bleeding doesn't stop.
	● Remind your doctor, dentist and pharmacist that you are taking warfarin, especially if they plan dental treatment or surgery.
	● Take your tablets at the same time each day; if you can, try to remember the dose and colour of your tablets (white 0.5 mg, brown 1 mg, blue 3 mg, pink 5 mg).
Don'ts	● Don't run out of tablets; ensure you have enough.
	● Don't take an extra dose of tablets if you cannot remember whether you've taken them already. It is best to miss the tablet. Try to document on a calendar whenever you've taken them.
	● Try not to miss a dose if possible; if you do, then take a note of the date and let the clinic know when you have your blood test. If you are pregnant, you must seek medical advice, as warfarin can affect the baby.

(continued)

Advice	Description
Don'ts (*cont.*)	• Don't take aspirin unless prescribed by a doctor who knows you are on warfarin. If in doubt, ask. Always inform the clinic of any new medicines, as they can affect your anticoagulant, e.g. antibiotics, cholesterol-lowering tablets, epilepsy drugs, sleeping tablets, liquid paraffin, certain herbal therapies.
	• Don't binge-eat or go on crash diets, as dietary change can affect your drug dosages. Avoid sudden increased intake of green vegetables, as they contain vitamin K, which is the antidote for warfarin. Avoid grapefruit, its juice and cranberry juice. Avoid drinking more than moderate amounts of alcohol, as this can be dangerous.

Practice discussing the above dos and don'ts with a patient, using lay terms as described above. This should cover the majority of marks to be gained in this OSCE station.

❏ **Discuss what INR means**

■ Explain that the target INR or international normalised ratio will vary for each patient, depending on the reason for anticoagulation.

■ In general, however, their regular blood tests should aim to check whether they are on the correct dose of warfarin; adjustments will be made according to this INR result.

■ If they are told their INR is too high, this means their blood is too thin and may result in easy bruising and bleeding, in which case their dose will be decreased or they would be asked to omit a dose.

■ If their INR is too low, then this means the blood is too thick, and this could result in a clot.

❏ **Stress importance of drug compliance**

■ Compliance is crucial in preventing the associated complications.

■ If needed, the patient can be offered transport to and from anticoagulation clinics; some GPs offer an anticoagulation service.

■ Stress that tablets need to be taken daily for the duration of treatment and that although initially daily, this may be altered to every other day or longer depending on the level of control achieved and their target INR.

■ If required, dosette boxes can be provided to help minimise confusion with tablets.

AUTHOR'S TOP TIP

We knew a colleague who had this very OSCE station in their exam and did not know many of the features stated here. She simply told the patient that she was unsure and that she would find out and let her know. And she still passed the station. This demonstrates that even if you do not know the answers, so long as you are honest and state that although you do not know, you will seek the correct information, you will pass the exam. Do not make stuff up; it will be very clear to the examiner that you do not know what you are talking about.

❏ **Offer the patient a copy of the yellow anticoagulant therapy record**

■ Advise them to keep this with them at all times and show to a doctor or healthcare professional, especially if starting new medicines.

- Whenever collecting medicines from the pharmacist, they should show this card so they can be advised accordingly.
- Document contact details if they need to seek medical advice.

❏ **Allow patient time for any queries**
- Answer any questions as fully as possible, if you are unsure state that you will find out for them from a more senior colleague.

Completion

This is a commonly tested OSCE, so make sure you have seen and are well versed with the yellow booklets, as this covers essentially what you need to discuss. *See* Chapter 12 on data interpretation for further information.

Case 4: Teaching a patient a technique/skill

Instructions: This young lady is a newly diagnosed asthmatic. Please demonstrate to her how to use the metered dose inhaler and how to assess her peak expiratory flow.

Key features to look out for

❏ **Gather information**
- Assess the patient's understanding of asthma, including the use of inhalers if any prior experience.
  - e.g. *'What do you know about inhalers? Have you ever seen a family member or friend use one before?'*

❏ **Discuss use of inhaler**
- Explain the inhaler's mechanism of action briefly.
  - e.g. *'The inhaler is a device which sends medicine into your airway so that it opens up and makes it easier for you to breathe.'*
- Explain the inhaler's indications: offer circumstances when the inhaler should be used, e.g. reliever just before exercise or regular inhaled steroids.

❏ **Demonstrate technique**
- Shake the inhaler device and remove the cap from the mouthpiece.
- Keep the inhaler close to the mouth, preparing to activate it when timed with inhalation in their respiratory cycle.
- Take a deep breath in and then exhale completely, and upon beginning the next breath, simultaneously activate the inhaler and continue breathing in.
- Keeping the mouth closed, hold this breath for about 10 seconds, then breathe out.
- Two puffs is usually enough to demonstrate; tell the patient that they can repeat as needed if symptoms are not relieved after 3–5 minutes.

Sometimes, the easiest way to explain to a patient is simply to show them. Of course, you mustn't actually put your mouth over their mouthpiece, but do describe what you wish for them to do as you go along.

❑ **Ask patient to demonstrate technique**
- Ask the patient to describe what they're doing as they go along and check to see if they are performing the task correctly; if not, then correct the patient as necessary.
- Explain that, if used correctly, the inhaler can provide fast and efficient relief of bronchospasm.
- If you note the patient has difficulty in coordinating inhalation and activation of the inhaler, then suggest the use of a spacer device.

❑ **Allow patient time for any queries**
- If the patient has any concerns or queries, attempt to answer them as fully as possible.
- Remember if you do not know, then say you will speak to a senior.

❑ **Offer patient support**
- If available, offer the patient leaflets summarising inhaler techniques to take home with them, reinforcing what they have just learnt.
- If this is not possible, leaflets of techniques can be found inside packaging for the inhalers themselves, as some models have slightly different techniques for use.
- Offer a follow-up appointment with either yourself or an asthma nurse specialist to check technique and monitor their condition.

Do not forget to perform the second part of this task, which is teaching the use of the peak flow meter. Remember to follow the above principles in explaining a task.

Peak flow meter demonstration

❑ **Discuss peak expiratory flow (PEFR) measurement**
- Explain the purpose of PEFR measurement; to assess control of asthma and allowing the physician the ability to adjust treatments as necessary based upon accurate recordings in the peak flow diary. Also, ask the patient to take note of their usual PEFR when well, as knowing this is useful whenever admitted to hospital for an acute asthma attack.
- Explain timing of PEFR measurement: the PEFR is measured first thing in the morning and before bed as well as at any other times when symptomatic; reading should ideally be taken at the same time each day.

❑ **Demonstrate technique**
- Ask the patient to stand up or, if unable, to sit up straight.
- Attach a new mouthpiece to the meter and slide the marker to the zero mark on the scale.
- Take a big deep breath in, and making as good a seal around the mouthpiece as possible, breath out as hard and as fast as possible, whilst keeping the meter horizontal.
- Take note of the reading, reset the marker and repeat so that there are three readings; take note of only the highest reading, and this is their PEFR.
- Record this number in the diary or enter this on the flow charts.

Ensure you have the correct-size peak flow meter as using a paediatric scale will clearly not be suitable for an adult.

❏ **Ask patient to demonstrate technique**
❏ **Allow patient time for any queries**
❏ **Offer patient support**

Completion

Note that this could equally be applied to teaching diabetic patients to check their own blood sugar.

Viva questions

Q1 This is the patient's PEFR diary. What can you ascertain from this?

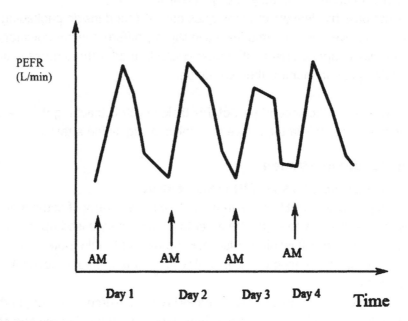

FIGURE 1.1 Peak flow chart

- There are wide diurnal variations, with early-morning dips.
- Patient may need stepping up of their treatment; however, you must always check inhaler technique, as poor technique is a common cause of poor control of asthma.
- The addition of steroids would decrease the wide diurnal variations.

Peak flow meters measure the maximum flow rate during the initial 2 milliseconds of expiration. Measurement is useful for disease monitoring and response to treatment. The predicted peak expiratory flow rate depends on the patient's age, sex and height and can be estimated using standardised charts. For example, a 1.8-m-tall 40-year-old man would have a predicted PEFR of approximately 600 L/minute. There is normally a diurnal variation, with a morning dip in asthmatics. It is the wide variation which alerts the candidate to the need for treatment optimisation.

Q2 What other information would you like to tell the patient?

- Ensure that patient understands that if using the salbutamol inhalers more than once a day and they are not on any regular inhaled steroids, they should contact their doctor for treatment optimisation.
- If they are taking high-dose regular inhaled steroids, they can sometimes get oral thrush. Therefore, advise them to wash their mouth after use.
- The steroid inhaler is not a reliever; the beta-agonist inhaler is typically blue (although not always) and is the inhaler to use when having an acute attack of asthma.
- If they wish to know about the side effects, the inhaler comes with a leaflet detailing these; otherwise, in general there are few systemic side effects from inhalers.
- Advise them to carry their reliever with them wherever they go, or have a spare at work/school.
- Advise them that should their symptoms not improve with their reliever, they should seek medical help urgently, calling an ambulance if required.
- Acute asthma can be life-threatening; this should not be taken lightly.

CHAPTER 2

Clinical histories

It is often said that the medical student history is thorough, detailed and comprehensive. However, in actual clinical practice you may find that time is very limited, preventing you from taking such a detailed and thorough history. The objective should be to identify the salient points needed to reach an accurate diagnosis. The best way to gauge how much information is required during the history-taking process in clinical practice is to present as often as the opportunity arises, preferably during a post-take ward round.

We advise being systematic but concise in order to elicit the relevant negative and positive points during the history-taking process. Your aim should be to take a focused history, in a busy environment such as the A&E department, within a set period of time. The time allowed for a history-taking station during the OSCE can range from 5 to 20 minutes, depending on your particular medical school. For those of you who think taking a history in 5 minutes is not possible, one of the author's third-year OSCEs involved doing just that. Although challenging, it is certainly possible, as long as you ask focused and clinically relevant questions.

Below, we describe a generic medical history-taking formula, which can be applied to any presenting symptom you may come across. More detailed systems-based histories can be found in their corresponding chapters, together with common cases that crop up in finals.

Medical history

General principles
❏ Introduce yourself and confirm that you are talking to the right patient
❏ Explain purpose of meeting, gain consent
  ▪ Introduce yourself; tell them your full name, grade and which team you work for.
  ▪ **Patient identity:** Clarify that you have the right patient by checking their name, and also confirm the identity of anybody else that they have brought with them.
  ▪ **Occupation:** Ask what they do or did for an occupation; this may have significance in identifying patterns within their presenting symptoms, such as boiler workmen who may have previous asbestos exposure and therefore an increased risk of mesothelioma.
  ▪ **Age:** Always clarify the age with the patient even if you have a date of birth, as sometimes these may have been entered incorrectly in the medical record or may alert you to a patient with confusion if they provide a clearly wrong answer or are unable to answer. Age is also important, as it allows you to risk-stratify the likelihood of certain diagnoses from within your working differentials.

❏ **Communication skills pertinent to history-taking**
- **Physical setting:** You should be seated at the same level as the patient, with no physical barriers such as a large table between you and the patient.
- **Question formats:** Start the conversation with an open-ended question, then move on to closed questions if needed. Avoid the use of single-answer yes-or-no questions.
- **Non-verbal communication:** Use appropriate gestures to maintain a friendly and attentive persona. Respond to non-verbal cues as appropriate.
- **Verbal communication:** React to the patient's concerns and expectations; try to be empathetic where appropriate. Periodically make use of summaries and signposting, as this helps clarify any queries the patient may have and gives the opportunity to add new information. This also provides you with a chance to think of any further questions you may want to ask in order to complete your history. Make good use of natural pauses in the conversation for this purpose.

The history

❏ **Presenting complaint**
- Start with an open-ended question that gives the patient an opportunity to freely express what has actually brought them to hospital, for example: *'What has brought you to see me today?'*
- Remember that patients do not present with a complaint of 'lung cancer' or 'pneumonia'; presenting complaints could be coughing up blood or increasing shortness of breath.

❏ **History of presenting complaint**
- **Pain:** For histories involving pain, use the mnemonic **SOCRATES** to help structure your history-taking:

TABLE 2.1 Pain history

	Description
Site	Where exactly is the pain? You can ask them to point to it, as this often helps if they are having difficulty explaining its site.
Onset	Did the pain start suddenly or gradually? Over what period of time? Have they had similar pain in the past? If so, how often do they get it?
Character	Can they describe the pain, whether is it sharp, heavy, burning or colicky? Can they rate the pain on a pain scale of 1–10, 1 being no pain and 10 the worst pain ever; does the pain wake them up at night? This will tell you about the severity of the pain.
Radiation	Does the pain move anywhere else?
Alleviating factors	What makes the pain better? For example, taking analgesia, adopting a certain position, rest or exercise.
Timing	When does the pain come on? Is it there all the time? Does it come and go? How long does it last for?
Exacerbating factors	What makes the pain worse? Movement, exercise, cold air, stress, breathing?
Associated **S**ymptoms	Ask about any symptoms associated with the pain, such as nausea or vomiting, diarrhoea?

For any given symptom, you must identify some key facts:

❑ **Symptom:** What is the symptom? Get them to describe it the best they can; give them possible options if they are struggling to express themselves.

❑ **Timeline:** Determine the timeline, e.g. when did it start, is this the first time they have had it?

❑ **Progression:** How has it changed or progressed over time in terms of frequency, severity?

❑ **Exacerbating/alleviating factors:** Does anything affect it, make it better or worse?

General features to question include:

❑ **Previous healthy state:** It is important to identify when the individual was last well, and what has been happening since, in a chronological manner.

❑ **Systems review:** You can ask for relevant symptoms according to the organ system involved (*see* below).

❑ **Previous symptoms:** It is important to ask whether they have had these symptoms before (you will not routinely be told this, but it is very important to ask as they may give you the answer!), and if so, were they investigated, were they given a diagnosis or any treatment at the time?

❑ **Risk-factor assessment:** This can be a very useful signpost in the exam; for example, whilst taking a history of cardiac chest pain, you can inform the patient that you would now like to assess for risk factors for heart disease. In doing so, you are also informing the examiner of what you are doing next and your intention. This can be adapted to almost any presenting complaint and is a list of important features that help you to assess the severity of a patient's diagnosis or risk stratification.

❑ **Past medical history**
  ▪ **Check for any pre-existing medical conditions**
  ▪ Sometimes, simply asking an individual whether they have any other medical problems will not give you any answers, as they may not understand what a medical problem is or consider any of their other co-morbidities to be medical illnesses (as the authors have all experienced many times).
  ▪ You will often need to dig deeper. Even if they have already given you a list of a few medical problems, they may have omitted something important, so always ask whether they have been in hospital before (you will find most people say yes), and if so, why and what were they diagnosed with? If they don't know the diagnosis, you may ask what they presented with to the hospital.
  ▪ Specifically in finals, ask about: tuberculosis, myocardial infarction, hypertension, diabetes, asthma/COPD and epilepsy.

❑ **Family history**
  ▪ This is an important question to ask in a history, especially if linked with the aetiology of the presenting complaint and the suspected diagnosis.
  ▪ Is there a family history of cancer, IBD, IHD, diabetes or MI at an early age?
  ▪ Ask if their parents are both alive; if not, what did they die of and at what age? What is the health of their siblings like? The death of multiple family members at young ages should trigger you to consider whether the same disease process is occurring in your patient.

❑ **Drug history & allergies**
  ▪ **Allergies:** Start by asking specifically about any allergies the patient has, and ask the

patient to describe what reaction they had to the medication, to help discern whether this is intolerance, drug side effects or a true allergy. Once you start working and writing up a patient's drug card, you will be asked to write down any drugs the patient is allergic to and the specific symptoms they get with this allergy. In practice, this becomes especially important when prescribing medications such as antibiotics where a patient informs you they have an allergy to penicillin, as this can severely limit the number of suitable antibiotics you are able to prescribe, especially if there is antibiotic resistance present.

- **Medications:** Specifically, enquire regarding:
  - **Drug name:** You may get some names you are unfamiliar with, as patients tend to use the trade names as opposed to generic names, e.g. Plavix for clopidogrel. If you hear a drug which you have not come across and are unsure what it is, sometimes asking the patient what they use the drug for can help you to narrow down the correct class of drug. Occasionally, the patient cannot pronounce the drug's name; again, finding out what they use the drug for can help you to suggest possible names and therefore narrow down the actual drug name.
  - **Frequency of administration & timing:** Is this once a day (od), twice a day (bd), thrice (tds), four times (qds), when required (prn), at night (nocte) or in the morning (mane)?
  - **Route:** Usually, self-taken medications are oral but can be subcutaneous, e.g. insulin.
  - **Compliance:** This is often missed when taking a drug history; classical examples include diuretics, which patients may have stopped taking due to the predictable effect of increased frequency of urine. This is especially true in elderly patients whose mobility is already reduced and who may suffer incontinence due to their inability to mobilise to the toilet in time.

To avoid all of this, you may simply ask if they have a copy of their repeat prescription from their GP. Some patients will carry a copy of this, so ask for the list and take a look. Note if any of the drugs on the prescription are for medical conditions the patient hasn't informed you of. A classic example is antihypertensives in a patient who says they have no medical problems; many patients do not consider hypertension to be a medical condition.

❏ **Social history**
- **Smoking:** Do they smoke? If yes, how much? And for how long? If they don't currently smoke, did they in the past? When did they stop, and how long did they smoke for? It is most useful and convenient to communicate number of cigarettes smoked in pack-years: **1 pack-year is 20 cigarettes per day for 1 year.**
- **Alcohol intake:** Ask them how much they drink a week; be specific and ask numbers of drinks and type. Many patients will say they don't drink much, but when directly questioned will reveal they are actually drinking over the recommended weekly allowance. It is best to work out number of units per week. The recommended limits of alcohol intake in the UK are 14 units/week for females and 21 units/week for males. For those who drink heavily, it may be easier to ask them what they drink in 1 day and multiply by 7. Another point to note is remembering to ask if patients have ever consumed alcohol heavily in the past. In the exam, they may often give you verbal clues, so listen out.

TABLE 2.2 Alcohol units

Drink	Units
Pint of beer (3%–5%)	2–3 units
Pint of cider	2–3 units
Small glass of wine, 125 mL (~12%)	1.5 units
Large glass of wine, 250 mL (~12%)	3 units
Bottle of wine, 750 mL	9 units
Glass of champagne, 125 mL	1.5 units
Alcopop bottle	1.5 units
Whisky, 25 mL (standard shot) (40%)	1 unit
Bottle of vodka, 750 mL	28 units

- **Accommodation:** Who do they live with? In a house/bungalow/flat? If elderly, how do they normally mobilise? Independently? Stick, frame? Do they have carers? Who does the cooking, cleaning and shopping? Do they still drive? (Important in cases of epilepsy and dementia).
❏ **Systems review**
  - There are often associated symptoms that occur commonly with the presenting complaint.
  - This also serves to form the basis of useful negative or positive symptoms which may help to differentiate between the various diagnoses:
    — **Cardiovascular:** chest pain, dyspnoea, orthopnoea, paroxysmal nocturnal dyspnoea, ankle oedema, palpitations, syncope
    — **Respiratory:** dyspnoea, cough, sputum, haemoptysis, wheeze
    — **GI tract:** indigestion, dyspepsia, dysphagia, odynophagia, abdominal pain/ discomfort, nausea, vomiting, haematemesis, change in bowel habit, tenesmus, urgency, rectal blood loss
    — **Neurological:** headaches, fits, faints, weakness, changes in vision or hearing
    — **Locomotor:** joint pain, stiffness or swelling?
    — **Genitourinary:** frequency, urgency, dysuria, haematuria, nocturia, incontinence
      - **Male:** hesitancy, poor stream, dribbling, urethral discharge
      - **Female:** last menstrual period or have they reached/going through the menopause; are they pregnant, any vaginal discharge
      - Sexual history (if applicable): same partner/new partner, protected/unprotected sexual intercourse.

Conclusion

❏ **Summarise:** Summarise back to the patient what they have just told you; this will ensure you have not missed their point or anything else important. This will also let the patient know that you have been listening (in addition to your usual communication skills during history-taking).
❏ **Anything patient wishes to add:** Always get into the habit of asking the patient to add anything that you have not covered in your summary which they feel is important or if they want to add something that you may not have asked them.

❑ **Offer a diagnosis/management plan:** If it is just a history-taking station, then to improve your marks for communication skills, you could tell the patient what you think the differential and likely diagnosis is and what the next steps will be. This could include detailing any examinations or investigations which you feel would help confirm or dispute your suspected diagnosis.

❑ **Answer any patient queries:** Ask the patient whether they have any questions for you. If they have, answer the best you can; if you do not know the answer, do not make something up. Be honest and say you do not know but that you will speak to a senior or your consultant and come back to them with the answer.

❑ **Offer a follow-up:** On ending the consultation, if deemed appropriate to your OSCE scenario, offer them a point of contact. This could be a consultant's secretary if the OSCE is set in an outpatient clinic or if set on the ward; identify a member of nursing staff who could bleep you.

❑ **Thank the patient**

❑ **Present your findings**

Finally, turn to the examiner and present your findings in a succinct manner, followed by a summary of your differential diagnosis and a plan. If it was a history-taking station, this will most certainly start with offering an examination of the relevant system involved, followed by tests which should start with simple bedside tests, non-invasive tests and escalating to more invasive and complex investigations.

AUTHOR'S TOP TIP

It is useful when presenting to list important positive and negative risk factors in your initial summary of findings and not always stick to the classical division of PC, HPC, PMH, etc. An example would be a patient with suspected cardiac chest pain, where after identifying the patient's name, age and presenting complaint, you should list whether they were a smoker, had any previous cardiac history or family history of cardiac disease, etc. This stratification of risk factors will show the examiner that you are interpreting the history in order to form a useful differential diagnosis, and not just regurgitating the history you have just taken verbatim.

CHAPTER 3

Cardiovascular

3.1 EXAMINATION OF THE CARDIOVASCULAR SYSTEM

This OSCE station is almost certainly guaranteed in finals, and you would be placing yourself at a great disadvantage if you were not well versed with its slick execution as well as a thorough understanding of the common cases that crop up. Below, we describe a schema to follow.

In general, OSCE stations will give clear instructions on what is expected of you. The majority will ask you to 'examine the cardiovascular system', in which case follow the schema below. Occasionally, you may have an instruction which simply says 'examine the heart' or 'listen to the heart'. These vague terms understandably add anxiety to an already pressured situation. In this case, we suggest you still follow the schema below, as the examiner will redirect if they wish for you to focus on simply 'listening to the heart'.

Clinical examination

Introduction

As for any clinical encounter (*see* Chapter 1, Section 3); specifically for this case:

❑ **Expose patient adequately:** The patient needs to have their chest and abdomen fully exposed. Ask for a chaperone if required.

AUTHOR'S TOP TIP

Female patients may not be comfortable removing bras, so use your discretion. In general, leaving the bra on and covering the patient up whenever exposure is not required is the best course of action. This leaves you appearing empathetic and caring for the patient's modesty.

❑ **Position patient appropriately:** The patient needs to be in a supine position, lying at 45 degrees, with the head resting on one pillow and their arms by their side; the level of the bed needs to be at an appropriate height to make the examination comfortable for the examiner from a standing position.

Inspection

❏ **Perform a general inspection from the end of the bed**

- **Paraphernalia:** Look around the bed for peripheral stigmata of disease, such as ECG leads, elastic compression stockings, oxygen masks, GTN spray.
- **Patient's demeanour:** Does the patient look comfortable? Or do they look like they are in pain? Is there a malar flush, as seen in mitral stenosis and pulmonary hypertension? Is there a syndromic appearance? Down's syndrome: ventricular septal defect (VSD); Turner's syndrome: coarctation, bicuspid aortic valve (AV), aortic stenosis (AS); Noonan's syndrome: pulmonary stenosis (PS).
- **Degree of illness:** Does the patient look well? Are they peripherally shut down, is there pallor (anaemia) or are they clammy? Cyanosis – peripheral or central (central could indicate congenital heart disease or end-stage heart failure). Breathing and respiratory rate – dyspnoea or wheezing (asthma, COPD, asthma, LV failure).
- **Scars** (*see* Viva Q3)
- **Listen carefully:** Occasionally, the patient may have had a metal heart-valve replacement, and so you may be able to hear the audible noise coming from this at the bedside.

AUTHOR'S TOP TIP

It is important to tell the patient exactly what you will be doing at each stage of the examination.

❏ **Examine the hands**

- **Inspect the nails**
  - Splinter haemorrhages: seen in infective endocarditis
  - Clubbing (*see* Chapter 9, Case 8)
  - Nicotine staining: indicative of smoking; a risk factor in IHD
- **Inspect the hands/arms**
  - **Peripheral cyanosis:** due to left-to-right shunts
  - **Signs associated with endocarditis:** Janeway lesions (non-tender flat erythematous macules on palmar aspect of hand); Osler's nodes (red-brown painful subcutaneous papules on fingertips)
  - Pallor of the palmar creases (anaemia); xanthoma (yellow deposits seen in hyperlipidaemia)
  - Puncture marks: signs of intravenous drug use; useful to know in a case of suspected subacute bacterial endocarditis (SBE)
- **Assess capillary refill time**
  - This is done by compressing the pulp of the fingertips and releasing to see how quickly the perfusion returns, giving you an indication of how well perfused the extremities are. You can also assess vein filling; if these are collapsed and empty, it suggests poor peripheral flow/perfusion.
  - Normally, this is equal to or less than 2 seconds.
- **Assess temperature of peripheries**
  - A quick assessment of peripheral temperature in the fingers and hands (unless in a very cold room) may indicate hypoperfusion and possible hypovolaemia.

❑ **Assess radial pulse**

■ The radial pulse can be found just lateral to the flexor carpi radialis tendon.

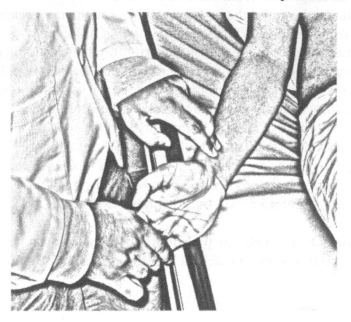

FIGURE 3.1 Assessing the radial pulse

TABLE 3.1A Pulse assessment

Assessment of pulse	Description
Rate	Count the radial pulse for 15 seconds and multiply by 4 to get the rate. Bradycardia if < 60 beats per min (bpm) most commonly due to beta-blocker therapy in the exam; a rate of > 100 is a tachycardia
Rhythm	Regular: a normal finding, called sinus rhythm
	Regularly irregular: heart block, ectopics
	Irregularly irregular: seen in AF
	(*See* Chapter 12, Table 12.11 Aetiology of tachycardias and bradycardia, for further details)
Delay	**Radial–radial delay:** assess the difference if any between the right and left radial pulses. Any delay may indicate atherosclerosis or aortic dissection
	Radio–femoral delay: assess difference if any between radial and femoral pulses; if present, this suggests coarctation of the aorta; a rare occurrence in finals but an important differential would be acute dissection
Pulse character	**Collapsing pulse:** this is seen in aortic regurgitation and persistent ductus arteriosus (PDA), although this is rare. This is best done by spreading the four fingers of your one hand over the distal radio-ulnar joint whilst palpating the radial pulse with the base of the fingers/forepalm as the hand is wrapped round the wrist; place the fingertips of your other hand over the brachial pulse and lift the arm straight up, feeling for the water-hammer pulse, with a brisk upstroke of the pulse and its sudden 'collapse' characteristically felt as a slap against your palm. If frank, it can feel like a bag of worms across your fingers. Ensure patient has no shoulder pain before doing this.
	(*See* Table 3.1B Further Pulse assessment below, for further details)

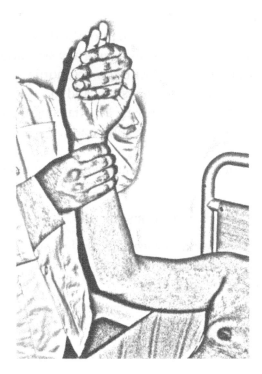

FIGURE 3.2 Assessing for a collapsing pulse

Although character and volume are features that need assessing as part of your assessment of the pulse, these are best examined using a central pulse, of which the carotid is most easily accessible. (*See* Table 3.1B)

AUTHOR'S TOP TIP

In the time before OSCEs, a common short case was to simply assess the pulse. In which case you would be expected to assess the aforementioned parameters alone.

AUTHOR'S TOP TIP

If you suspect AF on examining the radial rate, mention that it is useful to examine the apical rate by listening to the heartbeat. This ventricular rate is useful to know in patients with AF.

AUTHOR'S TOP TIP

Although likely to be atrial fibrillation in the exam, without an ECG you cannot say with certainty that an irregular pulse is AF.

❏ **Check the blood pressure**

■ Usually, this parameter is given to you as part of the doorway information; otherwise, ask the examiner for the BP in both arms, where any significant discrepancy (> 30 mmHg) is classically associated with thoracic aortic dissection.

■ The pulse pressure (difference between systolic and diastolic) can signify certain valvular disease; narrow pulse pressures are associated with aortic stenosis, whereas wide pulse pressures are seen in aortic regurgitation.

You may be required to perform this, so make sure you are confident in doing this manually.

AUTHOR'S TOP TIP

Blood pressure is easily forgotten, especially when presenting your findings. Remain vigilant to this, as blood pressure is an important aspect of the cardiovascular exam and is an easy mark to gain, given that usually the BP is given to you.

❏ **Inspect the eyes and face**

TABLE 3.2 Examination features

Feature	Assess for
Eyes	**Anaemia:** pull the lower eyelid of one eye down to assess for paleness; if found, assess for central cyanosis
	Sclera: blue sclera associated with Marfan's, Ehlers–Danlos syndrome; although rare, such patients have AR, ASD, mitral valve prolapse
	Fundoscopy: ophthalmoscopic findings of Roth spots (small red haemorrhages with a pale centre occurring in vasculitis; a feature of endocarditis); hypertensive and diabetic retinopathy
	Others: corneal arcus seen in hypercholesterolaemia
Face	**Central cyanosis:** look at the lips, mucous membranes and under the tongue for central cyanosis (congenital cyanotic heart disease)
	Cushingoid appearance: associated with hypertension
	Xanthelasma: these are periorbital deposits appearing as yellow plaques; highly suggestive of hypercholesterolaemia and diabetes

---

AUTHOR'S TOP TIP

Fundoscopy may not be practical in the setting of a 5-minute OSCE, and the examiner would certainly not expect you to perform this. However, do ensure you offer this at the end of your examination for the extra mark.

❏ **Assess the jugular venous pressure (JVP)**

Ask the patient to turn their head looking at the opposite wall, thereby exposing the right side of their neck.

■ **Anatomy:** JVP is assessed using the internal jugular vein (IJV); the right IJV is preferred

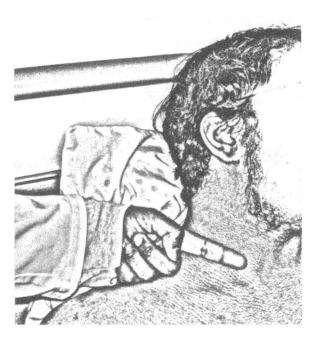

FIGURE 3.3 Assessing the JVP

as it runs an almost straight course from the lobule of the ear to the median end of the clavicle, lying in between the two heads of the sternocleidomastoid muscles; it is valveless (unlike the external jugular).

- **Physiology:** The IJV reflects the pressure and function of the right side of the heart and thoracic cavity, providing information on circulatory volume and right ventricular function.
- **JVP height:** At 45 degrees, the JVP should not be any higher than 3–4 cm from the sternal angle of Louis; if it is, then this suggests pathology (*see* Table 3.3).

TABLE 3.3 Causes of raised JVP

Cause	Description
Overfilled right atrium	Fluid overload, right ventricular failure, pregnancy
Right ventricular compression	Cardiac tamponade, constrictive pericarditis
Increased intrathoracic pressure leading to right heart failure	Pulmonary hypertension, pulmonary oedema, tension pneumothorax
Tricuspid valve disease	Stenosis, regurgitation, cardiac myxoma
Superior vena cava obstruction	Lung tumour, mediastinal masses, large thyroid goitre

A low jugular venous pressure may indicate that the heart is underfilled secondary to hypovolaemia from, for example, dehydration. This can be demonstrated in a patient when lying supine, whereby normally the JVP should be raised. In an underfilled patient, the JVP will not be visible in this position. Hence the importance of having the examining couch at 45 degrees in the cardiovascular examination, because at this angle the JVP should be just visible. If the JVP is very high, it may cause twitching of the ear lobe with the pulsations. In this scenario, the patient should be sat up to 90 degrees and the JVP reassessed.

You would not be expected to draw the venous waveform, although some understanding of the waveform will certainly impress any examiner.

■ **Perform the hepatojugular reflex**

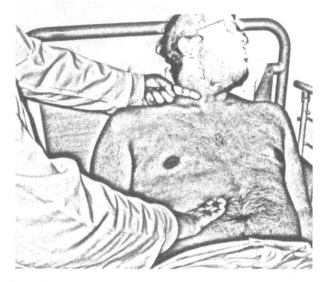

FIGURE 3.4 Hepatojugular reflex

— If the JVP is difficult to see, performing this test may help accentuate this.
— Ensure you ask about abdominal pain before you do this; press lightly over the liver in the right hypochondrium and look at the JVP for the expected rise. If the rise lasts > 5 seconds, this is suggestive of right heart failure.

❑ **Palpate the carotid pulse**
   ■ The carotid pulse is best felt with the pulp of your three fingers just lateral to the trachea; if difficult to locate, asking the patient to turn their head to the contralateral side may help.
   ■ Examine one side at a time and assess pulse volume and character.

TABLE 3.1B Further pulse assessment

Assessment	Description
Pulse volume	**Large volume:** suggestive of a hyperdynamic circulation such as sepsis, anaemia and CO_2 retention, aortic regurgitation
	Low volume: low cardiac output states such as CCF and hypovolaemia (where the pulse may be thin and thready in a shocked patient)
Character	**Slow-rising pulse:** sometimes called anacrotic pulse; is a feature of aortic stenosis
	Collapsing pulse: seen in aortic incompetence, amongst others (*see* Table 3.1A)
	Pulsus paradoxus: this is when there is a fall in pulse pressure to > 10 mmHg on inspiration. This is actually a misnomer, as this is an exaggerated physiological response and not in fact paradoxical. Classically seen in conditions whereby venous return is restricted, such as in severe acute asthma or cardiac tamponade, and thus unlikely to feature in the exam. This is diagnosed by using a manual blood pressure cuff and measuring the systolic pressure on inspiration and expiration
	Pulsus alternans: alternating large- and small-volume beats. Seen in aortic stenosis and severe left ventricular failure

❑ **Assess the thorax**
  ■ **Further inspection of anterior chest wall and axilla**
    — **Pacemaker:** You may see the pacemaker device; often found inferior to left lateral scapula but can also be on the right. (They are usually inserted on the non-dominant side, and thus can be found on the right also).

    — **Surgical scars:** Scars from the pacemaker insertion, thoracotomy (inframammary scar) in mitral valvotomy, median sternotomy from any number of open cardiac surgeries, e.g. CABG, valve replacement.
    — **Chest wall deformities.**
    — **Visible pulsations:** In thin patients, the apex beat may be visibly pulsating.

Palpation
❑ **Palpate for heaves and thrills**

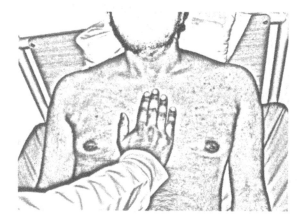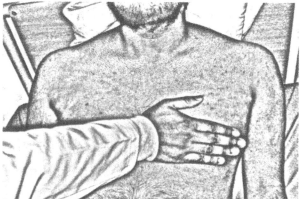

FIGURE 3.5A–B Heaves and thrills

TABLE 3.4 Heaves and thrills

Finding	Description
Heaves	**Technique:** feel with the flat of your hand placed vertically over the left sternal edge. A heave (forceful palpable impulse) will lift your hand off the chest wall.
	Pathology: right ventricular or left atrial hypertrophy
Thrills	**Technique:** place the flat of your hand transversely over the manubrium to feel for a thrill (felt as a vibration)
	Pathology: these are palpable murmurs caused by turbulent blood flow

❑ **Assess the apex beat**
   ▪ **Comment on its presence:** Identify its location.

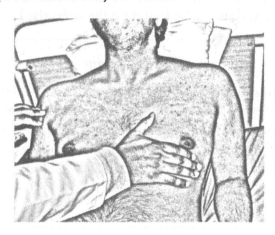

FIGURE 3.6 Apex beat

— Normally found in the fifth intercostal space in the midclavicular line; defined as the most inferior point where the cardiac impulse is still palpable.
— You must demonstrate the process of identifying the fifth intercostal space to the examiner.
— Begin by locating the angle of Louis at the manubriosternal joint (this is continuous with the second costal cartilage), inferior to this is the second intercostal space, count downwards to the fifth space and then move along to the midclavicular line by drawing an imaginary line from the midpoint of the left clavicle down to the 5th space.
— Place your hand here and feel for the apex beat.
— If difficult to feel, asking the patient to roll to the left slightly will make palpation easier as the apex is brought forward.
— If still difficult to feel, this may be because the apex is displaced (*see* Table 3.5), in which case you must identify the new location of the apex beat.
   • e.g. *'The apex beat is displaced to the 6th intercostal space in the anterior axillary line.'*

AUTHOR'S TOP TIP

If you cannot palpate the apex beat, then simply say so. The apex beat may not normally be palpable in some patients due to variations in body habitus.

You may choose instead to generally place your hand over where the apex beat should be and feel for the pulse, and then, working backwards, identify its exact location from here, rather than identify its expected location first, as explained above. This technique makes it easier to identify a displaced apex. Use whichever method you are comfortable with; both methods are acceptable.

- **Comment on the apex beat's features**

TABLE 3.5 Characteristic apex beat features

Feature	Description
Location	**Displaced:** this will be laterally and/or inferiorly displaced in cardiomegaly, often a sign of an incompetent valve
	Non-displaced: this is usually normal, but can be a feature of aortic and mitral stenosis
Character	**Strong/lifting:** mitral or aortic regurgitation
	Tapping apex beat: this is a palpable first heart sound, seen in mitral or tricuspid stenosis
	Sustained apex beat: aortic stenosis

AUTHOR'S TOP TIP

Some students prefer to palpate the apex beat before checking for heaves/thrills. We suggest you do this last as this brings you nicely onto auscultation of the mitral valve, as you have identified its location, and makes your examination look more slick.

Note that percussion of the heart has limited clinical value.

Auscultation

❑ **Identify the four areas for auscultation**

TABLE 3.6 SURFACE ANATOMY OF HEART VALVES

Valve	Surface location
Aortic	Right sternal edge, 2nd intercostal space
Pulmonary	Left sternal edge, 2nd intercostal space
Tricuspid	Left sternal edge, 4th intercostal space
Mitral	Midclavicular line, 5th intercostal space

AUTHOR'S TOP TIP

Note that you will be listening in turn over the four different areas where the heart sounds corresponding to each valve are best heard; these bear no actual anatomical meaning. These can be remembered with the mnemonic: A Place To Meet.

AUTHOR'S TOP TIP

We suggest you follow the order suggested below as this makes the examination of the heart look smooth and slick; rather than haphazardly checking a valve in a random fashion. Remember to use both the bell and diaphragm appropriately; the bell for low frequency murmurs and the diaphragm for high frequency sounds.

TABLE 3.7 Bell & diaphragm usage

Component	Description of use
Bell	Used for low-frequency murmurs, e.g. mitral stenosis – mid-diastolic murmur, S3
Diaphragm	High-frequency murmurs, e.g. ejection murmurs, clicks, aortic regurgitation – early diastolic murmur

---

AUTHOR'S TOP TIP

The surface location is useful to know, as this is commonly questioned in exams, so to avoid this question, physically demonstrate to the examiner your knowledge. This is best done by locating the angle of Louis, corresponding to the 2nd intercostal space, then the midclavicular line by dividing the clavicle in half and counting down the intercostal spaces with your fingers to identify the mitral valve or whichever valve you are auscultating. In actual practice, it is easiest just to demonstrate the mitral valve initially then move to each valve in turn from here, as this is the usual starting point.

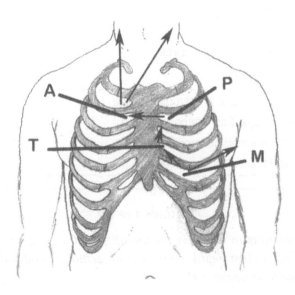

FIGURE 3.7 Surface anatomy of heart valves

Aortic, Pulmonary, Tricuspid & Mitral

❑ **Auscultate the mitral valve (the apex)**
- **Locate the valve**
  - You would have already identified the apex beat on palpation earlier; if the apex was non-displaced when you identified its location, this will be the 5th intercostal space, midclavicular line.
  - If you identify the location to be in the 6th intercostal space or more lateral than expected, this suggests the apex beat is displaced, and consequently you will need to auscultate in this position rather than the classical position.
- **Auscultate in this region**
  - Listen with the diaphragm of your stethoscope; followed by the bell placed lightly.
  - Listen for normal heart sounds, any added sounds and murmurs (*see* below).

If you hear a murmur, you must also perform the special manoeuvres below.

- **Special manoeuvres**

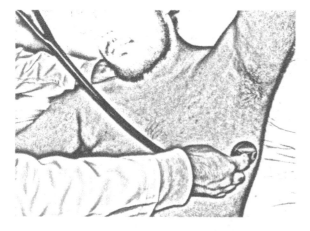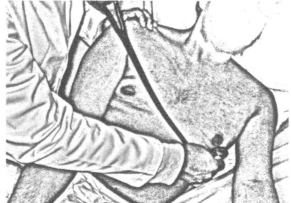

FIGURE 3.8A–B Special manoeuvres for mitral valve

— **Auscultate for radiation:** Listen in axilla with the diaphragm for an audible murmur which signifies radiation. The pansystolic murmur of mitral regurgitation radiates to the axilla.

— **Auscultate with patient in left lateral position:** This brings the apex closer to the chest wall. You may need to repalpate the apex, as its position would have moved, before listening again. Listen with the bell for the low-frequency mid-diastolic murmur of mitral stenosis.

— **Assess variation with respiration:** Listen with their breath held in end expiration (this will enhance mitral murmurs).

   • e.g. *'Can you please roll over to your left, slightly. Now take a deep breath in and then out and now hold your breath for a second. [Listen for a few seconds] Now breathe.'*

AUTHOR'S TOP TIP

It is important you remember to remind the patient it is OK for them to breathe again as some patients follow your instructions strictly and do not continue breathing again and turn blue! This also demonstrates that you have clearly done this before on a real patient as you would have come across this behaviour.

EXAMINER'S ANECDOTE

When I was a medical student, my colleagues had played a prank on me by placing gum into my stethoscope tubing so I couldn't hear a thing. Despite this, I still managed to pass finals without ever hearing any murmurs! Remember, it is your examination technique and sensible management plan that will get you out of trouble, even if you are deaf as a post!

❏ **Auscultate the tricuspid valve**
   ▪ **Locate the valve** (*see* Table 3.6)
   ▪ **Auscultate in this region:** Use the diaphragm
   ▪ **Special manoeuvres**

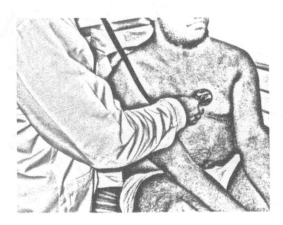

FIGURE 3.9 Special manoeuvres for AR

— Auscultate with patient sitting forward in expiration: this will amplify the high frequency diastolic murmur of aortic regurgitation if present.

Lie the patient back down again to 45 degrees to listen to the remaining two valves.

❏ **Auscultate the pulmonary valve:** Locate and auscultate the valve (*see* Table 3.6).

❏ **Auscultate the aortic valve:** Locate and auscultate the valve (*see* Table 3.6); if you hear a murmur, check for radiation by listening to the carotids (*see* below).

AUTHOR'S TOP TIP

Whenever you are listening to the four areas, keep in mind which valve you are listening to, as this helps you work out the pathology.

AUTHOR'S TOP TIP

Some prefer to listen to all four areas, before coming back to perform manoeuvres in the various individual areas. However, we feel it saves time by performing manoeuvres when initially auscultating each of the four areas, as in the heat of the exam you may forget to do this afterwards.

AUTHOR'S TOP TIP

Whilst auscultating the heart sounds of a patient, you should be forming a differential diagnosis in your mind and thinking about how best to present your finding such that it supports your diagnosis. By focusing on eliciting signs supportive of your diagnosis or collating signs you have already detected, you will find if you practise presenting in the same order in which you examine for these signs, your presentation will be convincing. This also helps focus your attention to actively look for these coexisting signs during the examination.

❏ **Assess the heart sounds**
  - **Auscultate for presence of two heart sounds (S1 & S2):** You should normally hear two heart sounds. You can time these with the pulse, S1 coinciding with the pulse.

TABLE 3.7 Normal heart sounds

First heart sound (S1)	Second heart sound (S2)
This occurs due to closure of the mitral valve.	This occurs due to closure of the aortic valve (A2) followed by the pulmonary valve (P2).
This can be loud in tachycardia and mitral stenosis.	These two sounds A2 and P2 comprise the second heart sound, i.e. it is normally split, although the timing of the split varies in certain conditions: widened normally in inspiration, fixed in atrial septal defects and can even be reversed.
This can be soft in bradycardia and heart block.	

  - **Auscultate for any added sounds.**

TABLE 3.8 Added heart sounds

Added sound	Description
Third heart sound (S3)	This occurs due to rapid left ventricular filling in diastole. Sometimes called a gallop rhythm.
	This can be a normal physiological finding in young healthy athletic adults and children. It is also seen in heart failure and mitral regurgitation.
Fourth heart sound (S4)	This occurs due to forceful atrial contraction against a stiff left ventricle. Its presence is always pathological and is associated with amyloidosis, aortic stenosis and hypertension, amongst others.
Others	Metallic heart sounds are unmistakeable when heard. *See* Viva Q7. Opening snap heard in mitral stenosis. Mid-systolic click in mitral valve prolapse. Pericardial rub seen in pericarditis.

❑ **Assess any murmurs:** Aim to describe the following:
- **Occurrence in systole or diastole**
  - Systolic murmurs occur between S1 and S2.
  - Diastolic murmurs occur between S2 and S3.

AUTHOR'S TOP TIP

Diastolic murmurs are notoriously difficult to hear. For finals, it is probably more than enough that you've heard the murmur for you to pass. Even if you are not sure if it's diastolic or systolic, in finals you are far more likely to hear a systolic murmur, therefore if you had to guess, guess systolic!

- **Murmur character**
  - Characteristic quality of a murmur is helpful in distinguishing the valvular lesion.
  - For example, is the murmur pansystolic, ejection systolic or a rumbling mid-diastolic murmur? (*See* Table 3.10 for further details)
- **Identify the region the murmur is heard best**
  - This may be at specific sites which are characteristic to the valvular lesion involved (*see* Table 3.10).
  - Occasionally, the murmur is so loud that it is heard all over the precordium.
- **Check for presence of radiation**
  - In systolic murmurs, routinely check the axilla and the carotids for radiation.
- **Assess variation with respiration**
  - This is performed in certain regions (*see* above) and will help identify the site of the lesion.

AUTHOR'S TOP TIP

Left-sided heart murmurs are heard loudest during expiration, as blood flow through the left side of the heart increases; whereas right-sided murmurs are exaggerated on inspiration, due to the increased flow of venous blood through the right side of the heart.

■ **Quantify the grade**
— If you are confident in your findings, you may quantify the murmurs as shown below.

TABLE 3.9 Grading of murmurs

Murmur grade	Description
Grade I	Very faint, only just audible with stethoscope
Grade II	Soft, audible with stethoscope
Grade III	Medium intensity, heard all over precordium
Grade IV	Loud, an associated thrill can be felt
Grade V	Louder, audible with stethoscope only partially touching the chest; easily palpable thrill
Grade VI	Very loud, audible without stethoscope

AUTHOR'S TOP TIP

There are other special manoeuvres that can augment difficult-to-hear murmurs, such as the Valsalva manoeuvre, exercise or by altering patient positioning from standing to squatting. Such manoeuvres are best avoided in finals, as they have potential for harm to the patient.

Typical murmurs you may come across include:

TABLE 3.10 Murmurs

Region	Characteristic murmurs
Mitral	**Mitral regurgitation (MR):** pansystolic murmur (PSM), radiating to the axilla (if very loud, can radiate across precordium)
	Mitral stenosis (MS): mid-diastolic; typically no radiation
Tricuspid	**Aortic regurgitation (AR):** early diastolic; radiating to apex
	Tricuspid regurgitation (TR): PSM
	Ventricular septal defect (VSD): ejection systolic murmur (ESM)
Pulmonary	**Pulmonary stenosis (PS):** ESM loudest on inspiration
Aortic	**Aortic stenosis (AS):** ESM loudest on expiration, radiating to carotids (if very loud, can radiate across precordium)
	Aortic sclerosis: ESM with no radiation

Although difficult to describe phonetically, the murmurs are best learnt by listening to as many hearts as you can in the build-up to finals. Below is a phonocardiogram of the commonly encountered murmurs.

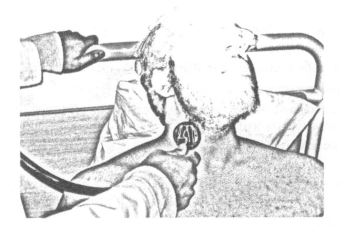

FIGURE 3.10 Phonocardiogram of murmurs

❑ **Auscultate for carotid bruits**

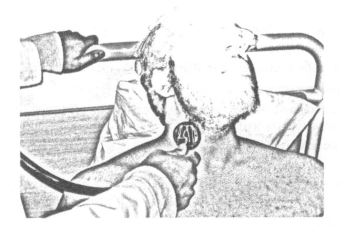

FIGURE 3.11 Carotid bruits

■ **Listen for bruits or radiation from an ESM**
  — Use the diaphragm of the stethoscope and listen to end expiration, bilaterally
    • *'Take a deep breath in, then out and now hold. [Listen] Now breathe normally.'*

Remember, a bruit is caused by turbulent blood flow through a narrowed artery giving rise to a characteristic audible noise.

❑ **Assess for oedema**
  - ■ **Check for pulmonary oedema**
    - — Ask the patient to lean forward so you can percuss and auscultate the lung bases for crackles as a sign of pulmonary oedema in left heart failure.
    - — It is best to take this opportunity to inspect further the posterior chest wall for any scars or deformities (ankylosing spondylitis is associated with AR).
  - ■ **Check for sacral oedema**
    - — After you have listened to the lungs, you are best positioned to examine the sacrum for oedema.
    - — This is best done by pressing firmly onto the sacrum for 10 seconds and releasing. A slowly resolving indentation is suggestive of pitting oedema.
  - ■ **Check for pedal oedema**
    - — Press firmly over the site of oedema for 10 seconds and release, looking for any indentations.
    - — Estimate the level of oedema, whether this is at the ankles, calves or knees, and whether the oedema is pitting.
    - — While you are examining the legs, you may inspect further for scars seen in vein harvesting for CABG.

Complete the examination

❑ **Further examination**
  - ■ *'To complete my exam, I would like to perform a brief examination of the abdomen, looking for hepatomegaly, a pulsatile liver (a feature of TR) and splenomegaly (seen in infective endocarditis).*
  - ■ *I would also like to perform a peripheral vascular examination, paying particular attention to peripheral pulses. I would also perform fundoscopy to assess for signs of SBE, hypertensive and diabetic retinopathy. I would also like to look at the chest radiograph, a 12-lead ECG, urine dip results for haematuria in infective endocarditis as well as examine any observation charts available: pulse, blood pressure, temperature.'*

AUTHOR'S TOP TIP

A PA chest radiograph is preferred, because the angle with which the X-ray beam hits the patient in an AP view results in an apparent cardiomegaly, and so heart size cannot be accurately commented on. Although the actual difference in heart size to the naked eyed between an AP and PA film is variable and may even be negligible in some cases, it is best to stick to the aforementioned rule in finals as the reasoning for disputing this is certainly not something you should be doing in finals.

Hepatosplenomegaly are signs of right-sided heart failure. If you heard a murmur, it is best to describe this murmur with all its characteristic features, e.g.:

'There was a grade III pansystolic murmur, best heard at the apex, radiating to the axilla. This is consistent with a mitral incompetence murmur.'

❑ Thank the patient
❑ Wash your hands
❑ Present your findings

Viva questions

Q1   How can the JVP be distinguished from the carotid pulse?
    'The JVP, unlike the arterial pulse:
    ■ *has a double pulsation (the 'a' and 'v' wave).*
    ■ *It is impalpable.*
    ■ *It can be obliterated by light pressure applied at the root of the neck.*
    ■ *The JVP rises momentarily with a hepatojugular reflex.*
    ■ *The height of pulsation varies with respiration, i.e. it falls with inspiration (as venous return increases).'*

Good answer

AUTHOR'S TOP TIP

This is a very common question in finals. It is important therefore that you are fully versed with this and can confidently distinguish between the JVP and carotid pulsation.

Do not confuse the JVP with the external jugular vein, which in some patients is easily visible. The JVP reflects right atrial pressure and consists of two main waveforms: the 'a' wave, representing atrial contraction, and the 'v' wave, representing venous return during tricuspid valve closure. The remaining three components of the waveform (c, x and y) are beyond the scope of this revision guide. The normal waveform is altered in certain conditions (*see* Viva Q2).

Q2   What is Kussmaul's sign, and when is it seen?

Difficult question

■ The JVP varies with the respiratory cycle.
■ The intrathoracic pressure becomes increasingly negative during inspiration, thereby increasing the flow of blood back to the heart, resulting in the JVP falling. During expiration, the reverse happens.
■ Kussmaul's sign is a paradoxical rise of the JVP occurring on inspiration. This occurs when the right atrium fails to accommodate the increased venous return on inspiration and is seen in, for example, constrictive pericarditis, cardiac tamponade and severe asthma.

Some characteristic JVP waveforms occur, for example, in atrial fibrillation, whereby the 'a' wave is lost due to ineffective atrial contraction. Cannon waves or giant 'a' waves occur in complete heart block.

AUTHOR'S TOP TIP

Although a detailed understanding of the JVP is not required, having a basic understanding of some of the abnormalities will make you stand out.

Q3 What are the common scars seen in the cardiovascular examination?

TABLE 3.11 Surgical scars

Scar	Description
Median sternotomy	Used in CABG, aortic or mitral valve replacement
Left thoracotomy scar	This is a diagonal scar running from under the left breast to left axilla
	Used in mitral valvotomy for mitral stenosis
Right parasternal	Used in aortic and mitral valve procedures
Upper hemisternotomy	Used in aortic and mitral valve procedures
Infraclavicular	Used for inserting a permanent pacemaker (PPM)

Q4 What are the causes of commonly heard murmurs?

TABLE 3.12 Aetiology of murmurs

Murmur	Common causes
Mitral incompetence	Endocarditis and rheumatic heart disease
	Rupture of chordate or papillae, e.g. following an MI
	Congenital, associated with ASD
Aortic Incompetence	Congenital causes such as bicuspid valve and Marfan's
	Endocarditis and rheumatic heart disease
	Connective tissue disorders such as rheumatoid arthritis
	Dissection and trauma
	Secondary to longstanding AS with a dilated heart
Pulmonary stenosis	Congenital and rheumatic heart disease
	Carcinoid
Tricuspid incompetence	Functional, rheumatic and carcinoid
	Endocarditis in IV drug users

Note that the terms incompetence and regurgitation are used interchangeably. For further details, see specific cases below.

Q5 What is reverse splitting of the second heart sound?

Honours question

■ This is a phenomenon which occurs when there is significant delay in left ventricular emptying such that the aortic valve closes after the pulmonary valve.

- It is detected when on auscultation the separate components of the second heart sounds are heard on expiration but come together on inspiration.
- **Aetiology:** left bundle branch block (LBBB), HOCM and right ventricular pacing.

This question was asked in one of the author's finals, and even if you weren't aware of the answer, having a brief understanding of physiological splitting will help you give a sensible answer to this difficult question. (*See* Clinical examination above for further details.)

Q6   Do you know of any indications of pacemakers?

Difficult question

- Most commonly due to atrioventricular (AV) block such as third-degree heart block with bradycardia or long periods of asystole, sick sinus syndrome with symptomatic bradycardia, symptomatic second-degree heart block.
- Symptoms include pre-syncope, syncope (Stokes–Adams), confusion and seizures; related to the bradycardia.

AUTHOR'S TOP TIP

You would not be expected to know any details of the pacemaker settings and the meaning of the symbols and codes. However knowing a few indications for having a pacemaker will stand you in good stead.

If you are ever asked what else would you look for on a CXR in a patient with a recently inserted pacemaker, say that although unlikely, some patients may have had an iatrogenic pneumothorax, and this would need to be treated as for any pneumothorax. (*See* Chapter 12, Viva Q3 for further details.) Other complications of pacemakers include: pacemaker failure, infection and electromagnetic interference, amongst others. Remember, there is an absolute contraindication to MRI scans, and this is something which you must actively check for and mention in the exam.

Q7   How would you recognise a mechanical heart valve clinically?

Honours question

- Aside from an audible click at the end of the bed and a midline sternotomy scar:

TABLE 3.13 Mechanical heart valves

Prosthetic	Clinical features
Mitral valve	**Signs:** metallic click at the first heart sound (closure of the prosthetic valve) and an opening click in diastole (opening of valve); normal S2
	Valve leakage: a PSM and heart failure suggest leakage
Aortic valve	**Signs:** normal S1, an ejection click (this is the opening of the prosthetic valve); an ESM and a second click on valve closure
	Valve leakage: early diastolic murmur and collapsing pulse

Even at honours level, you would not be expected to recognise leakage of a prosthetic valve; however, this shows you have spent a great deal of time on a cardiology ward and can recognise this important complication of prosthetic valves.

EXAMINER'S TOP TIP

I couldn't believe she turned round and told me her findings were completely normal. I asked her to stand next to the patient and listen carefully for the very loud and clearly audible sound coming from the metal heart valve! Clearly, she had never seen such a case before. Visit the cardiology ward – you will see plenty.

Other complications include: thromboembolism, infective endocarditis, leakage due to wear of the valve or infection or poor valve seating, obstruction or ball embolus. Haemolysis is a known complication of prosthetic aortic valves.

Other types of valves that can be used are bioprosthetic (cadaveric or a porcine tissue graft). Tissue valves do not cause clicks and have a limited life of up to 10 years, therefore are only really used in elderly patients. The main benefit is that long-term warfarin therapy is not required, as compared to metal heart valves, and the risk of endocarditis is less, although repeat operation rates are higher. It is also useful in patients in whom anticoagulation is not recommended.

Antibiotic prophylaxis is no longer routinely recommended in patients to prevent cases of infective endocarditis.

AUTHOR'S TOP TIP

Although you wouldn't be expected to know the details of prosthetic heart valves you must at the very least be aware of the need for anticoagulation and antibiotic indications. In fact this case came up in one of the author's finals; be prepared!

Q8   What are the signs of infective endocarditis on clinical examination?

TABLE 3.14 Features of endocarditis

Signs	Description
Hand	**Osler's nodes:** tender nodules on finger pulps;
	Janeway lesions: non-tender macules on the palms.
	These are both due to septic emboli and/or vasculitis
	Others: splinter haemorrhages, clubbing and digital infarct (from arterial emboli at end arteries leading to absent pulses)
Eyes	**Roth spots:** retinal vasculitis
	Subconjuctival haemorrhage
Abdomen	**Splenomegaly:** this occurs when the reticuloendothelial system is activated
	Haematuria

Endocarditis must be considered in any patient with a new heart murmur and fever, especially those with a *Staphylococcus aureus* sepsis with no known cause. High-risk patients include those with prosthetic heart valves, rheumatic heart disease, intravenous drug users and those who have had recent dental surgery, these patients should always have this diagnosis excluded, as overwhelming sepsis can lead to multiorgan failure and death. Although blood cultures and acute-phase reactants are useful in diagnosis, a transoesophageal echocardiograph is the definitive test available, demonstrating valvular vegetations. Organisms typically involved in native valves are *Streptococcus viridans*, *Staphylococcus* and *Haemophilus* species, amongst others. Prosthetic valves are affected usually by *Staphylococcus epidermidis* and *aureus*.

Case 1: Heart failure

Instructions: This 80-year-old woman presents with increasing SOB and leg swelling. Please examine the cardiovascular system.

Key features to look for

Inspection
❑ patient may be SOB
❑ poor peripheral perfusion with cool extremities with prolonged capillary refill
❑ central cyanosis may be present
❑ pitting oedema at sacrum and in legs
❑ **JVP:** raised

Palpation
❑ **Pulse:** jerky carotid pulse
❑ **Apex beat:** laterally displaced apex beat; its character may be forceful – signs of cardiac enlargement
❑ **Liver:** may be pulsatile and tender

Auscultation
❑ **Heart sounds:** 3rd heart sound, soft S1
❑ **Murmurs:** any murmur possible, most commonly PSM from mitral regurgitation, but can be any stenotic or incompetent valve
❑ **Lung bases:** bibasal coarse crackles indicative of pulmonary oedema; there may be wheeze

---

AUTHOR'S TOP TIP

The patient with heart failure may have more than one murmur. If you hear two murmurs then mention this to the examiner.

Complete the examination
❑ **Thank the patient**
❑ **Wash your hands**
❑ **Present your findings**

Heart failure affects 2% of the general population and nearly 20% of the elderly. As such, this is a very common case, as there are many stable patients with chronic heart failure who can come to the exam. Practice recognising such patients by visiting any general medical ward.

Viva questions

Q1   What pertinent features in the history would you be interested to know?
- **Age:** Those with heart failure secondary to ischaemic heart disease are typically middle-aged to elderly.
- **Presenting symptoms:** Increasing SOB, peripheral oedema or ascites. Orthopnea and cough productive of frothy white or pink phlegm due to pulmonary oedema.
- **Risk factors:** History of risk factors for IHD, such as smoking, hypertension, hypercholesterolaemia.
- **Medical history:** Previous myocardial infarctions and valve surgery (remember, failing valves cause failure). Screen for other causes; *see* Table 3.15 below.
- **Social history:** Smoking increases rates of IHD, which predisposes to cardiac disease. Excessive alcohol intake. Worsening exercise tolerance; try to quantify. How many pillows do they sleep with at night due to orthopnea?
- **Drug history:** Full drug history and compliance with medications, as poorly controlled hypertension can cause heart failure. History of use of diet pills; some diet pills in the past have been linked with pulmonary hypertension, which can lead to right heart failure.

AUTHOR'S TOP TIP

Don't forget that such patients are prone to side effects due to polypharmacy. You must consider the possibility that their symptoms may be a consequence of this, such as beta blockers causing lethargy, erectile dysfunction, SOB.

If you are aware of the various causes of heart failure, this will help focus your history:

TABLE 3.15 Aetiology of heart failure

Aetiology	Description
Ischaemic heart disease	Angina, myocardial infarction, coronary artery disease
Cardiac arrhythmias	Atrial fibrillation is commonly implicated
Volume & pressure overload	Incompetent valves, especially mitral and aortic. Hypertension is a common cause of pressure overload; aortic stenosis is another
Cor pulmonale	Patients with COPD can develop right heart failure, although multiple pulmonary emboli have also been implicated
Others	Anaemia, hyperthyroidism leading to high output failure; cardiomyopathy and endocarditis leading to valve dysfunction. Rarely, Paget's disease and beriberi

Q2   Do you know of any severity classification for heart failure?

Honours question

■ The New York Heart Association classifies heart failure into four classes based on symptomatology:

TABLE 3.16 Severity classification of heart failure

NYHA	Description
Class I	No limitation to physical activity
Class II	Some limitation to physical activity
Class III	Marked limitation of physical activity
Class IV	Symptoms present at rest

AUTHOR'S TOP TIP

Sometimes, it is very useful to see someone has taken the time to risk-stratify the patient in the exam. This shows to the examiner that you are thinking about the long-term management of the patient.

Note that by the time a patient reaches Class IV, their LVEF is < 35%.

Q3   What pertinent investigations would you request?
■ **Routine blood tests**
— **FBC:** anaemia can cause heart failure
— **U&Es and albumin:** to assess whether fluid overload seen is due to renal failure or low albumin, as opposed to actual heart failure leading to pulmonary oedema
— **Cholesterol & glucose:** to address modifiable risk factors such as diabetes
— **TFTs:** thyrotoxicosis can cause high-output heart failure
■ The following tests are recommended in all suspected heart-failure patients; if normal, then heart failure is unlikely. If abnormal, patients should go on to have a transthoracic echo (TTE).
— **Specialist blood test:** raised B-type natriuretic peptide (BNP)
— **ECG:** signs of ischaemia, old MI or hypertrophy, arrhythmias, especially AF
— **CXR:** cardiomegaly, pleural effusion, dilated upper-lobe vessels, interstitial oedema (often in batwing distribution), Kerley B lines (*see* Chapter 12, Case 6)
■ **Transthoracic echo:** Gold-standard test and investigation of choice used to quantify heart and valve function and degree of failure; degree of left ventricular systolic dysfunction important to know as well as the left ventricular ejection fraction (LVEF); normally > 65% in healthy individuals, higher in hyperdynamic states such as sepsis. This test will help exclude heart failure if not present.

Q4   How would you treat this patient?
Treatment depends upon whether this is acute left ventricular failure (*see* Chapter 11, Emergencies) or chronic heart failure. For chronic heart failure:

- Conservative
  - **Lifestyle changes:** Smoking cessation, healthy diet, weight loss, low-salt diet, avoidance of strenuous exercise (advanced-stage heart failure).
  - **Risk-factor modification:** Manage hypertension and diabetes if present; influenza immunisations.
  - **Avoid precipitating drugs:** Any drugs which cause fluid retention should be stopped, e.g. NSAIDs, calcium channel blockers, corticosteroids and any negative inotropic agents.
  - **Fluid restriction:** For those with advanced-stage heart failure, fluids should be limited to no more than 2 L daily, sometimes less.
- Medical

TABLE 3.17 Treatment of heart failure

Class of drug	Description
ACE inhibitors	This is a crucial drug and all patients should be on this unless contraindicated, as strong evidence exists that it improves outcome.
Beta blockers	These are negative inotropic drugs, and so should be used in chronic heart failure only when patients are stable clinically. Proven to improve outcome in non-advanced-stage (i.e. excluding Class IV) disease, and should be given to all patients who currently take ACE inhibitors. The paradox here is that despite improving prognosis, they may not offer symptomatic relief to patients. Cardioselective ones are preferred, e.g. bisoprolol, carvedilol.
Diuretics	Patients with fluid retention and sodium retention benefit most from these through improved symptoms. Examples include thiazide and loop diuretics.
Spironolactone	This should be added to patients already on diuretics and ACE inhibitors, in low dose. Is useful in those with dyspnoea at rest. Patients require regular U&Es to check for hyperkalaemia.
Digoxin	Patients who also have AF who require a rate-controlling drug would most benefit from this. Patients who are still symptomatic despite being on all the above drugs would also benefit from digoxin.

AUTHOR'S TOP TIP

A useful way to remember these drugs is ABD and Spiro Dig.

All these drugs, except digoxin and diuretics, have been proven to improve prognosis and should be given to all patients unless contraindicated.

- **Surgical:** Cardiac resynchronisation therapy, pacemakers and defibrillators; CABG in patients with angina and heart failure is controversial.

AUTHOR'S TOP TIP

It is important you distinguish between the acute or chronic presentation of the patient as your management differs. This shows to the examiner that you are thinking in practical terms.

Q5 In what situation would you not use ACE inhibitors?

- **Patient intolerance:** Classically, patients complain of a dry cough due to inhibition of bradykinin, in which case an alternative is angiotensin II receptor blockers (ARBs).
- **Renal artery stenosis:** Therefore, check renal function, and auscultate for a renal bruit.

Q6 How would you distinguish right from left heart failure?

Difficult question

TABLE 3.18 Left versus right heart failure

Type	Description
Left ventricular failure	**Symptoms:** lethargy, SOB, orthopnea, paroxysmal nocturnal dyspnoea (PND), cough (especially at night)
	Signs: resting tachycardia, bibasal crepitations on lung auscultation, presence of S3 (gallop rhythm)
Right ventricular failure	**Symptoms:** ankle swelling
	Signs: pulsatile liver (liver congestion), which may also be tender; peripheral and sacral oedema; raised JVP

Case 2: Aortic stenosis

Instructions: Please examine the cardiovascular system of this 76-year-old man who has been increasingly SOB on exertion with syncopal episodes.

Key features to look for

Inspection
❑ Patient appears breathless

Palpation
❑ **BP:** narrow pulse pressure
❑ **Pulse:** low volume, slow-rising character to pulse
❑ **Apex beat:** non-displaced apex beat but heaving (due to pressure overload)
❑ **Heaves/thrills:** left ventricular heave

Auscultation
❑ **Heart sounds:** S4, reversed S2, soft S2 (signs seen in severe stenosis)
❑ **Murmurs:** loud ejection systolic murmur heard best in aortic area, often radiating to the carotids; loudest on inspiration

---

AUTHOR'S TOP TIP

Remember your differential diagnosis of such a murmur includes MR, HOCM and pulmonary stenosis.

Complete the examination

❑ **Further examination**
  ■ *'To complete my exam, I would like to assess for left ventricular failure.'*
❑ **Thank the patient**
❑ **Wash your hands**
❑ **Present your findings**

This is an important diagnosis not to miss, as the patient needs assessment for valve replacement. Aortic stenosis is caused by rheumatic heart disease, age-related valvular degeneration and calcification, a congenital bicuspid valve or endocarditis.

A loud murmur does not necessarily imply severe aortic stenosis and is related more to the cardiac output and turbulence around the valve. Indeed, a soft murmur may occur due to minimal flow across the valve in severe heart failure and may be a sign of severe disease.

Viva questions

Q1   What salient features in the history would you be interested to know?
  ■ **Age:** if elderly, diagnosis is most likely to be senile calcification causing aortic sclerosis; if middle-aged, likely to be congenital bicuspid valve
  ■ **Presenting symptoms:** classically, **SAD** – syncope, angina and dyspnoea (these symptoms alone are an indication for valve surgery). Patient may have pre-syncope, acute heart failure
  ■ **Social history:** Worsening exercise tolerance

Q2   What pertinent investigations would you request?
  ■ **ECG:** left axis deviation (LAD), LVH with strain, P mitrale; may have LBBB
  ■ **CXR:** LVH, may be able to see calcified aortic valve, pulmonary oedema if in heart failure
  ■ **Echo:** used to estimate gradient, valve area and jet velocity
  ■ **Cardiac catheterisation:** can be used to assess gradient, ventricular function and coronary artery disease

---

AUTHOR'S TOP TIP

Although a peak-to-peak gradient > 50 mmHg, valve area < 0.5 cm², or jet velocity of > 4 m/ second are indications for referral for valve replacement, symptomatic patients without these findings should still be referred for valve replacement.

AUTHOR'S TOP TIP

Those being assessed for aortic valve surgery will need a preoperative angiogram to review the need for synchronous CABG.

Cardiac exercise testing must be avoided in such patients as it may be fatal.

Q3 How would you treat this patient?

Difficult question

- **Conservative:** avoid strenuous exercise; avoid ACEi and nitrates as they increase the gradient across the valve
- **Medical:** beta blockers
- **Surgical:** valve replacement, balloon dilatation of valve

Asymptomatic patients with valvular gradient < 50 mmHg can be followed up, as surgery is not recommended. If a patient is symptomatic, however, surgery is indicated.

Q4 How would you distinguish between aortic stenosis and aortic sclerosis?

Difficult question

As opposed to aortic stenosis, aortic sclerosis has the following features:

TABLE 3.19 Aortic sclerosis versus stenosis

Feature	Distinguishing aspect
Age	Commonly seen in the elderly
Apex beat	Non-displaced
Pulse	Pulse volume is normal
Murmur	The ESM does not radiate to the carotids

Case 3: Rheumatic fever

Instructions: This 18-year-old Indian man was visiting his family in England and has presented with pyrexia, joint pain and increasing SOB following a sore throat 2 weeks ago. Please perform a cardiovascular examination.

Key features to look for

Inspection

❏ **Rash:** erythema marginatum, a red raised edge rash with a clear centre, on the trunk, thighs and arms

❏ **Sydenham's chorea:** (occurs late) involuntary semi-purposeful movements (uncommon)

Palpation

❑ **Pulse:** tachycardia

Auscultation

❑ **Heart sounds:** pericardial rub
❑ **Murmurs:** new-onset murmur, particularly mitral stenosis and aortic regurgitation murmurs

---

AUTHOR'S TOP TIP

Remember that rheumatic heart disease can cause mitral stenosis, and mitral, atrial and tricuspid regurgitation. So any murmur is possible, however most commonly in this country, mitral stenosis.

Complete the examination

❑ **Further examination**
- *'To complete my exam, I would like to assess for the presence of any major or minor diagnostic criteria for rheumatic heart disease, such as a fever, and the presence of polyarthritis.'*

A recent sore throat coupled with a fleeting polyarthritis affecting the large joints should alert you to this diagnosis even before you enter the room.

❑ **Thank the patient**
❑ **Wash your hands**
❑ **Present your findings**

AUTHOR'S TOP TIP

This is an example of where reading the information given to you before you enter the OSCE station can help give you the diagnosis, even if your signs do not add up to a unifying diagnosis. Make use of the minute or so you are given to read the instructions.

EXAMINER'S TOP TIP

Students who don't take the time to read the instructions prior to coming into the station commonly perform the wrong task. If you forget the instructions in the pressure of the exam, there will be a copy of the instructions available to you, simply ask and we will give it to you to re-read. Avoid wasting valuable time during the OSCE by doing this BEFORE you enter.

Viva questions

Q1 What features in the history would you be interested to know?
- **Ethnicity:** rare in developed countries, patients often from developing countries
- **Presenting symptoms:** initial sore throat and fever (pharyngeal infection with Lancefield group A beta-haemolytic streptococcal bacterium); patients present 2–4 weeks later when there is antigen cross-reactivity with valve tissue

Q2 How would you investigate this patient?
- **Throat swab:** positive growth
- **Bloods:** raised CRP/ESR, ASOT +ve, blood cultures
- **ECG:** conduction defects, with prolonged PR interval
- **Echo:** commonly, there is incompetence of mitral and aortic valves, less commonly tricuspid and pulmonary

Treatment is with bed rest, antibiotics (benzyl penicillin) and benzodiazepines for those with chorea. Occasionally, valve replacement is required.

Q3 What are the diagnostic criteria for rheumatic fever?

Honours question

- These are the Jones major and minor criteria; whereby the presence of two major criteria or two minor plus one major criteria, in the presence of group A streptococcal infection suggests rheumatic fever.

TABLE 3.20 Jones criteria

Criteria	Features
Major	Fleeting polyarthritis, erythema marginatum, chorea, subcutaneous nodules
Minor	Fever, raised acute-phase reactants, arthralgias and prolonged PR interval

Case 4: Mitral stenosis

Instructions: This elderly lady with a past history of rheumatic fever presents with SOB on exertion. Please perform a cardiovascular examination.

Key features to look for

Inspection
- ❑ **Gender:** female, as incidence is F > M (2 : 1)
- ❑ **Rash:** malar rash
- ❑ **JVP:** prominent 'a' wave in the presence of pulmonary hypertension; may be raised
- ❑ **Scars:** previous mitral valve surgery leaving a left-sided thoracotomy scar

Palpation
- ❑ **Pulse:** irregularly irregular (AF), may be sinus rhythm

❑ **Apex beat:** tapping, non-displaced
❑ **Heaves/thrills:** left parasternal heave

AUTHOR'S TOP TIP

In the presence of pulmonary hypertension, there may be a palpable P2. If you are able to feel this, you will be commended for picking this sign up. Occasionally, if there is mixed valvular disease, there may be a displaced apex beat. This is when MR predominates.

Auscultation
❑ **Heart sounds:** the following may be heard:

TABLE 3.21 Heart sounds in mitral stenosis

Heart sounds	Description
Opening snap	This high-pitched sound is due to the mitral valve snapping open as a result of the large left atrial pressures.
Loud S1	The stenotic valve causes left atrial pressures to be high, and the loud S1 occurs due to the mobile mitral valve leaflets closing against this high pressure.
Loud S2	This is largely due to the P2 aspect as a consequence of pulmonary hypertension.

❑ **Murmurs:** low-pitched 'rumbling' diastolic murmur, best heard at the end of expiration at the apex, with the patient in the left lateral position; the longer the murmur duration, the greater the severity of disease

Complete the examination
❑ **Further examination**
   ▪ *'To complete my exam, I would like to assess for the presence of endocarditis, rheumatic fever and/or pulmonary hypertension.'*

Pulmonary hypertension with right heart failure is a sign of severity and in most cases is irreversible.
❑ **Thank the patient**
❑ **Wash your hands**
❑ **Present your findings**

AUTHOR'S TOP TIP

A lot of the signs seen in mitral stenosis can be difficult to pick up on; examiners know this, as they themselves find it difficult to pick these up! Therefore, don't worry about facing a case like this. As long as you can describe what you have seen and have a differential diagnosis, you will do well.

Viva questions

Q1   What are the causes of mitral stenosis?
- rheumatic heart disease (by far the most common cause)
- congenital mitral stenosis
- rheumatoid arthritis, lupus and rarely left atrial myxomas

Aside from symptoms suggestive of rheumatic heart disease and exertional dyspnoea, rarely patients may exhibit Ortner's phenomenon; this is hoarseness due to left atrial enlargement causing recurrent laryngeal nerve damage.

ECG may show broad bifid P waves (called P mitrale), or AF in severe disease. CXR may reveal an enlarged left atrium with an obtuse carinal angle. Echo is diagnostic, whereby severity of disease can be judged and the need for surgery. Indications for surgery include a diastolic gradient drop of > 5 mmHg between the left atrium and left ventricular end-diastolic pressures. Surgical measures include mitral valvotomy, which can be performed percutaneously, valvuloplasty or mitral valve replacement with prosthesis. Anticoagulation is indicated to prevent thromboembolic disease, especially stroke.

Other valvular heart disease you should be aware of:

TABLE 3.22 Classical features of valvular heart disease

Valvular disease	Classical clinical signs to aid diagnosis
Mitral regurgitation	Displaced apex beat (no signs of AR)
	PSM, best heard at apex, radiating to axilla
Mitral stenosis	AF or sinus rhythm, non-displaced apex beat
	'Rumbling' diastolic murmur, best heard at the end of expiration at the apex, with the patient in the left lateral position
Aortic stenosis	Slow-rising pulse, low-volume pulse; narrow pulse pressure, heave, non-displaced apex. ESM best heard in aortic area, radiating to carotids
Aortic regurgitation	Collapsing pulse, large-volume pulse, wide pulse pressure, displaced apex beat, diastolic murmur best heard at left sternal edge

---

AUTHOR'S TOP TIP

If you remember the key facts outlined in the table above, you should be able to accurately identify the majority of murmurs you will come across in finals and beyond.

Whenever you're describing a murmur in your exam, it is best to say all the classical features of the valve abnormality you think it is (*see* table above). That way, the examiner knows that you are describing a specific valvular lesion without actually saying what the lesion is, till your diagnosis at the end. For example, saying that you heard an ejection systolic murmur radiating to the carotids or a pansystolic murmur radiating into the axilla will alert the examiner that you know what you're talking about and are trying to unify your examination findings.

Case 4: Hypertrophic obstructive cardiomyopathy (HOCM) – difficult case

Instructions: Please examine this 25-year-old man who collapsed whilst playing rugby.

Key features to look for

Inspection
❑ **JVP:** presence of an 'a' wave

Palpation
❑ **Pulse:** jerky carotid pulse, sometimes referred to as bifid
❑ **Apex beat:** double-tap apex beat (due to presystolic ventricular expansion from atrial systole)
❑ **Heaves/thrills:** systolic thrill at left lower sternal edge; systolic heave may be seen also

Auscultation
❑ **Heart sounds:** 4th heart sound due to atrial systole
❑ **Murmurs:**

TABLE 3.23 Characteristic HOCM murmurs

Murmur	Description
Late ejection systolic murmur (ESM)	This is the most characteristic feature of HOCM
	Heard at left sternal edge (due to obstruction)
	This can be accentuated by asking the patient to perform a Valsalva manoeuvre
	The Valsalva increases dynamic obstruction, and the release of Valsalva accentuates this murmur
Pansystolic murmur (PSM)	At the apex
	MR is commonly seen in HOCM

AUTHOR'S TOP TIP

The easiest way to perform a Valsalva in the exam would be to ask the patient to strain; squatting is an alternative. Do whatever is quickest and slickest for you, however in the exam it is best to avoid any special manoeuvres unless directed to do so by the examiner, simply mentioning these would gain you marks. Remember Valsalva involves four phases, of which you need to be aware of two, the strain and release.

Complete the examination

Your main objective after recognition would be to asses the severity of HOCM through clinical history, particularly the age of onset, presence of syncopal episodes and family history of sudden death, as these features risk-stratify HOCM.
❑ **Thank the patient**
❑ **Wash your hands**
❑ **Present your findings**

HOCM is the most common cause of sudden cardiac death in young adults. There is a mutation in the genetic coding for contractile proteins found in the myocardium, resulting in myocardial fibre disarray leading to left ventricular outflow tract obstruction and asymmetrical hypertrophy of the septum. This leads to late systolic obstruction, stiffness of cardiac muscle and diastolic dysfunction. Sudden death occurs most likely from conduction defects. Dilated cardiomyopathy can also be inherited, but can be due to alcohol, thiamine deficiency or an inflammatory reaction. The dilated ventricle leads to systolic dysfunction. Restrictive cardio-myopathy may be caused by amyloidosis and sarcoidosis leading to diastolic dysfunction and conduction defects. Patients demonstrate Kussmaul's sign and may be breathless.

Viva questions

Q1 What features in the history would you be interested to know?

Difficult question

- **Presenting symptoms:** Angina, palpitations, syncopal episodes (collapse), shortness of breath on exertion, sudden death; this may be the patient's first presentation to hospital
- **Family history:** Ask about family history of HOCM. Half are inherited, most commonly autosomal dominant, the remaining 50% are sporadic. If patient is not sure, you must ask about family history of syncope and sudden death in young adults

Q2 What investigations would you request?
- **ECG:** LVH, deep Q waves in inferior and lateral leads, LAD, T-wave inversion; conduction defects
- **CXR:** may be normal or cardiac hypertrophy
- **Echo:** asymmetric septal hypertrophy, systolic anterior movement of mitral valve and MR

Q3 How would you treat this patient?
- **Conservative measures:** avoid strenuous exercise; family counselling
- **Medical**
  — drugs: beta blockers, calcium channel blockers (verapamil), anticoagulation if arrhythmias, amiodarone (first choice for arrhythmias); prophylaxis for endocarditis
  — septal ablation: alcohol
  — dual chamber pacing may be needed if patient symptomatic, an implantable cardiac defibrillator (ICD) is indicated especially if episodes of VT
- **Surgical:** myomectomy of septum

Drugs which reduce preload are contraindicated, e.g. diuretics and nitrates. Patients will require emotional counselling and be encouraged to join patient self-help groups.

Q4 What is the Valsalva manoeuvre?

Honours question

- This is simply a test of the baroreceptor reflex.
- There are four phases.
- Involves getting the patient to breath out forcefully though a closed larynx – the straining bit (phase 1).
- This results in raised intrathoracic pressure.
- On release (phase 3), the BP and CO fall.

AUTHOR'S TOP TIP

This is an example of where you can get yourself into trouble. If you mention anything in the exam, you should expect to be questioned about it; this is fair game. If you do not understand the principles of something, do not mention it.

3.2 CARDIOVASCULAR HISTORIES

By far the most likely case you will come across in finals will be cardiac chest pain. It is important that you are fluent with this history. *See* Chapter 2 for the general history-taking schema described. Here, we focus on specific points related to the cardiovascular system.

History Case 1: Chest pain

Instructions: This 55-year-old diabetic hypertensive smoker presents with a 15-minute hi: of central crushing chest pain. Please take a focused clinical history.

Key features to look for
☐ **Note the patient's age/sex**
- The risk of atherosclerosis and IHD increases with age.
- Age also increases the risk of the patient suffering co-morbidities.
- Males are more likely to have cardiac chest pain.

☐ **Occupation**
- Specific occupations are associated with certain cardiac diseases:
  - publicans – alcoholic cardiomyopathy
  - working with organic solvents – arrhythmias
  - deep-sea divers – embolism through foramen ovale
  - outdoor workers – cold exposure can cause angina symptoms.

☐ **Cardiac chest pain**
- **Site:** Cardiac pain could be central or left-sided. Between the shoulder blades co suggest aortic dissection. Epigastrium can suggest oesophageal reflux.
- **Onset:** Acute onset due to acute MI, a pneumothorax, aortic dissection; gradual onset such as angina, pneumonia.
- **Character:** A sharp pain worse on movement is likely to be pericarditis, a tight crushing pain MI, pressure like pain seen in angina, tearing in aortic dissection, burning in oesophageal reflux and peptic ulcer disease.

- **Radiation:** MI pain classically radiates to the shoulders, typically the left shoulder and down the arm; aortic dissection pain radiates into the back.
- **Alleviating factors:** Pain that is relieved on sitting forward is seen in pericarditis, relief on use of antacids suggests oesophageal reflux, relief on use of GTN spray is seen with angina but can also be a feature of oesophageal spasm. Relief on stopping exercise or exertion can be seen in stable angina.
- **Timing:** If the pain lasts for longer than 30 minutes and is constant, this is an infarct until proven otherwise.
- **Exacerbating factors:** Angina can be brought on by exercise, emotional stress, cold weather; chest pain worse on inspiration is called pleuritic pain and is a feature of pericarditis, rib fractures and respiratory causes of chest pain; pain related to meals should prompt consideration of peptic ulcer disease.
- **Scale:** If severe, you should consider MI or aortic dissection.

❑ **Associated symptoms**
- **Dyspnea:** Could be a sign of heart failure, acute myocardial infarction, angina or PE, cardiac causes of shortness of breath may be on exertion.
- **Cough:** More likely to be a feature of respiratory causes of chest pain.
- **Palpitations:** This could indicate a skipped beat, ectopics or a tachyarrhythmia such as AF, atrial flutter or SVT. Ask about duration of symptoms and any precipitating or relieving factors.
- **Swelling:** Peripheral oedema could indicate congestive cardiac failure, right-sided heart failure or constrictive pericarditis.
- **Syncope/pre-syncope:** Feature of aortic stenosis, HOCM, AR, bradyarrhythmias, orthostatic hypotension; could be due to neurological causes.
- **Fever/vomiting:** Fever can occur with cardiac chest pain such as MI and pericarditis, although you should consider other infective causes. Vomiting is classically associated with acute MI chest pain.

AUTHOR'S TOP TIP

If your patient complains of palpitations, ask them to tap out the rhythm that they can sense. This will help distinguish whether they have had a skipped beat or are having a tachyarrhythmia such as AF.

❑ **Risk-factor assessment**
- **Diabetes:** Can lead to coronary artery disease.
- **High cholesterol:** High risk of atheromatous coronary arteries.
- **Hypertension**
- **Smoking:** If yes, how many and for how long? Smoking is an important aetiological factor in the development of cardiovascular disease. Calculate the pack-years:
  - One pack-year is equivalent to 20 cigarettes a day for 1 year
  - Therefore, 10 cigarettes a day for 2 years is equal to 1 pack-year.

❑ **Past medical history**
- **Previous history:** Patients who have had an MI in the past are likely to have another one. Equally, those with a history of angina, whether stable or not, should be considered to be having cardiac chest pain. It is important to ask whether this chest pain is different to their normal angina pain.
- **Past medical history of:**
  - hypertension
  - rheumatic fever – as a child; this is very rare in developed countries with access to antibiotics
  - hyperthyroidism – AF, acute heart failure if severe
  - amyloid – cardiomyopathy, constrictive pericarditis
  - Marfan's – AR, dilation of the aortic root
  - Down's syndrome – ventricular septal defect (VSD)
  - Turner's syndrome – coarctation, bicuspid aortic valve (AV), aortic stenosis (AS)
  - Noonan's syndrome – pulmonary stenosis (PS).

❑ **Drug history**
- This is important to note, as some medications can cause cardiac symptoms and others can exacerbate symptoms.

TABLE 3.24 Drugs and associated symptoms

Symptoms/condition	Associated drug
Dyspnoea	Beta blockers and NSAIDs in patients with asthma, exacerbation of heart failure by beta blockers
Dizziness	Alpha blockers such as doxazosin which leads to vasodilation and therefore can lead to peripheral pooling and reduced venous return to the heart
	ACE inhibitors and nitrates both act to peripherally vasodilate
Palpitations	Thyroxine, salbutamol, diuretics leading to hypokalaemia
Oedema	NSAIDs, steroids, calcium channel blockers
Heart failure	NSAIDs and steroids causing fluid retention

- Reviewing a list of medications taken by the patient can also reveal chronic conditions the patient may have forgotten to mention.

❑ **Family history**
- This is important, because some conditions are inherited and many have strong genetic correlation.
- Ask specifically about premature heart disease in a first-degree relative < 55 years in a non-smoking female, < 50 years in a non-smoking male.
- Any history of sudden unexplained death which may indicate a cardiomyopathy.

❑ **Social history**
- **Alcohol consumption:** Excessive consumption is associated with AF, hypertension and cardiomyopathy.
- **Recreational drugs:** Amphetamines and especially cocaine can lead to cardiac pain due to tachycardia and coronary vasospasm.
- **Exercise tolerance:** This is used in the determination of the degree of heart failure.

> **Completion**
>
> You are almost certain to have a case of chest pain in the history-taking section of your exam. The key is in differentiating between cardiac chest pain and other causes, such as respiratory. Taking a focused clinical history will help distinguish between your differentials.

Viva questions

Q1 What are the causes of chest pain?
- There are many causes of chest pain.
- They can be divided into cardiovascular, respiratory, gastrointestinal and other causes:

TABLE 3.25 Causes of chest pain

Classification	Aetiology
Cardiovascular	Acute MI, angina
	Aortic dissection
	Pericarditis
Respiratory	Pneumothorax
	Pneumonia
	Pulmonary embolism
Gastrointestinal	Peptic ulcer disease, oesophagitis
	Oesophageal spasm
Others	Rib fracture
	Costochondritis
	Anxiety/panic attacks

Note: This list is not exhaustive, as there are many causes.

Q2 What investigations would you request?

It is important to mention to the examiner that you will tailor your investigations to the findings of your clinical history and examination. A clinical examination is always your first investigative step. In general, however, the following tests may be useful:
- **Simple blood tests:** Full blood count to check the Hb, as anaemia can cause chest pain. A raised WCC could point towards a pneumonia, but can also be seen in an acute myocardial infarction
- **Cardiac enzymes:** Troponin I or T tests can be performed to check for a rise indicative of an MI. The test needs to be taken at certain times after the onset of symptoms, usually 6 hours but this varies between hospital labs.
- **ECG:** There are typical changes depending on the location, ischaemia and infarction on an ECG; *see* Chapter 12, Data interpretation, for further details. Angina can cause ischaemia and consequent ST depression with T-wave inversion. Infarcts will cause ST elevation and Q waves. A PE causes the classic S1Q3T3 pattern, i.e. an S wave in lead I, Q wave in lead III and an inverted T in lead III,

indicating right heart strain. However, the most common ECG finding in PE is a sinus tachycardia.

- **CXR:** This is usually done to consider any life-threatening causes of chest pain, such as aortic dissection, as part of the many differentials. You may also see rib fractures as causes of chest pain, a wedge-shaped shadow in PE, areas of consolidation in a pneumonia or absent lung markings in a pneumothorax.

TABLE 3.26 Differential diagnosis of common cardiology conditions

Diagnosis	Main Features
Angina (stable)	Chest pain associated with exercise and exertion
	Chest pain settles on rest
Angina (unstable)	Chest pain that can occur at rest as well as on exertion
	May not settle on resting
	Determine if attacks are getting more frequent (crescendo) and how often they occur at rest
Myocardial infarction	Central crushing chest pain
	Tight chest with associated feeling of shortness of breath
	Radiating commonly into neck and arms
	Diaphoresis (sweating), nausea and vomiting, syncope
Pericarditis	Constant central pain
	Often made worse on laying flat or on deep breathing
	Relieved by sitting forward
	Can be associated with SOB or syncope, fever
Aortic dissection	Tearing-like pain radiating through to the back
	Discordant blood pressures in arms
	May be proceeded by trauma
	May occur in patients with connective tissue disease such as Ethlers–Danlos and Marfan's
Tachyarrthymias, e.g. paroxysmal AF	Feeling of palpitations sometimes with associated anxiety; syncope and pre-syncope
	Can have associated chest pain in patients with coronary artery disease
Heart failure	Leg swelling
	Inability to lay flat due to breathlessness
	Worsening exercise tolerance
	Often history of MI or long-standing hypertension
	May have obviously elevated JVP

CHAPTER 4

Respiratory system

4.1 EXAMINATION OF THE RESPIRATORY SYSTEM

This is one of the primary core examination systems, and you should expect to be examined on this in finals. The majority of cases tend to be patients with stable chronic obstructive or fibrotic lung disease, although occasionally you may get a patient who has been in hospital recently with an effusion.

This is a notoriously long examination routine to perform in a standard 5-minute OSCE station. Many struggle to complete the exam in its entirety within this time frame; you must therefore practice this and be slick in your execution. In reality, you may however be asked to skip things for the sake of time, as the examiners would like to ask you some questions. Usually, if they can see you performing a thorough examination executed well, they will be happy to do this. However, if your examination routine is poor, they will pick up on this and concentrate on it rather than ask you questions. The viva questions are part of the overall mark, so any time lost due to your slow examination may work against you. Of course, this varies between medical schools, and in some schools all candidates are stopped at a specified time which is allotted specifically for questions.

EXAMINER'S ANECDOTE

I once saw a candidate finish the entire respiratory examination in 3 minutes. He was so fast that he was actually short of breath himself when he was presenting his findings! Speed is not of the essence here; you need to show you are a kind and considerate physician to your patients, and rushing them through an examination for the sake of getting all the marks is not an excuse.

Of note, some candidates prefer to examine the entire anterior side of the respiratory examination, beginning with palpation and ending with auscultation, before going onto the posterior aspect. This is of personal choice; do whatever you feel comfortable with, so long as you remember to examine both sides. For purposes of clarity, we will adopt the former method.

Clinical examination

Introduction

As for any clinical encounter (*see* Chapter 1, Section 3), specifically for this case:

❑ **Expose patient adequately**

■ The patient needs to have their chest and abdomen fully exposed. Ask for a chaperone if required; in general, female patients should keep their bras on and be exposed only when necessary and covered whenever not.

❑ **Position patient appropriately**

■ The patient needs to be in a supine position, lying at 45 degrees, with the head resting on one pillow and their arms by their side; the level of the bed needs to be at an appropriate height to make the examination comfortable for the examiner from a standing position.

AUTHOR'S TOP TIP

If the patient gives you a verbal response to any of your instructions, listen to the quality of their voice; a hoarse voice could indicate laryngeal nerve palsy that can occur in throat and apical lung cancers.

Inspection

❑ **Perform a general inspection from the end of the bed**

■ **Paraphernalia:** Look around the bed for peripheral stigmata of disease, such as nebuliser delivery units, oxygen tubing/masks, inhalers, peak flow meter. Comment on each of these to the examiner.

■ **Patient's demeanour:** Do they look comfortable at rest or dyspnoeic with an increased respiratory rate? On general observation, do they look cachectic? A sign of possible malignancy. Bruises on the skin may indicate thin, delicate skin from repeated steroid courses, such as in COPD or asthma. Remember to comment on the Cushingoid appearance of chronic steroid use if you think it is present.

■ **Degree of illness:** Are they pale/cyanosed/suffused? Central cyanosis can be seen in such conditions as COPD, pneumonia, PE, severe pulmonary fibrosis and bronchial asthma.

■ **Chest wall deformities:** Are there any obvious deformities of the chest wall, such as a barrel or hyperinflated chest? Is there pectus excavatum (funnel chest), where the sternum is depressed? This is usually congenital and idiopathic, but can be associated with Marfan's syndrome. Is there pectus carinatum (pigeon chest), where the sternum and costal cartilages project outwards? This is a feature seen in children with rickets or chronic respiratory disease such as chronic childhood asthma, or it may be idiopathic. There may be an increased AP diameter, seen in emphysema and referred to as a barrel chest.

■ **Scars:** From thoracotomy, lobectomy, pneumonectomy or old TB treatment.

■ **Accessory muscle breathing:** What muscles are they using for respiration? Is this mainly diaphragmatic, or are they using accessory muscles?

❑ **Assess chest expansion**

■ This is a sensitive test to help localise the side of the pathology. Ask the patient to take a deep breath in and out and observe for:

— **Expansion:** assess whether bilaterally equal, or reduced unilaterally (*see* table below)

- Muscle groups involved in respiration
  - **Diaphragmatic:** may indicate a problem with the chest wall, such as pleural pain or ankylosing spondylolitis
  - **Intercostal muscles:** may indicate paralysis of the diaphragm, a distended abdomen or peritonitis
- **Paradoxical movements**
  - **Abdominal:** if the diaphragm is paralysed, the anterior abdominal wall will move in rather than out on inspiration
  - **Chest:** if a patient is tetraplegic and has chest wall paralysis, you will see the chest wall move in on inspiration as the diaphragm descends

TABLE 4.1 Causes of reduced unilateral chest wall movements

Findings	Aetiology
Reduced expansion unilaterally	Pleural effusion, empyema
	Collapse
	Consolidation
	Fibrosis
	Tension pneumothorax
	Pneumothorax

❏ **Examine the hands**
  - Inspect the nails

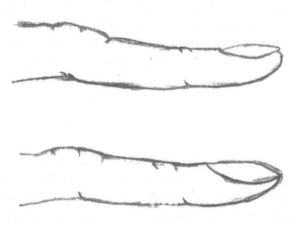

FIGURE 4.1 Digital clubbing

TABLE 4.2 Signs of clubbing

Four signs of clubbing
1. Loss of the angle of the nail bed
2. Drumstick-like appearance
3. Boggy nail bed
4. Increased curvature of the nail

— **Clubbing** (*see* Chapter 9, Case 8)

— **Tar staining** (yellow nails): indicative of smoking and an important cause of COPD and bronchial carcinoma

- **Inspect the hands/arms**
  - **Peripheral cyanosis**
  - **Pallor of the palmar creases**
  - **Skin changes:** thin skin or bruising both indicative of long-term steroid use
  - **Deformities:** features of rheumatoid disease may be seen, which is linked to fibrosing alveolitis
- **Assess temperature of peripheries**
  - A quick assessment of peripheral temperature in the fingers and hands may indicate warmth, a feature in sepsis, and may indicate CO_2 retention.

❑ **Assess for tremor and asterixis**

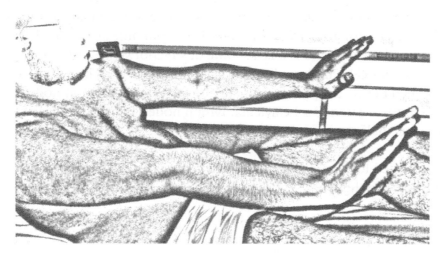

FIGURE 4.2 Flap

- **Check for tremor:** Ask the patient to hold both arms straight out (showing them can make it easier to understand), and look for a fine tremor. This is associated with nebulised salbutamol (beta agonist) therapy, which is used in the treatment of asthma and COPD.
- **Check for CO_2 retention flap:** Ask the patient to extend their wrists back (you might need to gently do this for them), and observe for a flap for 15–30 seconds. The patients you see in the OSCE bay will not display this sign, as it indicates severe CO_2 retention; however, it forms an important part of a complete respiratory examination.

❑ **Respiratory rate and pulse**

- **Radial pulse:** Palpate the radial pulse, which may be bounding (as in CO_2 retention) or tachycardic (in an acutely unwell patient with an asthma exacerbation or sepsis from pneumonia).
- **Respiratory rate:** Whilst palpating the pulse, also calculate the respiratory rate as subtly as possible; this is so as not to artificially increase the patient's respiratory rate. Count for 30 seconds and multiply by two; the normal rate is 12–20 respiratory cycles per minute.

AUTHOR'S TOP TIP

Tachypnoea is a very sensitive but often non specific test for pathology, i.e. an abnormal respiratory rate implies that something abnormal is happening!

❏ **Assess the head and neck**
- **Evaluate the eyes:** Check for evidence of Horner's syndrome (ptosis, meiosis, anhydrosis and enopthalmos). Pull down the lower eyelid of one eye, look to see if the conjunctiva are pale (anaemia), look for suffusion, a sign of SVC obstruction that can occur with enlarged mediastinal lymph nodes secondary to a bronchial malignancy.
- **Mouth:** Look under the tongue for central cyanosis.
- **Assess the JVP:** With the head and neck relaxed on a pillow, ask the patient to look towards the left. Respiratory causes of a raised JVP include SVC obstruction, where distended neck veins are also seen, pulmonary oedema secondary to CCF, pulmonary hypertension resulting from COPD, PE or RVF. A pulsatile and raised JVP implies cor pulmonale, whereas a fixed JVP is a feature of superior vena caval obstruction.
- **Palpate the cervical lymph nodes:** Ideally, standing behind the patient, or if not possible then beside the patient, palpate the seven cervical lymph node chains, in addition to the infra- and subclavicular lymph nodes. Enlarged nodes may indicate an intrathoracic malignancy.

Note that an enlarged left supraclavicular node (Virchow's node or Troisier's sign) may indicate an intrathoracic malignancy.

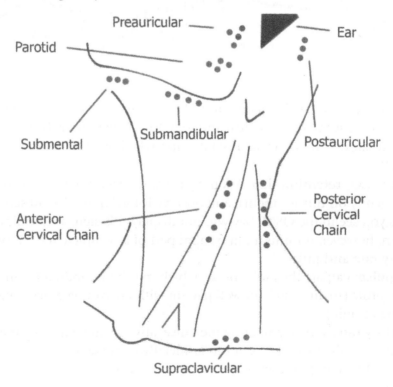

FIGURE 4.3 Cervical lymph node chains

❑ **Assess the trachea**

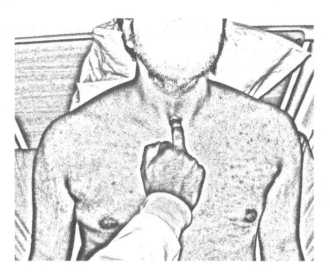

FIGURE 4.4 Assessing the trachea

- **Assess tracheal deviation:** Place the index and ring finger of your right hand either side of the trachea, with your middle finger on the surface of the trachea, and palpate lightly to ensure it is central. If it is not, your middle finger will slip towards the opposite side of the deviation (due to the now-empty space left by the normally central trachea).
- **Assess for tracheal tug:** A tracheal tug is seen in a hyperinflated chest. This is done by estimating the cricosternal notch distance, which would be decreased.

Remember that both these are intrusive examination techniques, so tell the patient what you are going to do, as some may find it uncomfortable.

TABLE 4.3 Causes of a displaced trachea

Tracheal deviation	*Causes*
Towards (the pathological side)	Collapse due to infection, fibrosis (caused by old TB commonly), or obstruction
Away (from the pathological side)	A space-occupying lesion, e.g lymphoma, malignancy
	Tension pneumothorax (this is an emergency, and should not be sitting in the OSCE bay) Large pleural effusion

---

AUTHOR'S TOP TIP

An enlarged thyroid goitre may cause tracheal deviation so assess for this, or mention this in your differentials.

❑ **Detailed inspection of the chest wall**
In addition to the above, repeated as necessary, specifically evaluate for:
- **Scars:** supraclavicular scars from phrenic nerve crush

- **Radiotherapy tattoos** (will often appear as small inked blue dots)
- **Deformity**
- **Use of accessory muscles of respiration:** use of shoulder and neck muscles to increase intrathoracic volume
- **Distended veins** (signs of SVC obstruction)
- **Listen to the breathing** (without a stethoscope)
  — Listen for any noisy breathing such as inspiratory stridor, a high-pitched sound from upper-airway obstruction which may occur secondary to secretions or vocal cord palsies.
  — Listen for stertor, which is lower-pitched then stridor and caused by obstruction above the larynx, e.g. in severe tonsillitis.
  — There may be an obvious expiratory wheeze (implying airflow limitation) in COPD.

Palpation

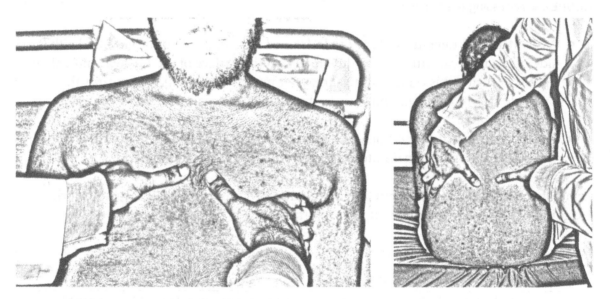

FIGURE 4.5A–B Assessing chest wall expansion anteriorly and posteriorly

❏ **Chest wall palpation** ('bucket handle' technique)
  - Place only the fingertips of both hands on either side of the chest wall over the ribcage, pressing firmly, and stretch your hands such that the thumbs meet in the middle.
  - The thumbs should be floating and not touching the chest wall surface.
  - Ask the patient to take a deep breath in, and watch your thumbs as they move apart; the degree to which they move apart will indicate how well the chest wall is expanding.
  - Ideally, this needs to be performed twice, once over the upper part of the ribcage and then over the lower half.
  - Also ensure that you palpate anteriorly and posteriorly.

Another technique some prefer is to place the palmar aspect of both their hands over the patient's chest wall and ask the patient to take a deep breath in and out, whilst assessing the degree with which the chest wall rises. We suggest you avoid this, as this is simply a repeat of the initial inspection assessment of expansion, with only your hand placed over the chest wall as a modification; there is little added information gained from this method.

AUTHOR'S TOP TIP

Subcutaneous emphysema may be detected on chest wall palpation. It feels like crackling when palpating the chest wall and is caused by air in the subcutaneous tissues. It is a common complication of chest drain insertion for a pneumothorax.

❑ **Assess chest wall expansion**
  ■ Assess for chest wall movement, whether this is reduced or normal and if there is a difference on either side.
  ■ **Reduced expansion**
    — **Unilateral:** Occurs on the side with the pathology and implies that air cannot enter the affected side. Causes include pneumothorax, pleural effusion, consolidation and collapse.
    — **Bilateral:** Reduced chest wall expansion is difficult to detect clinically unless severely reduced, and in some cases is due to poor respiratory effort on the patient's part.

Percussion
❑ **Percuss anteriorly**

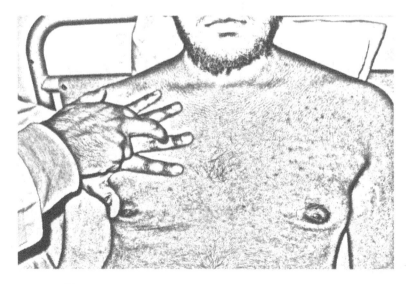

FIGURE 4.6 Finger percussion

  ■ **Percussion technique:** Good percussion takes practice; ensure you have short nails.
    — Place your left hand horizontally on the chest wall over the intercostal spaces, ensuring the fingers are all widely spaced out and hyperextended.
    — Using the middle finger of your right hand, tap lightly over the middle phalanx of the left middle finger using the tip of the right middle phalanx; this movement should come at the wrist.

— Upon contact, your finger should spring away.

The number of taps you perform in sequence is of personal preference; commonly a double tap is performed, although some candidates prefer triple taps. Classically, percussion is performed using a single digit; however, the use of two fingers to elicit percussion has been seen and is acceptable.

AUTHOR'S TOP TIP

Good percussion does not mean hitting as hard as you can but ensuring you press firmly with your hand resting on the chest wall and having a staccato nature to the tap that will give you the most informative feedback.

■ Starting at the clavicle (for apical lung percussion), percuss down, comparing both sides at each level as you go along, ensuring you do not forget the axillae.

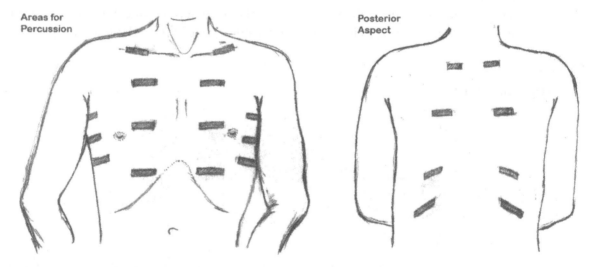

FIGURE 4.7A–B Suggested areas for percussion

In the exam, it is probably best that you do not percuss in every single intercostal space, as this is time-consuming and rarely required. In clinical practice, four levels anteriorly and posteriorly including the axilla and clavicle is adequate, unless an abnormality is found, in which case further delineation will be required.

AUTHOR'S TOP TIP

Some candidates choose to percuss down the entire right-hand side then the left. This is not advisable, as it makes it more difficult to appreciate any differences in percussion note on either side, and therefore more likely that you will miss localised pathology. We suggest you percuss the left-hand side then right at each individual level as you move down the chest.

For left handed candidates, we appreciate that percussion can be difficult with your non-dominant hand; it is perfectly acceptable to use your left hand in the exam. However, in practice left-handers tend to percuss patients most easily by standing on the left-hand side of the patient beginning with the right side of the chest, i.e. the side furthest away from you. The majority of OSCE stations' logistical setup would have the examining couch against the wall such that the candidate would be on the right-hand side of the patient. Therefore, you must be able to adapt to the situation, at least for the exam. Once the exam is over, it doesn't really matter which side you examine the patient from.

- **Percussion assessment:** You need to note whether the percussion note is normal, hyperresonant, dull or stony dull (*see* table below).

Percussion enables determination of the underlying lung tissue density and hence differentiation between air-filled, fluid-filled or solid tissue mass.

TABLE 4.4 Abnormal percussion notes

Note	Description
Resonant	Normal lung
Hyperresonant	Suggests AIR, hyperinflated chest wall, pneumothorax, emphysema, asthma
Dull	Suggests FLUID/SOLID, collapse, consolidation, fibrosis
Stony dull	Classically suggests FLUID from a pleural effusion, haemothorax

---

AUTHOR'S TOP TIP

In actual clinical practice, relying solely on the audible noise you elicit from percussion for detection of pathology would be inadequate. This is for a number of reasons, ranging from poor percussion technique to an often loud and noisy ward making it difficult to hear. We suggest therefore that you not only have an appreciation for the percussion note but also of the resistance and 'springing' away you feel when percussing. Springing away can be likened to hitting a drum with a stick and that stick tends to bounce or rebound back up, whereas hitting a stick against a concrete wall does not. A lot of resistance to your percussion with poor spring would be in keeping with dullness, whereas less resistance and more springiness with resonance and hyperresonance.

❑ **Percuss posteriorly** (repeated as above)

Some candidates prefer to finish with the anterior side by performing auscultation also and then go on to examine the posterior aspect with percussion then auscultation, etc. Do whatever you are most comfortable with. Be vigilant however, as percussion of the back is often forgotten and is an easy mark to obtain in the exam. Indeed, some mark schemes will award you a mark for performing percussion on both sides and no marks for only a single side completed.

Of note, most physicians in clinical practice would prefer to examine the posterior chest wall in favour of and sometimes instead of the anterior chest wall, as it is more informative in terms of pathology. This is because anatomically you get easy access to the lower lung lobes, including the axilla for access to the right middle lobe. The upper lobes are best examined anteriorly; there are only a handful of pathologies that tend to affect the upper lobes.

Auscultation

❑ **Auscultation technique**

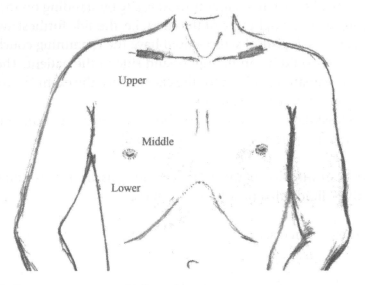

FIGURE 4.8 Auscultation zones: upper, middle and lower zones

- Starting by placing the bell of the stethoscope in the apex, listen whilst asking the patient to take a deep breath in and out through their mouth.
- It may be easier to show the patient exactly what you mean to make it easier for them to copy.
- Listen in all the same areas that you performed percussion: over the apex, upper, middle and lower zones and then in the axilla on the right to assess the middle lobe.

❑ **Assess breath sounds**

- Listen carefully for normal breath sounds, described as vesicular breathing.
- Also for abnormal breath sounds, known as bronchial breathing. Bronchial breathing is a harsh sound, which has an equal inspiratory and expiratory time.

AUTHOR'S TOP TIP

If you place your stethoscope over your trachea and listen to your own breath sounds you will hear what bronchial breathing sounds like. Bronchial breathing sounds like breath sounds heard over the larynx.

TABLE 4.5 Causes of bronchial breathing

	Causes
Bronchial breathing	Pneumonic consolidation
	Collapsed lung/lobe
	Pulmonary fibrosis, e.g. chronic suppurative pneumonia

- Note whether breath sounds are absent or reduced such as in a pneumothorax, effusion or collapse.

❏ **Assess for added sounds**
   ■ Added sounds may be heard in inspiration and/or expiration; note in which component they occur
   ■ Added sounds may be:

TABLE 4.6 Added sounds on auscultation

Findings	Description
Crackles	**Fine crackles**
	These are high-pitched sounds created by the 'popping' open of the small airways that have prematurely closed at the end of the last expiratory cycle.
	They typically represent pulmonary fibrosis, in which case they are end-inspiratory crackles and would be expected to be heard at both lung bases.
	Other causes include pulmonary oedema due to CCF.
	Coarse crackles
	These occur due to fluid resting in larger bronchi. The sound has been described as similar to Velcro being pulled apart.
	Can be heard in a myriad of conditions, usually during inspiration; they can be classified according to the phase of inspiration in which they occur:
	● **early inspiratory** – bronchiectasis, chronic bronchitis
	● **late inspiratory** – pneumonia, fibrosis or LVF
	To further help differentiate the cause, note that localised crackles can be caused by conditions such as consolidation and bronchiectasis, whereas pulmonary oedema and fibrosis are more widespread.
Wheeze	Heard mainly in expiration. They represent localised airway narrowing and are commonly heard in COPD and asthma.
	Remember to comment on whether they occur in the inspiratory or expiratory component and whether they are mono- or polyphonic.
Pleural rub	Heard when inflamed pleural surfaces rub together. Its sound has been likened to someone treading on freshly fallen snow. It is usually a localised sound.
	Causes include pneumonia, rib fractures and pulmonary embolism.
	Due to the inflammation present, there is often associated pain in the same area on breathing (pleuritic pain).

Don't forget to listen in the axilla, especially on the right for the middle lobe. The middle lobe of the lung can only be auscultated from the axilla and back of the patient. The left lung has no middle lobe; instead, its counterpart is the so-called lingular lobe. This is due to the anatomical location of the heart. Note that crackles are occasionally referred to as crepitations.

AUTHOR'S TOP TIP

If you are finding it difficult to distinguish between low-pitched wheeze, coarse crackles or a pleural rub, then ask the patient to cough forcefully and listen again following this.

❏ **Perform vocal or tactile fremitus**

When lung tissue has become solid and lost its normal consistency, the sounds are transmitted more easily. This is translated into the palpable/audible vibrations or fremitus transmitted through the chest wall on speaking.

You need to decide if you want to do tactile or vocal fremitus, as you do not need to do both. We suggest vocal fremitus, as you have already auscultated the lungs, so it looks slicker to perform at this stage, as opposed to tactile fremitus, which is technically palpation and ideally performed earlier in your examination routine. Vocal resonance is perhaps easier to appreciate, as hearing is more sensitive and easier to detect than the sense of touch in the exam.

TABLE 4.7 Technique for performing fremitus

Method	Description
Tactile fremitus	Place the ulnar border of your hands in the intercostal spaces. Starting from the clavicles and moving downwards, ask the patient to say '99' each time you place your hand on their chest wall. Note where the fremitus is increased or decreased.
	Increased tactile fremitus: consolidation or fibrosis
	Reduced tactile fremitus: fluid or collapse
Vocal fremitus	This is performed by asking the patient to say '99' each time you place your stethoscope on the chest wall over the same sites you originally placed them for breath-sound auscultation.

Ask the patient to sit forward, so you can repeat everything on their back. You may want to ask them to bend their knees and sit with their arms folded across their legs; this may make the examination easier for you and make it more comfortable for the patient.

Complete the examination

It is particularly important when you've finished to cover the patient up to protect their modesty, especially in the exposed female patient.

❏ **Further examination**

- *'To complete my exam, I would like to check for sacral and peripheral oedema.'*
- *'I would also like to examine the sputum pot, peak flow reading, oxygen saturations and look at the temperature chart and chest radiograph.'*

AUTHOR'S TOP TIP

These additional tests can be remembered by 'SPOT X' (Sputum, Peak flow, Oxygen sats, Temperature and CXR).

Peripheral oedema suggests right heart failure from pulmonary hypertension due to chronic lung disease, specifically in conditions whereby lung compliance is reduced.

❏ **Thank the patient**

❏ **Wash your hands**

❏ **Present your findings**

TABLE 4.8 Common clinical examination findings

Pathology	Tracheal position	Chest movement	Percussion note	Breath sounds	Additional sounds
Collapse	Central or towards	Reduced	Dull	Reduced	
COPD	Central, (shortened cricosternal length)	Reduced	Increased resonance	Reduced	Wheeze (polyphonic) Crackles
Consolidation	Central	Reduced	Dull	Bronchial breathing	Wheeze Crackles
Effusion	Central or away	Reduced	Stony dull	Reduced	
Fibrosis	Central	Reduced	Normal	Reduced or bronchial	Fine end-inspiratory crackles
Pneumothorax	Central or away	Reduced	Increased resonance	Reduced	

Note that although fibrosis reduces lung expansion, it usually occurs symmetrically, such that tracheal deviation does not occur.

Viva questions

Q1 What are the respiratory causes of clubbing?
- carcinoma of the bronchus
- suppurative lung diseases, e.g. cystic fibrosis, empyema, lung abscess, bronchiectasis
- mesothelioma
- fibrosing alveolitis

This is a very common question, so ensure you know this well (*see* Chapter 9 for further details).

Q2 How would you identify Horner's syndrome and what are the causes?

Difficult question

- Horner's syndrome is caused by interruption of the face's sympathetic supply.
- **Signs include:**
  — ptosis (drooping of the eyelid)
  — miosis (constricted pupil)
  — anhydrosis (loss of sweating, affecting the ipsilateral side)
- **Aetiology:** It is useful to classify causes anatomically along the sympathetic chain:

TABLE 4.9 Causes of Horner's syndrome

Classification	Causes
(1st-order neuron) Brainstem & spinal cord	Demyelination, stroke, trauma, syringomyelia
(2nd-order neuron) Preganglionic	Pancoast tumour, thyroid and mediastinal pathology, cervical rib, carotid endarterectomy
(3rd-order neuron) Postganglionic	Orbital disease, cavernous sinus disease, carotid artery dissection

Honours response

Q3   What are the causes of enlarged cervical lymph nodes?

TABLE 4.10 Causes of lymphadenopathy

Classification	Causes
Malignancy	Lymphoma, chronic lymphocytic leukaemia, local metastatic cancer spread
Viral	Infectious mononucleosis, CMV, HIV, local viral infection
Bacterial	TB, syphilis, brucellosis, local bacterial infection

Case 1: Chronic obstructive pulmonary disease (COPD)

Instructions: Please examine this 60-year-old man who has presented with increasing SOB and wheeze.

Key features to look for

Inspection

❑ **General features at bedside:** SOB, wheeze, cough, using accessory muscles of respiration; you may see inhalers and peak flow meter at bedside

❑ **Hands/arms:** CO_2 retention flap if toxic levels in bloodstream and dilated warm peripheries with a bounding pulse; tar staining on fingers

❑ **Face/neck:** may have central cyanosis (seen under tongue), pursed lip breathing, a shortened ($< 3\,cm$) cricosternal distance (due to lung hyperexpansion)

❑ **Chest expansion:** an increased anteroposterior (AP) diameter (barrel chest)

AUTHOR'S TOP TIP

If a patient is breathless, as this patient is likely to be, ensure you count and state to the examiner the patient's respiratory rate.

Palpation

❑ **Chest expansion:** reduced

❑ **Percussion note:** hyperresonant

Auscultation

❑ **Air entry:** reduced throughout the chest

❑ **Added sounds:** monophonic expiratory wheeze; crepitations may be heard if concomitant infective process

Others: peripheral oedema if cor pulmonale present

Complete the examination

❑ **Further examination**

- *'To complete my examination, I would like to assess the severity of disease by looking for the presence of cor pulmonale, CO_2 retention and look at the sputum pot.'*

Cor pulmonale is right ventricular enlargement and subsequent failure due to pulmonary disease leading to the development of pulmonary hypertension. Signs associated with cor pulmonale include peripheral oedema, a tender pulsatile enlarged liver, 'v' waves in the JVP, pulmonary and/or tricuspid regurgitation with a right ventricular heave on heart examination and the presence of a loud pulmonary component of S2.

❑ **Thank the patient**

❑ **Present your findings**

COPD is a progressive lung disease affecting 5% of the population, and is characterised by spirometric signs of obstructive lung disease and airflow limitation, which is poorly reversible by bronchodilators. COPD is most commonly caused by chronic habitual smoking; unfortunately, despite knowing the negative effects of smoking, many patients continue to smoke. Smoking cessation advice is therefore an important part of management. There used to be a significant mortality associated with this condition before the advent of non-invasive ventilation (NIV) techniques. Other causes you may be questioned about include alpha 1-antitrypsin deficiency; consider this as a cause in those who are non-smokers or patients exposed to environmental/occupational hazards such as pollution or in coal workers.

Viva questions

Q1   What investigations would you request?

- **Bloods:** polycythaemia on FBC
- **Peak expiratory flow rate (PEFR):** reduced
- **Spirometry:** FEV1 < 80%, FEV1/FVC ratio is < 0.7 (*see* Chapter 12, Data interpretation, for further details)
- **ECG:** right axis deviation (RAD), right atrial and ventricular hypertrophy, RBBB, p pulmonale
- **CXR:** hyperexpanded lung fields (> 6 anterior ribs visible on PA film), flattened diaphragm, bullae and prominent pulmonary vasculature
- **Sputum:** cultures sent to rule out an infective exacerbation
- **Arterial blood gas (ABG):** *see* Chapter 12, Data interpretation

Q2   Define chronic bronchitis and emphysema.

TABLE 4.11 Definitions of terms

Term	Definition
Chronic bronchitis	A productive cough on most days for at least 3 months in 2 consecutive years without any other clear cause.
	This is a clinical definition.
Emphysema	An abnormal permanent enlargement of the airway distal to the terminal bronchiole. This is a pathological definition.

AUTHOR'S TOP TIP

These are very specific definitions, which we would advise you to learn verbatim.

COPD was traditionally classified into two types: the so-called blue bloaters and pink puffers. This is a crude division, as there is much overlap between the two, and so patients are no longer grouped this way. However, you may still be asked to define these terms in the exam, should you ever mention them. As such, you cannot really diagnose emphysema without pathological evidence. We suggest therefore that if you suspect COPD in the exam, then say the patient has COPD, rather than use the above terms.

Q3   How would you treat this patient?

Management can be divided into the acute management of an exacerbation of COPD (*see* Chapter 11) or management of chronic COPD.

TABLE 4.12 Management of chronic COPD

Classification	Description
Conservative	**Pulmonary rehabilitation:** smoking cessation, exercise, weight loss and patient education
	Vaccinations: regular influenza and pneumococcal vaccines
	Depression: this is common and may be a contributory factor to poor compliance; patients may benefit from antidepressants and/or referral to psychiatric services
Medical	**Inhaled bronchodilators:** short- and long-acting beta agonists
	Inhaled glucocorticoid: high-dose inhaled steroids in moderate to severe COPD has been shown to be prognostically beneficial
	Inhaled long-acting antimuscarinic: e.g. tiotropium (Spiriva)
	Oral steroids, nebulisers
	Theophylline and mucolytics: e.g. carbocysteine
Surgical	**Lung volume reduction surgery:** improves function
	Bullectomy: improves gas exchange and airflow
	Lung transplant

(continued)

Classification	Description
Oxygen therapy	Evidence shows that long-term oxygen therapy (LTOT) benefits those who are chronically hypoxic, i.e.:

- $PaO_2 < 7.3$ kPa when measured twice on ABG analysis at least 3 weeks apart, or
- $PaO_2 < 8$ kPa with pulmonary hypertension and cor pulmonale
- FEV1 < 1.5 L

Such patients demonstrate a reduction in mortality if PaO_2 is maintained at > 8 kPa for more than 15 hours a day with oxygen administered via nasal cannula at 2–4 L/minute.

Such patients are eligible for LTOT.

Testing candidates for oxygen therapy should ideally be done in the outpatient setting where medical COPD treatment has been optimised.

AUTHOR'S TOP TIP

For detailed management, we suggest you read up on the latest NICE, BTS or GOLD guidelines; detailed knowledge of which will certainly impress any examiner and is worthy of an honours response.

There are specific pulmonary rehabilitation programmes set up to help patients achieve goals of conservative treatment. For those not in such a programme, you should still offer such advice whenever possible, e.g. smoking cessation, weight reduction, etc. Enlist the help of their GP to reinforce behavioural changes.

Case 2: Asthma

Instructions: Please examine this 17-year-old girl who has come into the GP surgery with nocturnal cough, wheeze and SOB.

Key features to look for

Inspection

❑ **General features at bedside:** SOB with tachypnoea, wheeze, cough, using accessory muscles of respiration; you may see inhalers and peak flow meter at bedside; unable to talk if severe

❑ **Hands/arms:** beta-agonist tremor if requiring regular nebs, tachycardia, pulsus paradoxus (unlikely in finals)

AUTHOR'S TOP TIP

If a patient is coughing during the exam, this may be part of the case aimed to aid your diagnosis. This should certainly be mentioned to the examiner, as audible clues are part and parcel of the clinical examination, especially in asthma, where an inability to talk in full sentences is an ominous sign. You could say, 'I can see that the patient is breathless at rest with a respiratory rate of 24, there is an audible cough . . .', etc.

Palpation

❏ **Percussion note:** hyperresonant

Auscultation

❏ **Air entry:** reduced throughout the chest
❏ **Added sounds:** widespread expiratory wheeze; crepitations may be heard if underlying pneumonia

Others: fever if concomitant infective process

Complete the examination

❏ **Further examination**
- *'To complete my examination, I would like to assess the severity of disease by assessing her observations and PEFR.'*

You are unlikely to get a severe asthmatic in the exam, but this may form part of a viva question regarding managing an acutely unwell asthmatic (*see* Chapter 11).

❏ **Thank the patient**
❏ **Present your findings**

Asthma is a reversible airways disease characterised by hyperresponsive airways to various stimuli, leading to narrowing.

Viva questions

Q1 What pertinent features in the history would you like to know?
- **Presenting symptoms:** breathlessness, recurrent cough, wheeze, tight chest; is it reversible? i.e. improves with bronchodilators
- **Cough:** productive or not (may be a recent infection; ask about fever); cough pattern, especially nocturnal cough and its diurnal variation, is pattern worsening?
- **PEFR:** do they know their normal PEFR and whether they keep a PEFR chart? (expect to see a morning dip)
- **Past medical history:** previous A&E attendances or admissions for asthma, were any to ITU/HDU?; have they ever been intubated?; ask about other atopic disease
- **Occupational/environmental:** occupational asthma in dusty environments, e.g. baker with flour; new pets in the house, e.g. birds; a travel history is important to elicit
- **Known trigger factors:** ask if they know what makes their asthma worse, e.g. exercise, cigarette smoke, cold air, pollen, dog/cat allergens, dust mites, NSAIDs, season
- **Family history:** history of atopy, i.e. hayfever, asthma, eczema, various allergies
- **Social history:** smoking, although it can exacerbate asthma and most asthmatics do not smoke, some still do, although this cohort probably represents a very mild form of asthma

- **Activities of daily living:** the impact of disease on daily life is important to quantify and how asthma has interfered with any of their usual activities, i.e. any difficulty sleeping due to cough, how much absenteeism from work/school, inability to do normal hobbies, sports, etc.
- **Drug history:** gauge compliance with current medication (many patients are school aged and are poorly compliant for various reasons), any recent antibiotics/ steroid courses; medications used so far and ascertain which treatment step they are on (*see* Viva Q3)

Honours response

AUTHOR'S TOP TIP

Although some asthmatics can use NSAIDs without any problems, for finals purposes, NSAIDs and beta blockers are contraindicated in asthmatics.

The term 'atopy' implies that the patient tends to respond to environmental triggers with an allergic antibody response with IgE.

Q2 What investigations would you request?
- **PEFR:** less than predicted; less than the usual PEFR for the patient
- **ECG:** sinus tachycardia if unwell
- **CXR:** hyperexpanded lung fields
- **Bloods:** raised CRP/WBC if signs of lung infection; may be a viral exacerbation
- **ABG analysis:** only really required if acutely unwell (*see* Chapter 12, Data interpretation)

Normally in a chronic asthmatic, clinical examination and PEFR assessment is all that is required. However, be careful as asthmatics are notorious for being well one minute and then moribund the next. Always treat asthmatics with caution and prolonged observation, particularly those with brittle asthma.

Q3 How would you manage this patient?
The management of asthma depends upon whether the patient is acutely unwell with an exacerbation or if the patient is stable. For emergency management, *see* Chapter 11.

The management of chronic asthma requires a multidisciplinary team approach with input from the GP, the practice nurse or the asthma specialist nurses, patient education leaflets, and if severe or brittle asthma, then respiratory physician input may be sought; however, in general, patients should start from step 1 and move up. Note that the treatment is generally cumulative, i.e. a patient on step 3 is also taking medications suggested in steps 1 and 2.

TABLE 4.13 Management of chronic asthma in adults

Management	Description
Step 1	Inhaled short-acting beta-2 agonists PRN for symptom relief, e.g. salbutamol, terbutaline
	If patient requires more than twice weekly, step up
Step 2	Regular inhaled corticosteroid, e.g. budesonide, beclometasone
Step 3	Inhaled long-acting bronchodilator (this is preferred), e.g. salmeterol
	High-dose inhaled steroid given via a volumatic spacer
Step 4	High-dose inhaled steroid
	Oral leukotriene receptor antagonist, e.g. montelukast
	Theophylline as oral sustained modified release
	Oral beta-2 agonist (modified release)
	Cromoglicate, in selected cases
Step 5	Regular oral steroids; in refractory cases
	Specialist referral to a respiratory consultant/asthma clinic

Long-term follow-up with GP and practice nurse is important, as management involves:
- Identification of trigger factors and their avoidance, e.g. smoking, exercise, pets, etc.
- **Patient education:** inhaler technique, individualised management plans so patients can alter their own treatment to manage symptoms, which enables autonomy and a degree of freedom for the patient. Advice to seek urgent medical attention if worsening symptoms, especially if severe enough to attend A&E or call an ambulance. To keep a rescue short-acting beta agonist such as salbutamol with them in case needed for acute symptomatic relief; referred to by some patients as the 'reliever'
- **Appropriate inhaler delivery devices**, e.g. there is no point giving a metered-dose inhaler to a child who will not comply; perhaps a volume spacer is more ideal. There are numerous devices available on the market to meet patients' needs
- Regular monitoring of patient (PEFR charts), with appropriate changes in management step whenever required, including stepping down.

Honours response

For detailed management, refer to either the BTS or NICE guidelines.

AUTHOR'S TOP TIP

If a chronic asthmatic's symptoms are becoming increasingly difficult to control when they have been previously stable, in the absence of an obvious exacerbation with a potential trigger or infective process, you should consider poor compliance or poor inhaler technique. Therefore always check the patient's inhaler technique as often as you can, especially newly diagnosed patients. If needed refer to the asthma practice nurse specialist for follow up with patient education leaflets.

Case 3: Pleural effusion

Instructions: Please examine this 60-year-old man who has presented with increasing SOB.

Key features to look for

Inspection
❏ **General features:** SOB with reduced chest expansion on affected side

Palpation
❏ **Chest expansion:** reduced on affected side
❏ **Tracheal position:** deviation of the trachea away from affected side, if the effusion is very large

Percussion
❏ stony dull percussion note

Auscultation
❏ decreased vocal resonance
❏ reduced breath sounds
❏ bronchial breathing at surface of effusion

Complete the examination
❏ **Further examination**
  ■ *'To complete my examination I would like to view the chest radiograph.'*
❏ **Thank the patient**
❏ **Present your findings**

Remember, although an effusion is the most likely diagnosis, your differential diagnosis would include consolidation, atelectasis, pleural thickening, subphrenic abscess collection or on the right, hepatomegaly leading to a raised hemidiaphragm. It is possible to differentiate between some of the above on clinical examination, for example, in consolidation the vocal resonance would be increased rather than decreased as seen in an effusion (*see* Table 4.8 above).

AUTHOR'S TOP TIP

Remember, 500 ml of pleural fluid needs to be present for it to be detected on clinical examination.

Patients usually present with progressive shortness of breath over a period of days to weeks, rather than acutely in hours. However, many patients can be asymptomatic if the effusion is small and discovered as an incidental finding on imaging. A history of a significant underlying disorder should always be sought, such as lung cancer (weight loss, smoking, haemoptysis, etc.) amongst many other causes.

Viva questions

Q1   What investigations would you request?
- **CXR:** used to quantify the size and location of effusions; large effusions may fill the entire lung, whereas small effusions may just blunt the costophrenic angle (this is the earliest radiological sign of an effusion; *see* Chapter 12, Radiology); at least 300 ml of fluid needs to be present for this to occur
- **CT chest/abdo/pelvis:** to look for an underlying cause particularly malignancy
- **USS chest:** it is now recommended that ultrasound is used to guide pleural taps and drain insertion
- **Pleural biopsy:** for mycobacterial and histopathological examination
- **Pleural aspiration:** fluid sent off for:
  - **microscopy** – highly cellular aspirate suggests an exudate
  - **cytology** – malignant cells in cancer; blood can be seen in cancer, TB or pulmonary embolism; a high neutrophil count in a parapneumonic effusion; a high lymphocyte count in cancer, TB and SLE/RA
  - **fluid pH** – a pH < 7.1 is highly suggestive of an exudate and is often used when looking for an empyema complicating a pneumonia
  - **biochemistry** – LDH and protein levels compared to serum levels (*see* below).
- There is a highly sensitive test based on certain criteria which can further help diagnose an exudative effusion over a transudate, Light's criteria, which states that for an exudate the:
  1. pleural fluid protein : serum protein ratio is > 0.5
  2. pleural fluid LDH : serum LDH ratio is > 0.6
  3. pleural fluid LDH is more than two thirds the upper limit of normal for serum LDH.

Further specialist tests will depend on the likely causes, for example, a bronchoscopy in a patient likely to have lung cancer, rheumatoid factor and ANAs in possible cases of SLE or rheumatoid-induced effusions. Pleural fluid can also be sent off for further specialist tests, which again will depend on the likely diagnosis, for example, fluid amylase or fat levels in cases of pancreatitis and chylous effusions, respectively.

Honours response

Q2   What are the causes of an effusion?
The causes of a pleural effusion can be divided into whether the pleural aspirate is an exudate or a transudate:
- A transudate contains < 3 g/L of protein and can be caused by increased venous pressure in combination with hypoproteinaemia.
- An exudate contains > 3 g/L protein and is generally due to increased pleural capillary permeability.

TABLE 4.14 Causes of a pleural effusion

Effusion	Aetiology
Transudate	**Cardiac:** left ventricular failure, constrictive pericarditis
	Hepatic: liver cirrhosis, chronic liver failure
	Renal: glomerulonephritis, nephrotic syndrome
	Gut: malabsorption
	Other: hypothyroidism (myxoedema), pulmonary embolus, peritoneal dialysis, Meigs' syndrome (ovarian cancer)
Exudate	**Lung infection:** pneumonia, TB and less commonly viral or fungal
	Malignancy: primary lung cancer, mesothelioma, metastatic lung cancer, lymphoma
	Trauma: haemothorax, ruptured oesophagus
	Inflammation and vasculitides: rheumatoid arthritis, SLE, Sjögren's, Wegener's granulomatosis, pancreatitis
	Others: pulmonary embolism, Dressler's syndrome, subphrenic abscess

Q3   What are the principles of treatment?
- **Aetiology:** Determine underlying cause and manage.
- Management depends on the size of the effusion and the presence of symptoms.
  - **Conservative:** If small and asymptomatic, management involves observation with repeat imaging.
  - **Medical:** This will require aspiration with a chest drain +/– pleurodesis; pleurodesis is commonly used in malignant effusions in an effort to reduce recurrence.
  - **Surgical.**

4.2   RESPIRATORY HISTORIES

By far the most likely case you will come across in finals will be cough. It is important that you are fluent with this history. Cardinal respiratory system symptoms include shortness of breath, cough, haemoptysis and chest pain. *See* Chapter 2 for the general history-taking schema described; here, we focus on specific points related to the respiratory system.

History Case 1: Cough

Instructions: This 25-year-old smoker presents with cough. Please take a focused clinical history.

Key features to look for

❏ **Note the patient's age**
- For a young patient with a chronic cough, you should consider asthma, or in an older age group pneumonia or COPD.

❏ **Occupation**
- Enquire as to what job they do or what they did in the past. Certain occupations increase the risk of specific respiratory diseases.
- Ask if respiratory symptoms are associated with their occupation, and if they resolve on leaving such an environment.

TABLE 4.15 Occupational lung diseases

Occupation	Description
Asbestos exposure	Examples: dock worker, pipe lagger, industrial applications, etc. Disease: mesothelioma
Farmer or pigeon keeper	Farmer's lung: exposure to fungal spores in mouldy hay Pigeon fancier's lung Both are forms of extrinsic allergic alveolitis
Baker, chemical worker, plastics	Occupational asthma
Highly radioactive areas	Lung cancer
Coal miner, cotton picker	Pneumoconiosis
Bar/club worker	Passive smoking – lung cancer (however many bars/clubs in the UK are smoke-free by law)

❑ **Assess features of cough**

TABLE 4.16 Features of cough

Feature	Description
Timescale	When did it start? Is it getting better or worse? Worse in the morning and especially at night is characteristic of asthma Is it constant?
Sputum	Dry cough seen in asthma, early viral and bacterial infections, pharyngitis, cancer Productive cough and/or haemoptysis (*see* below)
Exacerbation	Cold air, smoke, perfumes, dust (all known precipitants for bronchospasm in conditions such as asthma)
Relief	Does your normal inhaler help to control the cough? In asthma, increased usage of salbutamol inhalers may indicate an oncoming exacerbation
Medications	ACE inhibitors may induce cough due to accumulation of bradykinin
Other symptoms	**Nasal drip:** may indicate rhinitis, which is a cause of chronic cough **Fever:** may indicate an infective process such as pneumonia

❑ **Productive cough**
  ▪ If the patient has a productive cough (sputum), you need to ascertain the following:
    — **volume:** those with bronchiectasis can often cough up multiple cupfuls every day
    — **frequency**
    — **viscosity**
    — **colour and character:** green/yellow may indicate pneumonia, bloodstained may indicate haemoptysis (*see* below)
    — **purulent:** infection, may be acute or chronic
    — **mucoid:** grey-white in chronic bronchitis
    — **serous:** clear, may be pink-tinged in pulmonary oedema or pulmonary embolism.
❑ **Haemoptysis**
  ▪ **True haemoptysis:** Discern whether this is aspirated haematemesis or nasal bleeding which is being coughed up. This is a serious symptom and should not being taken lightly if present, as it may indicate an underlying malignancy.

- **Frequency, volume**
- **Fresh, clotted, specks in sputum**
- **Characteristics** – certain features make specific diagnoses more likely:

TABLE 4.17 Characteristics of haemoptysis

Characteristic	Suggested diagnosis
Frank haemoptysis	Bronchiectasis, TB, aspergilloma, lung cancer
Bloodstained sputum	Lung abscess, lung cancer
Blood-streaked sputum	Lung cancer
Rusty sputum	Pneumococcal pneumonia

❏ **Chest pain**
- **Take a pain history:** in the SOCRATES format, i.e. **S**ite, **O**nset, **C**haracteristic, **R**adiation, **T**ime scale, **E**xacerbating/Relieving, **S**everity scale
- **Pleuritic in nature:** worse on movement and inspiration, sharp stabbing pain, can be extremely severe and cause patients to hypoventilate. Can be confused with musculoskeletal pain. Caused by inflammation of the pleura; common causes include PE and infection

---

AUTHOR'S TOP TIP

Reproduction of pleuritic-sounding chest pain by palpation of the chest wall does not indicate that the diagnosis is definitely musculoskeletal.

AUTHOR'S TOP TIP

Remember to think of other causes of chest pain, such as gastritis/reflux, angina/myocardial infarction. Bone pain in sickle-cell crisis can also have a pleuritic nature and cause hypoventilation. Remember that GTN spray in some people may relieve the pain of reflux.

❏ **Shortness of breath (dyspnoea)**
- **Timescale:** acute versus chronic SOB can have many causes:

TABLE 4.18 Duration of dyspnoea

Timescale	Conditions
Minutes	Pneumothorax, cardiac-related, e.g. pulmonary oedema, arrhythmias, myocardial infarction
	Pulmonary embolism, foreign body
	Laryngeal oedema

(continued)

Timescale	Conditions
Hours	Asthma, exacerbation of COPD
	Pneumonia
Days	Pneumonia, left heart failure
Weeks	Pulmonary effusion, lung cancer
	muscle weakness, anaemia
Months	Pulmonary fibrosis, thyrotoxicosis
	Muscle weakness
Years	COPD, interstitial lung disease

- ■ **Exacerbating and relieving factors**
  - — **Environment:** if it occurs mainly at work, it may be due to occupational factors such as dust or chemicals.
  - — **Wheeze:** suggests COPD/asthma
  - — **Seasonal:** worse in spring/summer months suggests mild asthma
  - — **Exercise tolerance:** assess their normal exercise tolerance and how this has changed with the disease. A simple form of assessing this is asking how many stairs they can climb without stopping. You need to determine that it is the dyspnoea that is limiting their exercise tolerance and not other symptoms, such as angina or hip pain from osteoarthritis.
- ❑ **Past medical history**
  - ■ **Previous history:** known asthma/COPD or bronchiectasis

---

AUTHOR'S TOP TIP

It is important to ask asthma and COPD patients how often they get exacerbations of their condition and if they have ever been to ITU or been intubated, as a positive answer to either of these points to a more severe disease state and the necessity to be extra vigilant.

- ■ **Past medical history of:**
  - — **atopy:** eczema, hay fever may be present in asthmatic patient or their family
  - — **known or previous TB:** immunisation with BCG vaccine does not give 100% protection against all strains of TB
  - — **GORD:** chronic cough
  - — **rheumatological or autoimmune conditions:** can have associated pulmonary fibrosis and vasculitis destruction of lungs
  - — recurrent chest infection history, aspirated objects and measles in childhood can lead to bronchiectasis
  - — previous thromboembolic disease, i.e. PE/DVT.
- ■ **Previous surgical history of:**
  - — **lung transplant:** e.g. COPD, pulmonary fibrosis, cystic fibrosis
  - — **lung cancer:** pneumonectomy, lobectomy
  - — **pulmonary hypertension:** heart and lung transplant
  - — **bronchiectasis:** may have lobectomy

- **aspergilloma:** may have thoracic surgery
- **emphysema:** bullectomy, lobectomy; allows less damaged lung to expand and function better.

❑ **Drug history**
- **Inhalers:** Ask about inhalers prescribed, when they are used and how often they are needed. This is especially important for the blue inhaler in determining severity of exacerbations of asthma and to a lesser extent COPD.
  - blue inhaler: reliever; salbutamol, beta agonist
  - brown inhaler: preventer; beclometasone or equivalent, steroid
- **Known COPD/asthma:** Ask specifically about any recent antibiotic and steroid courses. Some patients may stay on a low-dose permanent dose of steroid that will need doubling when they become unwell. A multiple course of steroids also points to more brittle forms of the diseases.
- **ACE inhibitors:** ACEi-induced cough.

❑ **Social history**
- **Smoking:** Smokers are more likely to get chest infections; asthmatics tend not to smoke, as it exacerbates their symptoms.
- **Pets:** Cough or SOB may be exacerbated by pets with fur dander, such as cats and dogs or birds.
- **Foreign travel:** In patients who normally reside in other countries and are visiting, consider TB, especially in those from developing countries. Those who work in areas with standing water or air conditioning, consider legionnaires' infection. Ask about any recent contact with others who are unwell, or those who are known to have TB.
- **Recreational drugs:** Smoking illicit drugs can cause SOB, cough or pneumonia.
- **Exercise tolerance:** If SOB, this is useful to quantify the effect this has on the patient's activities of daily living.

Completion

Cough is a common presenting complaint in the OSCEs, of which pneumonia is the most likely diagnosis in the exam. You must be proficient at taking such a history quickly and succinctly.

Viva questions

Q1   How would you manage a patient with pneumonia?
- You must always mention you will take a focused history, followed by clinical examination and undertake investigations tailored to your findings.

In general
- **Investigations:** FBC may demonstrate a raised WCC, and a raised CRP, blood cultures, CXR may demonstrate consolidation.
- **Need for admission:** Some patients can easily be managed at home with oral antibiotics. You need to determine who needs admission; this is achieved using prognostic indicators as determined by the CURB-65 score.
- **CURB-65 score:** This determines whether patient needs HDU/ITU care. In addition to

age > 65 years, the presence of Confusion, a raised Urea, a Respiratory rate > 30, and a BP < 90 systolic indicates the patient should be admitted to hospital for intravenous antibiotics.

- **Antibiotics:** You should follow local hospital guidelines, but generally broad-spectrum antibiotics including typically a penicillin and macrolide.
- **Consider HIV test:** This should be considered in young patients and any at-risk groups.
- **Follow-up:** For those patients discharged home on presentation, a 6-week post-treatment repeat CXR is required in at-risk patients. This is to ensure resolution of signs. If there is no resolution, you should consider underlying bronchogenic carcinoma.

With the recent epidemics of swine flu, more and more patients are being admitted to HDU/ITU with severe pneumonia. Your treatment therefore must include the possibility they may have swine flu in addition to any atypical organisms such as *Mycoplasma pneumoniae*, *Chlamydia pneumoniae*, *Chlamydia psittaci*, *Legionella* and *Coxiella*. This highlights the importance of taking a thorough history.

Common organisms in community acquired pneumonia include *Streptococcus pneumoniae*, followed by *Haemophilus influenzae*. Streptococcal pneumonia is common in winter and is characterised by fever with rigors, lobar consolidation and herpetic cold sores. Non-resolving pneumonia should prompt you to consider lung cancer.

CHAPTER 5

Endocrinology

This chapter will focus on spot diagnoses and their more detailed examinations, such as in a patient with acromegaly, wherein a candidate would be expected to either offer or simply examine the patient's visual field for a bitemporal hemianopia, a well-known associated sign. Other typical cases include Cushing's syndrome and thyroid disease. Diabetes will be covered thoroughly due to its impact and incidence in today's society and clinical medicine; this will be in the form of a newly diagnosed diabetic, a case you will likely see as part of a history station in the exam.

Due to the nature of the disease profiles, a lot of the pathological signs include obvious facial and skin abnormalities. As such, this lends itself to picture-recognition stations in the exam. And so in the absence of an actual patient, you must still be able to recognise what other features you may wish to examine or look for, so as to impress the examiner.

EXAMINER'S ANECDOTE

The downfall of many candidates when presented with an obvious case of acromegaly is that they simply state the patient has acromegaly. What the candidates fail to appreciate is that this case may be an entire station on its own and that they need something more to either examine or discuss. After all, simply stating 'acromegaly' will gain you at the very most a single mark.

This chapter helps to teach the candidate that by being aware of these commonly associated signs or symptoms, they will score much more highly than they would have otherwise. Using the knowledge and skills contained in this chapter will thus enable the keen student to capitalise on this fact and score highly in the exam scenario.

The stations' instruction sheet is an important tool in aiding your diagnosis and performance in the exam. Often the examination of an endocrinological disorder is multisystemic, so examiners cannot direct you to one organ system to examine over another. Often a vague instruction such as 'Look at this picture or patient and examine as you see fit' or 'Please examine his face' will give you a clue that this is likely to be an endocrine case and is more about recognition of the phenotypic characteristic of the various syndromes. Occasionally, you will be given a short case, whereby the examiner may give you a brief history and expect you to come up with pertinent examination findings and discuss brief aetiology; endocrinology lends itself very well to this format, due to the number of conditions with overt clinical signs. This may be seen in a station where there are multiple cases for you to assess and time is of the essence. It is important therefore that you answer exactly what the examiner asks of you and do not waffle, as this will only irritate them. Remember, they are trying to help you to pass, so remember to help yourself!

AUTHOR'S TOP TIP

Remember, recognition of the syndrome is often not difficult. But to gain all the marks available, you must be able to recognise the associated features and complications.

AUTHOR'S TOP TIP

On the whole, the examination routine focuses on inspection, as most of the signs are detectable on inspection alone. You must therefore say what you see. Be careful not to offend a patient, as some of the commonly used terms to describe endocrine signs, e.g. 'buffalo hump' in Cushing's syndrome, may not be welcomed by the patient. We advise you to therefore use the medical terms (thoracocervical fat pads) or generalise your findings into 'features of corticosteroid excess'. The examiner will be aware that you are trying to be professional and courteous to your patients, and your patients will be appreciative also.

The important exception to these general rules is the thyroid examination, as it has its own specific examination routine, and only a handful of cases can really come up in finals. Thus, the thyroid examination will also be covered in this chapter. Although one may attribute this to a surgical clinical finals case, it may also be seen in medical finals, whereby different aspects of disease management are examined, particularly the medical management. Thyroid disease is managed by both physicians and surgeons.

Of note, an extensive examination routine and discussion of the thyroid gland has been covered in our companion book, *The Ultimate Guide to Passing Surgical Clinical Finals*; we will focus our endeavours on the medical aspects of the examination only.

5.1   EXAMINATION OF THE THYROID

Clinical examination

Introduction

As for any clinical encounter (*see* Chapter 1, Section 3). Specifically for this case:

❑ **Position patient appropriately** [The patient is sitting on a chair, with space for you to stand behind them]

AUTHOR'S TOP TIP

Some examiners like to challenge candidates by placing the chair against a wall. It is perfectly acceptable to ask the patient to stand, and move their chair forward for them to sit.

❏ **Build rapport** [Inform patient of what you are doing as you go along; remember you are going to be feeling the patient's neck, with your hand around their airway; this can be an intrusive exam which may well be uncomfortable, so ask about pain as necessary]

Inspection

The patient may appear restless or anxious, i.e. signs of hyperthyroidism.
❏ **Inspect the hands**
  - warm and sweaty, fine tremor (hyperthyroidism)
  - palmar erythema, seen in hyperthyroidism
  - dry, cool and rough with non-pitting swelling (hypothyroidism)
  - assess for thyroid acropachy, seen in Graves' disease
  - feel the pulse; are they tachycardic or in AF (hyperthyroidism), bradycardia (hypothyroidism)?
❏ **Inspect the facies**
  - **complexion:** peaches and cream in hypothyroidism
  - **myxoedematous:** thick and coarse facial features with periorbital swelling/puffiness
  - **eyebrows:** loss of the outer third in hypothyroidism
  - **dry thinning hair:** seen classically in hypothyroidism
❏ **Inspect the eyes**
  - Inspect for exophthalmos (Graves' disease) from above the patient and the side. This is due to retro-orbital fat/muscle inflammation and infiltration by lymphocytes. This can lead to chemosis, corneal ulcerations and ophthalmoplegia.

AUTHOR'S TOP TIP

Make a point of looking from the front, side and back of the patient for exophthalmos.

  - Look for lid retraction or lid lag. Ask the patient to follow your finger with their eyes, but keeping their head still; move your index finger first up and then down and look for lid lag.
❏ **Inspect the neck**
  - **Scars:** Look for a horizontal scar at the baseline of the neck. This is also called a collar incision or visor scar and may indicate a previous thyroidectomy.
  - **Skin changes:** Erythema, which can be seen in suppurative thyroiditis.
  - **Obvious lump:** Look at the neck for any visible lumps; if you see one, note where it is and roughly how large.
  - **Tracheal deviation:** Difficult to see unless gross.
  - **Tongue protrusion test:** Ask the patient to protrude their tongue; a thyroglossal cyst will rise as the tongue is protruded; the thyroid will not.

AUTHOR'S TOP TIP

If you ask the patient to tilt their head back as they do this it becomes a lot easier to see this sign.

- ■ **Swallow test:** Next, hand the patient a glass of water and ask them to take a mouthful and hold it. Then move the glass away and observe the neck for a swelling as you ask them to swallow. Do any lumps become more visible on swallowing? Do they move on swallowing? On swallowing, a goitre or thyroglossal cyst will rise due to attachment to the larynx and trachea.
- ❑ **Palpate the thyroid swelling**
  - ■ Palpate from behind. Warn the patient you will be standing behind them and before you put your hands on their neck.
  - ■ Palpate for the thyroid: place the flat of your four fingers over the left lobe and palpate the right lobe to begin with, feeling the upper, middle and lower lobes; ask them to swallow.
  - ■ Now repeat this, keeping the flat of your right hand still and palpating with the left-hand fingers.
  - ■ If you feel a lump, describe it as you would describe any lump:
    - — site, size, shape, surface and consistency
    - — edges: whether well demarcated or diffuse
    - — fluctuance and pulsatility
    - — reducibility and whether it is fixed to deeper structures.

It is probably easier to describe what you are feeling at this stage, as you may not recall all the details at the end of the examination.
  - ■ e.g *'I can palpate a 2x2 cm hemispherical non-tender lump in the upper lobe of the right thyroid; it is soft with well-defined edges. It is fluctuant but non-reducible or compressible. It is not fixed to the overlying skin, which is not inflamed. My diagnosis is a cyst of the right thyroid; however, this could also be . . .'*
- ❑ **Palpate the lymph nodes**
  - ■ Examine all the lymph nodes in the neck starting in a systematic fashion: the preauricular, postauricular, occipital, superficial cervical, deep cervical, submandibular and anterior cervical chains.

Percussion
- ❑ **Check for retrosternal extension**
  - ■ If you find a diffusely enlarged thyroid, percuss for retrosternal extension.

Auscultation
- ❑ **Auscultate for a bruit in Graves' disease**

Complete the examination
- ❑ **Thank the patient**
- ❑ **Wash your hands**
- ❑ **Further examination**
  - ■ *'To complete my examination, I would like to assess the patient's thyroid status and ask some questions.'*

If you have time, you can assess for slow-relaxing reflexes, seen in hypothyroidism.
- ❑ **Present your findings**

TABLE 5.1 Common neck lumps in finals

Neck lump	Description
Parotid tumour/ enlargement	**Parotid tumour:** Warthin's tumour (pleiomorphic adenoma) (commonest)
	Enlargement: can be caused by infections such as mumps and TB, parotid stones, inflammatory conditions such as sarcoid and Sjögren's, endocrine disease, e.g. diabetes, Cushing's disease, drugs, e.g. thiouracil, isoprenaline and in chronic alcohol abuse
Swollen submandibular glands	Usually caused by malignancy (adenoid cystic is the commonest), non-Hodgkin's lymphoma
	Metastasis from facial cancers or stones
Thyroglossal cyst	Centrally located on the neck; elevates with protrusion of the tongue
	Common in those under 20 years
Thyroid nodule	Nodular disease is a common problem and is usually benign. Factors associated with benign lesions:
	• smooth, mobile and soft
	• pain or tenderness on palpation
	• family history of benign thyroid masses or goitre
	• autoimmune thyroid disease or presence of thyroid dysfunction
	Raise your index of suspicion for malignancy if:
	• firm, hard or immobile with presence of cervical lymphadenopathy
	• history of thyroid cancer or neck irradiation
	• younger than 20 or older than 70 years
	• dysphonia or dysphagia present
Branchial cyst	Usually occurs in teenagers, fluctuant and difficult to excise, found in anterior triangle

Short Case 1: Non-toxic goitre

Case history: A 24-year-old pregnant female presents with a slowly growing lump in the midline of her neck with no associated symptoms. She does not smoke or consume any alcohol. Please examine her.

Key features to look for

Clinical examination

❑ **Thyroid:** diffusely enlarged thyroid gland, smooth and non-tender. No retrosternal extension or Graves' bruit, no associated lymphadenopathy

❑ **Patient thyroid status:** euthyroid

Clinical impression

❑ **Diffuse non-toxic simple goitre:** hypertrophy occurring as a result of a reduction in T_3 and T_4 production. The thyroid enlargement results from increased TRH and TSH from the reduced T_3 and T_4.

❑ A differential diagnosis would include Graves' disease or Hashimoto's, both of which are also seen in a euthyroid state.

The most likely cause here is due to increased physiological needs secondary to pregnancy resulting in the goitre. This may progress to becoming a multinodular goitre, which can cause local pressure symptoms such as dysphagia, stridor or even SVC obstruction and in some instances toxicity.

Viva questions

Q1   What are the causes of a non-toxic simple goitre?
- **Physiological:** pregnancy, puberty
- **Dietary iodine deficiency:** traditionally seen in people from the Himalayas or Andes
- **Treated Graves' disease:** in such patients, there is a bruit and exophthalmos, but otherwise clinically euthyroid
- Hereditary defects in thyroid metabolism

Short Case 2: Solitary nodule – thyroid cancer

Case history: A 33-year-old female presents with an enlarging neck mass which has been present for the past 4 months. There are no other associated symptoms, and clinically she is euthyroid. Of note, as a child the patient had a history of irradiation to the neck.

Key features to look for

Clinical examination
❑ **Thyroid:** palpable, firm non-tender lump over the right lobe of the thyroid, non-fluctuant, reducible or pulsatile. No retrosternal extension or bruit. No associated lymphadenopathy in the neck.

Clinical impression
❑ Most likely diagnosis is that of a **papillary carcinoma** due to its enlarging nature in addition to the past history of irradiation to the neck.
❑ However, this could also be a cyst, an adenoma or a prominent nodule in a multinodular goitre.

AUTHOR'S TOP TIP

If you felt a nodule in a thyroid examination, remember that half are prominent nodules as part of a much larger multinodular goitre. The remaining are solitary thyroid nodules which could be due to a cyst, cancer or an adenoma.

Viva questions

Q1   What are the four main types of thyroid cancers?

Difficult question

TABLE 5.2 Different types of thyroid cancers

Type	Description
Follicular	More common in females
	Metastasises to the lung and bone
	If resectable, prognosis is good
Papillary	Commonest form of thyroid cancer. Found in younger patients, can be associated with a history of neck irradiation, usually local spread with a good prognosis
Medullary	Usually part of the MEN syndrome (*see* below), local and metastatic spread, poor prognosis
Anaplastic	Very aggressive tumour carrying the worst prognosis

Q2   In which instances are FNA not definitive?

Difficult question

- If you suspect a follicular carcinoma.
- This is because the FNA results will not be able to distinguish benign from malignant.
- Therefore, histology is needed and a hemithyroidectomy is normally performed.

Case 1: Graves' disease – thyrotoxicosis

Instructions: Please examine this 40-year-old woman with a history of type 1 diabetes who presents with reduced heat tolerance, irritability and protuberant eyes.

Key features to look for

Signs of hyperthyroidism
❑ tremor, restlessness
❑ warm sweaty hands, with palmar erythema
❑ tachycardia or AF
❑ thyroid bruit: seen exclusively in Graves' disease
❑ thyroid goitre; scar from previous surgical resection

Eye signs
❑ **Exophthalmos:** this is virtually pathognomonic of Graves' disease
❑ **Ophthalmoplegia:** occurs due to inflammatory infiltration and enlargement of retro-orbital muscles
❑ **Proptosis, lid lag and retraction**

AUTHOR'S TOP TIP

Ophthalmoplegia in thyroid disease can occur in any autoimmune thyroid disease, most commonly Graves'.

Skin changes
❑ **Pretibial myxoedema:** elevated lesions found on the shins bilaterally. It has a shiny peau d'orange appearance (although differing opinions exist as to the exact description). The lesions may or may not be tender. This is pathognomonic of Graves' disease
❑ **Nails:** thyroid acropachy, onycholysis

Complete the examination
❑ **Thank the patient**
❑ **Wash your hands**
❑ **Further examination**
   ▪ *'To complete my exam, I would like to assess for evidence of decompensation.'*

Features in Graves' disease that would suggest decompensation include: a fixed painful gaze, which requires steroids with or without surgical correction due to the risk of optic nerve damage and blindness; high output heart failure; and thyroid storm.

❑ **Present your findings**
Graves' disease is an autoimmune disease with antibodies stimulating TSH receptors causing excessive TSH and T₄ and T₃. Patients are often hyperthyroid at presentation, but may later become hypo- or euthyroid. In pregnancy, TSH receptor antibodies can cross the placenta and cause foetal hyperthyroidism. The presence of a goitre, ophthalmopathy and pretibial myxoedema are features of Graves' disease.

Viva questions

Q1   What pertinent features in the history would you look for?
   ▪ **Symptoms:** gritty eyes, excessive lacrimation or blurred vision, sometimes with diplopia. May have a history of hyperthyroid symptoms, such as heat intolerance, increased energy, irritability, weight loss despite increased appetite, diarrhoea, thyroiditis (tender goitre)
   ▪ **Past history:** it is associated with other autoimmune conditions, so ask if the patient has, e.g. vitiligo, type1 diabetes, Addison's disease, coeliac disease, pernicious anaemia

Q2 What investigations would you carry out to investigate hyperthyroidism?

- **Bloods:** TSH/T$_4$/T$_3$, autoantibodies (antimicrosomal, thyroid peroxidase [TPO], antithyroglobulin); these are seen in Graves' disease, as well as TSH receptor antibodies
- **Radioisotope scanning:** high uptake in hot nodules, low uptake in cold nodules and cancer; high diffuse uptake in Graves' disease
- **USS scan:** look for masses, cysts and thyroid size
- **Eye tests:** visual fields, acuity and eye gait

Good response

Q3 What is the treatment for hyperthyroidism?

TABLE 5.3 Treatment for Graves' disease

Treatment	Description
Medical	**Beta blockers:** propranolol for symptomatic relief
	Antithyroid medication: this can be titrated to reduce hyperthyroidism or used in a block-and-replace regime, e.g. carbimazole/propylthiouracil. Antithyroid medication can also cross the placenta and cause foetal hypothyroidism. Patients on carbimazole must be warned of agranulocytosis, and the presence of a sore throat should alert them to seek medical advice, as life-threatening neutropenia can occur. There is a high rate of relapse of disease upon discontinuation of drugs
Radioiodine	Can be used in hot lesions which rapidly uptake the radioiodine. Unfortunately, half of patients will subsequently end up hypothyroid and require lifelong thyroxine replacement
	Contraindications: iodine allergy, breastfeeding, pregnancy and active eye disease as it can exacerbate symptoms
Surgical	**Thyroidectomy:** indicated when radioiodine is not possible, or if there is a large symptomatic goitre. Surgery can be partial or total and usually results in permanent resolution of symptoms. However, lifelong thyroxine replacement is required

In addition, if the patient also has thyroid eye disease (fixed gaze, visual loss), in general they will require:

- ophthalmological specialist input
- high-dose steroids, orbital radiotherapy, surgical decompression

If the patient cannot fully close their eyelids, this requires urgent referral, as the normally protected eye is now at risk of exposure keratitis. Note that radioiodine and surgery are extremely effective treatments and both result in permanent cure.

Once treated, patients will require annual TFTs to monitor resolution; more frequently if any treatment regimens are altered. Note that it takes several weeks for changes to be biochemically detectable on TFTs. It is important to advise patients with hyperthyroidism to stop smoking.

Honours response

You do not need to be fully versed with the block-and-replace regimens, as this is considered postgraduate level and beyond the scope of this revision guide.

Q4 What is a thyroid storm?
- Thyroid crisis or thyroid storm is a rare complication of hyperthyroidism that consists of the following features:
  — hyperpyrexia
  — tachycardia
  — restlessness.

It carries a mortality of 10% and can be precipitated by infection, surgery, stress or radioiodine therapy.

Case 2: Acromegaly

Instructions: This 50-year-old man has presented with problems putting his hat on. Please examine him as you see fit.

Key features to look for

Inspection

❑ **Hands**
- sweaty, spade-like hands (feet are also very large)
- wasting of thenar eminence and paraesthesia in those with associated carpal tunnel syndrome
- thick rubbery skin

AUTHOR'S TOP TIP

Sweaty dough-like hands will be obvious upon shaking the patient's hands on your introduction.

AUTHOR'S TOP TIP

A quick screen for carpal tunnel syndrome may be elicited by performing Tinel's test, whereby tapping over the flexor retinaculum reproduces symptoms.

❑ **Face**
- **Macroglossia:** soft tissue enlargement of the tongue; often the nose and ears are also enlarged
- **Prominent supraorbital ridges**
- **Prognathism:** protrusion of the lower jaw, leading to an overbite
- **Widespread teeth:** increased interdental spaces; clenching of the teeth will enhance this feature

❑ **Other**
- Deep, husky voice: you may ask the patient to repeat a sentence to you or simply ask how the patient is feeling today to ascertain this feature

- hypertension
- gynaecomastia; thyroid goitre
- bitemporal hemianopia on visual field testing, optic atrophy on fundoscopy
- spine: kyphosis
- gastrointestinal: hepatosplenomegaly
- type 2 diabetes
- acanthosis nigricans

Complete the examination

- ❑ **Thank the patient**
- ❑ **Wash your hands**
- ❑ **Further examination**
  - *'To complete my exam, I would like to take the blood pressure, check the blood sugar, assess for carpal tunnel syndrome and assess the risk of colorectal cancer and sleep apnoea.'*

This is an honours response, as you have considered all of the associated conditions that carry increased morbidity and mortality. Cardiac and respiratory disease in combination with malignancy account for the increased mortality associated with acromegaly.

❑ **Present your findings**

Acromegaly is usually caused by increased growth hormone (GH) secretion due to a pituitary tumour (macroadenoma) and in very rare cases by carcinoid tumours. This induces increased insulin-like growth factor production in the body (IGF-1), leading to excessive soft tissue growth. It is one of three anterior pituitary tumours, the other two being a microadenoma precipitating release of excessive ACTH, causing Cushing's disease, and a prolactinoma. Macroadenomas such as those seen in acromegaly may also secrete prolactin. Prolactin release is normally inhibited by dopamine, which is derived from the hypothalamus. Patients may therefore demonstrate signs and symptoms of hyperprolactinaemia. It is worthwhile noting that in a man, the patient may initially present with erectile dysfunction, a sign of hypogonadism.

AUTHOR'S TOP TIP

It is possible that you may be simply shown a photo of a patient with acromegaly. You cannot of course examine these patients, but it is still important to mention what you would be looking for. If you do have a patient in the exam, quickly examining for a bitemporal hemianopia would be impressive, time permitting.

Viva questions

Q1   What are the presenting symptoms and associated complications of acromegaly?
- **Symptoms**
    — excessive sweating and headache
    — patient normally notices poorly fitting clothes due to change in soft tissue mass (poorly fitting shoes, gloves, hats and rings)
    — relatives and friends, especially those who don't frequently see the patient, may also note coarsening of facial features and spreading of teeth
    — patient may complain of impairment of vision due to the local compression of the optic tract by the enlarged pituitary gland (*see* Chapter 7, neuro-ophthalmology)
- **Complications**
    — cardiomegaly, hypertension, cardiomyopathy and heart failure (most significant in morbidity and mortality)
    — pituitary insufficiency
    — osteoarthritis of joints
    — sleep apnoea
    — carpal tunnel syndrome, diabetes or incidental high BM on regular check-ups
    — may be associated with multiple endocrine neoplasia syndrome

Note that patients may initially present with the associated complications and then upon further investigations be found to have acromegaly.

EXAMINERS ANECDOTE

I once knew of a medical student who worked in a store and noted a customer who looked like they had acromegaly. He boldly told the patient to get tested, and it turned out he did indeed have acromegaly. If you suspect a diagnosis based upon a patient's facial features, do not be afraid to voice your concerns, even if you risk offending a patient. You are after all a healthcare professional, and most patients will understand your genuine concern for their well-being. However, please be tactful in doing so!

AUTHOR'S TOP TIP

Sometimes, the examiner may ask you to ask the patient some pertinent questions. In this case, what they are referring to is the insidious development of acromegaly, whereby some patients are not even aware of their symptoms for many years. In this situation, you can ask if the patient has an old photograph of themselves to compare how much they have changed in appearance; classically, whether or not the patient's favourite top hat no longer fits, or if their wedding ring or shoe is now too small for them to wear.

The most common causes of death in acromegalics are heart failure and the mass effect from tumour expansion. The associated cardiovascular risks with hypertension and diabetes also play a role in increased mortality.

Q2 What MEN syndromes do you know of?

Difficult question

- MEN stands for multiple endocrine neoplasia which are essentially clinical syndromes whereby multiple malignant or benign endocrine cancers coexist.

TABLE 5.4 MEN syndromes

Classification	Description
MEN1	**Gene affected:** menin gene, chromosome 11
	Associated neoplasia:
	Parathyroid hyperplasia or adenoma; with associated hypercalcaemia
	Pancreatic tumours, gastrinoma, insulinoma (rarely somatostatinoma, glucagonoma or VIPoma)
	Pituitary adenoma
	Adrenal and carcinoid tumours
MEN2	**Gene affected:** *ret* proto-oncogene, chr10
	Associated neoplasia:
	MEN2a / **MEN2b**
	MEN2a: Medullary thyroid cancer — MEN2b: MEN2a features and Marfanoid appearance
	MEN2a: Phaeochromocytoma (usually bilateral) — MEN2b: Neuroendocrine tumours
	MEN2a: Parathyroid hyperplasia

All MEN syndromes are autosomal dominant, so there will be a positive family history. They are also all associated with hypercalcaemia and may even be the initial presenting feature, especially in MEN1.

Q3 How would you investigate this patient?
- **Bloods:** raised GH, raised IGF-1 levels. Fasting blood glucose for diabetes or impaired glucose tolerance. Prolactin, thyroxine, luteinising hormone and testosterone levels will also need to be requested (there may be hypopituitary function, with associated hyperprolactinaemia and testosterone deficiency)
- **Specialist tests:**
  — **Oral glucose tolerance test:** 75 g of glucose is given to the patient, and if there is a failure to suppress GH production to < 2 mU/L, then this confirms acromegaly
- **CXR/echo/ECG:** cardiomegaly, cardiomyopathy, hypertensive ECG changes
- **MRI pituitary fossa:** enlarged pituitary gland
- **Visual field testing:** bitemporal hemianopia
- **Old and new photos:** so as to compare the patient's physical appearance

> **AUTHOR'S TOP TIP**
>
> *Visual fields will need formal perimetry assessment and mapping. Some patients may be commercial drivers, and this may affect their work.*

Q4 What are the principles of treatment?
- **Medical**
  - **somatostatin analogues:** these are preferred to dopamine agonists. They work by inhibiting GH secretion and can be given as monthly depot injections, e.g. octreotide, lanreotide
  - **dopamine agonists:** used to reduce GH secretion, e.g. cabergoline and bromocriptine
  - **GH antagonist:** a GH-receptor antagonist; used in cases unresponsive to surgery/ traditional medical therapy, e.g. pegvisomant

With traditional drug therapy, significant shrinkage of the tumour does not occur, and so most patients go on to surgery.
- **Radiotherapy**
  - given routinely after surgery to prevent recurrence
  - can be given alone in patients not suitable for surgery, but takes many years to achieve any effects; may cause hypopituitarism
- **Surgical**
  - **Transphenoidal hypophysectomy surgery:** this is first-line treatment
  - **Transcranial** is an alternative route if there is suprasellar extension of the tumour
  - Complications of surgery include a transient diabetes insipidus, residual GH excess and persistent signs and symptoms of acromegaly

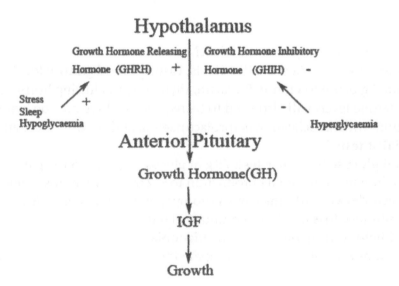

FIGURE 5.1 Growth hormone synthesis

It is important to remind the patient that even if surgery is successful, the excess soft tissue growth will not revert back to normal. If, however, GH levels are brought back to normal, there should be resolution of symptoms of excessive sweating and peripheral oedema.

Q5 What features would suggest disease activity?

Difficult question

- evidence of glycosuria
- hypertension
- sweating
- others: headache, poor vision

Case 3: Cushing's syndrome

Instructions: This 60-year-old woman has presented with polyuria and pigmented marks across her abdomen. Please look at this patients' face and examine as you see fit.

Key features to look for

Signs of excessive corticosteroids
- ❏ the so called moon-face appearance may be apparent
- ❏ skin: thin with prominent pigmented striae on abdomen, easy bruising
- ❏ hirsutism, acne
- ❏ centripetal distribution of fat
- ❏ supraclavicular and thoracocervical fat pads

Other signs
- ❏ hypertension
- ❏ poor wound healing
- ❏ proximal myopathy

Complete the examination
- ❏ **Thank the patient**
- ❏ **Wash your hands**
- ❏ **Further examination**
  - *'To complete my exam, I would like to assess the blood pressure, check the blood glucose for diabetes and examine for a proximal myopathy.'*
- ❏ **Present your findings**

You may also choose to take a brief history to ascertain whether the patient is taking any corticosteroids. Often, these are patients who are likely to be on long-term steroids, such as those with COPD, inflammatory bowel disease or transplant cases. Patients may present with weight gain, altered mood (depression, irritability), proximal muscle weakness, acne, hirsutism, irregular menses in women and impotence in men. They may also complain of symptoms relating to diabetes due to increased blood sugar levels. Patients are also at risk of osteoporosis.

Viva questions

Q1 What is the difference between Cushing's syndrome and disease?
- Cushing's syndrome refers to a state of chronic cortisol (glucocorticoid) excess in the body due to any cause.
- The commonest cause is exogenous steroid treatment, i.e. iatrogenic, with the commonest endogenous cause being Cushing's disease.
- Cushing's disease itself occurs due to a specific cause: a pituitary microadenoma secreting ACTH.

Endogenous causes can be divided into whether they are ACTH-driven or ACTH-independent. They can also be divided into whether the cause is pituitary, adrenal or ectopic.

TABLE 5.5 Causes of Cushing's syndrome

Aetiology	Description
Increased ACTH	**Cushing's disease:** pituitary microadenoma secreting ACTH leading to bilateral adrenal hyperplasia; most common non-drug-induced cause
	Ectopic ACTH production: common causes include small cell lung cancer and bronchial carcinoid
	Ectopic CRH production: very rare
Decreased ACTH	**Increased glucocorticoids:** exogenous steroid administration
	Adrenal adenoma: some secrete cortisol and androgens
	Adrenal hyperplasia

Q2 How would you investigate this patient?
- **Bloods:** hypokalaemia, hyperglycaemia
- **Screening tests**
  — 24-hour free urinary cortisol levels
  — Overnight dexamethasone suppression test
  - Patient is given dexamethasone (a synthetic glucocorticoid) at midnight.
  - Cortisol should be normally suppressed in this situation.
  - However, the 9 a.m. cortisol levels are high and midnight cortisol is high in a positive test.
- **Diagnostic tests**
  — **Low- or high-dose dexamethasone test:** This is used to ascertain whether the ACTH secretion is from the pituitary gland (Cushing's disease) or from an ectopic site. Ectopic ACTH does not suppress (usually, although there are exceptions), whereas pituitary adenomas will suppress, at least partially.
  — Imaging with bilateral inferior petrosal sinus sampling measuring ACTH levels after CRH stimulation can be done but is technically difficult.

Note that traditional imaging techniques may be difficult to interpret, as the tumour may be a few millimetres in size and therefore difficult to see.

Good response

AUTHOR'S TOP TIP

Reciting these tests in an exam situation can become confusing both to yourself and to the examiner. If you keep things simple and do not go into detail about low-dose dexamethasone testing, etc., you should be able to describe generally to the examiner the tests used in diagnosing Cushing's syndrome.

These suppression tests work on the understanding that cortisol levels follow a circadian rhythm, rising in the morning and falling to half their levels around late afternoon, and to an all-time low level at midnight. Isolated levels of a hormone are therefore meaningless. Remember, most hormones are regulated by negative feedback loops or by other hormones. These dynamic tests can help in the diagnosis of many conditions you will come across in endocrinology. This remains a commonly confusing area for medical school finalists. In general, it is useful to remember that a suppression test is used to detect a condition with an excessive amount of hormone, whereas a stimulation test can be used to detect a hormone deficiency.

Q3 How would you treat this patient?

Treatment will depend on whether the driver for increased glucocorticoid levels is exogenous, pituitary, adrenal or ectopic, i.e. it depends on whether it is Cushing's disease/syndrome and its cause. In general, however:

- **Conservative:** stop exogenous steroid administration; may not always be possible in some cases
- **Medical:** radiotherapy; metyrapone
- **Surgical:** once tumour location identified, surgical removal is advised usually via transphenoidal hypophysectomy.

Of note, there is a risk of developing Nelson's syndrome upon bilateral adrenalectomy for Cushing's disease, which can lead to an aggressive pituitary tumour due to the lack of feedback previously caused by high cortisol levels. Melanin-induced hyperpigmentation occurs.

AUTHOR'S TOP TIP

The main cause of morbidity and mortality is the increased risk of infection. Patients with untreated Cushing's syndrome most commonly die from sepsis.

Case 4: Addison's disease

Instructions: Please examine this 60-year-old woman who has presented with diarrhoea, low mood and lethargy.

Key features to look for

Inspection

❏ **Increased pigmentation:** hyperpigmented buccal mucosa, palmar and elbow creases (due to high ACTH levels); any surgical scars may also be hyperpigmented

❏ **Paucity of hair:** especially axillary in males

❏ **Vitiligo:** seen in 20% of cases (*see* Chapter 9)

Other

❏ **Blood pressure:** there may be postural hypotension.

Complete the examination

❏ **Thank the patient**

❏ **Wash your hands**

❏ **Further examination**

■ *'To complete my exam, I would like to assess for an abdominal scar.'*

AUTHOR'S TOP TIP

If there is an abdominal scar suggestive of bilateral adrenalectomy, then offer Nelson's syndrome as a differential diagnosis and offer to examine the visual fields for a temporal field defect. This would however be considered an honours response.

❏ **Present your findings**

Addison's disease is due to adrenal (glucocorticoid) insufficiency and also mineralocorticoid deficiency. The disease is sometimes referred to as hypoadrenalism.

Conn's disease is a form of primary hyperaldosteronism leading to mineralocorticoid excess, whereby renin levels are suppressed. This leads to hypokalaemia, hypertension and an alkalosis. Treatment is with spironolactone or amiloride; an adenoma will require surgical resection.

Q1 What are the causes of Addison's disease?
  ▪ Causes can be divided into primary causes and secondary causes:

TABLE 5.6 Causes of Addison's

Classification	Aetiology
Primary	Autoimmune (most common cause in UK)
	TB (most common cause worldwide)
	Adrenal haemorrhage
	HIV
	Amyloid
	Fungal infiltration, e.g. histoplasmosis
Secondary	Anterior pituitary disease
	Long term exogenous steroid administration – with sudden withdrawal
	Hypotension causing infarction from poor perfusion and ischaemia

Hypoadrenalism is commonly seen in critically ill patients. Indeed, infarction of the adrenals due to meningococcal septicaemia is a well-recognised cause, referred to as Waterhouse–Friderichsen syndrome.

Q2 Would you like to ask the patient any questions?
This is a subtle hint for you to take a brief focused history for symptoms related to Addison's disease, helping you to confirm your initial diagnosis.
  ▪ **Presenting symptoms:** Non-specific if not in an acute crisis; generalised fatigue, malaise, dizziness, myalgia, arthralgias, weight loss. Can have low mood/depression, diarrhoea, constipation, abdominal pain, nausea and vomiting.
  ▪ **Drug history:** Ask about steroid use; especially those on long-term steroids that have been stopped recently or abruptly. This can also occur in patients who take multiple frequent courses of steroids, e.g. brittle asthma or COPD.

Patients may present acutely if unstable in what is called an Addisonian crisis; features include confusion, pyrexia, metabolic disturbance and shock. Hypoadrenalism is seen in critically unwell patients, particularly in sepsis, and recognition of this hypoadrenalism is part of the well-known Surviving Sepsis Campaign care bundle, something you will come across once you start clinical practice.

Q3 What investigations would you request?
  ▪ **Bloods:** hyperkalaemia, hyponatraemia, high urea, hypercalcaemia, hypoglycaemia, eosinophilia, lymphocytosis, normocytic anaemia, raised TSH
  ▪ **ABG:** hyperchloraemic metabolic acidosis
  ▪ **Adrenal autoantibodies:** present in more than 75% of autoimmune causes
  ▪ **CXR:** signs of pulmonary TB
  ▪ **Specialist test:** short synacthen test
    — This is an ACTH **stimulation test** using tetracosactide (a synthetic ACTH).

— Normally, the synthetic ACTH should stimulate an appropriate rise in cortisol levels (> 550 nmol/L).

— Plasma cortisol levels are measured pre- and 30 minutes post-administration. If cortisol levels are > 550 nmol/L, it excludes Addison's disease.

— If there is a poor or negative response to the stimulation, then this suggests Addison's disease.

Q4   How would you treat this patient?

In general, treatment involves treating the underlying cause and replacing deficiencies in mineralocorticoid and corticosteroids. Specific treatment can be divided into whether the patient is stable or unstable:

■ **Stable:** oral hydrocortisone and may need fludrocortisone for the correction of postural hypotension. Patients will need a steroid card and MedicAlert bracelet

■ **Emergency treatment (Addisonian crisis):** IV hydrocortisone, fluid resuscitation and electrolyte correction.

Good response

AUTHOR'S TOP TIP

The metabolic and haemodynamic instability seen in Addisonian crises is life-threatening and should be managed as a medical emergency, beginning with airway, breathing and circulation. Remember to state this in your answer to the examiner.

Q5   What is a typical patient's daily steroid requirement?

Difficult question

■ Normal daily requirements are between 15 and 25 mg of hydrocortisone.
■ This dose can be doubled if unwell.
■ A typical regime involves:
  — 10 mg morning
  — 5 mg lunchtime
  — 5 mg dinnertime.

Steroid doses if given too late in the evening can lead to insomnia and are best avoided.

5.2 ENDOCRINE HISTORIES

By far the most likely case you will come across in finals will be a chronic or newly diagnosed diabetic patient. *See* Chapter 2 for the general history-taking schema described. Here, we focus on specific points related to the endocrine system.

History Case 1: Diabetes

Instructions: This 17-year-old woman presents with polyuria, polydipsia and weight loss. Please take a focused clinical history.

Key features to look for

❏ **Classical features of type of diabetes**

TABLE 5.7 Features of diabetes

Classification	Description
Type I diabetes	**Age:** often present young, < 20 years **Ethnicity:** more common in Caucasians **Clinical features:** • weight loss • polyuria (esp. nocturia) • polydipsia • blurred vision • occasionally with peripheral neuropathy. **Other:** Initial or subsequent presentations may be with diabetic ketoacidosis (DKA): abdominal pain, vomiting, high sugars, metabolic acidosis, decreased GCS and confusion. May have other associated autoimmune diseases, e.g. pernicious anaemia, coeliac, autoimmune thyroid disease.
Type II diabetes	**Age:** tends to occur in middle-aged to elderly, although now is being seen in younger age groups **Ethnicity:** all racial groups, especially Asian/African **Clinical features:** • weight loss • polyuria (especially nocturia), polydipsia • blurred vision • recurrent infections – fungal/yeast • peripheral neuropathy, retinopathy or nephropathy • associated with obesity. **Other:** Initial or subsequent presentations may be with hyperosmolar non-ketotic acidosis (HONK) due to insulin presence but resistance in the body. Glucose levels rise without the associated ketone production. Patients present with very high blood sugar levels, e.g. $> 30\,mmol/L$.

❏ **Pertinent features in known diabetics**

The following are features you should ascertain in any diabetic:

TABLE 5.8 Pertinent features in a diabetic history

Feature	Description
Duration	The longer the patient has had the condition, the more likely they have had complications or hospital admissions. This will also help gauge how well controlled the diabetes is, especially if their HbA1c is poor and they have had diabetes for many years.
Type of diabetes	Occasionally, some patients are aware of the type of diabetes they have. In general, T1DM go straight onto treatment with insulin.
Medications	Take note of any current oral hypoglycaemics being used, and if used previously, if any side effects.
	Ask about insulin use, what type of insulin (the name, e.g. Mixtard), the dose and regimen, whether short-acting/long-acting.
	Ask about compliance with medications.
	Specifically, ask about ACEi and ARB; these will be for complications associated with diabetes (*see* Viva Q3 below).
Glucose monitoring	Need to ask about normal sugar control and how often they test their blood sugar levels, what their normal readings are.
	How often do they have hypoglycaemic attacks, and have they had a hypoglycaemic coma?
Diet	Ask about their diet; lots of sweet sugary foods often makes glycaemic control harder than slow-release complex carbohydrate foods.
Assess for complications	Ask how regularly they get their eyes, blood pressure and renal function checked.
	If they have peripheral neuropathy, whether they see a chiropodist. Have they ever had any ulcers or joint disruption?
	Ask specifically about macrovascular complications, such as a history of MI, stroke, hypertension, peripheral vascular disease.

Completion

Occasionally, you may be presented with a patient that is known to have diabetes, in which case the above pertinent points are worth exploring in your history. A young patient makes type 1 diabetes (T1DM) more likely. If the patient were much older and presented with progressive deterioration in vision with numbness of his feet and ankles, type II diabetes (T2DM) is more likely.

T1DM is caused by the autoimmune destruction of pancreatic beta islet cells, which causes the patient to be insulin **deficient**. All patients eventually go on to develop micro- and macrovascular complications. T2DM is more common than type 1 and is due to increased insulin **resistance** in the body rather than insulin deficiency. T2DM may often go undiagnosed for a longer period than type 1. T2DM is becoming one of the world's major health problems, due to the globally increasing rates of obesity. There are HLA-DR3 and DR4 inheritance links in over 90% of patients with T1DM, whereas there are no known HLA links in T2DM.

Viva questions

Q1   What is diabetes?
■ This is a condition characterised by a state of chronic hyperglycaemia as a result of a state of relative insulin deficiency, increased insulin resistance or both.
■ It can be primary or secondary.
■ Primary diabetes is divided into type 1 and type 2.
■ Secondary diabetes is due to many causes, including pancreatectomy, Cushing's syndrome, corticosteroid-induced, amongst others.

Q2   How do you define diabetes?
The WHO has defined diabetes mellitus as either:
■ two diagnostic blood glucose tests on separate days, in **asymptomatic** patients
■ one diagnostic blood glucose measurement, in a **symptomatic** patient.

The following represent what diagnostic blood glucose measurements are:

TABLE 5.9 Diagnostic blood glucose results

Test	Diagnostic result
Fasting venous	Plasma glucose ≥ 7.0 mmol/L
Random venous	Plasma glucose ≥ 11.1 mmol/L
OGTT	2-hour venous plasma glucose ≥ 11.1 mmol/L

Impaired fasting glucose is when fasting venous plasma glucose is ≥ 6.1 to < 7.0 mmol/L; these patients should have a 75-g oral glucose tolerance test (OGTT). The term impaired glucose tolerance (IGT) is used when patients initially have a fasting venous plasma glucose < 7 mmol/L and once they have had an OGTT their 2-hour results are ≥ 7.8 mmol/L but ≤ 11.1 mmol/L.

Q3   What are the complications of diabetes?
These can be microvascular or macrovascular:

TABLE 5.10 Diabetic complications

Complications	Description
Macrovascular	**Hypertension:** blood pressure should be tightly controlled in diabetics, with an optimal target pressure of < 140/80 mmHg. The first-line antihypertensives that tend to be favoured in diabetics are ACE inhibitors
	Atherosclerosis: leading onto ischaemic heart disease, silent myocardial infarction, stroke and peripheral vascular disease
	Dyslipidaemia: again increasing the risks for the above conditions. Most patients require statins

(continued)

Complications	Description
Microvascular	**Diabetic nephropathy**
	Chronic kidney disease (CKD) is suggested by the presence of proteinuria. The use of ACE inhibitors (ACEi) and angiotensin receptor blockers (ARB) has been shown to slow progression of albuminuria and nephropathy. End-stage renal failure is commonly caused by diabetes.
	Diabetic neuropathy
	These complications are thought to occur because of nerve ischaemia due to occlusion of the vasa vasorum leading to disruption of the function and structure of the nerve. Complications such as sensory neuropathies (glove-and-stocking distribution), painful acute neuropathies, Charcot's joints, diabetic mononeuropathy, e.g. carpal tunnel syndrome or diabetic amyotrophy, can occur.
	Diabetic foot: This is a significant cause of morbidity and mortality in diabetics. Meticulous foot care can avoid ulcers as a possible source of infection, ischaemia and eventually tissue necrosis and amputations.
	Autonomic neuropathy: this may manifest as postural hypotension, erectile dysfunction, the neuropathic bladder and gastroparesis leading to nausea and vomiting.
	Diabetic retinopathy
	The prevalence of diabetic eye disease is falling; however, 5% of diabetics in the UK still become blind. It is therefore an important and significant complication in diabetics, and nearly one third will go on to develop some form of visual problems. These can range from background retinopathy, to maculopathy, preproliferative and proliferative retinopathy, including cataracts, glaucoma and ocular nerve palsies. *See* Chapter 8.

Diabetics are also more prone to infections, with TB being more commonly seen in diabetics. The infection may lead to poor glycaemic control, and patients may present with ketoacidosis. There are various skin disorders associated with diabetes, such as acanthosis nigricans, necrobiosis lipoidica diabeticorum, vitiligo, granuloma annulare, fungal and bacterial infections, amongst many others.

Honours response

Q4   What is the basis of management of a chronic diabetic?

Difficult question

The management of diabetes involves a multidisciplinary approach. In general, the following features need to be addressed:
- **Patient education:** patients need to be informed of the chronic nature of their condition and treatment goals, including dietary advice with referral to a dietician. Diet alone may be enough in some patients. Foot care with involvement of chiropodist if necessary. Patients need to be aware of signs and symptoms of hyperglycaemia, hypoglycaemia and its management. The importance of regular self-monitoring with urine or blood glucose testing should be encouraged; also the importance of recognition of acute intercurrent illness and the need to increase insulin dose or seek medical advice. Regular exercise and control of obesity should be encouraged. Patients who are being treated for diabetes will need to inform the DVLA regarding their driving status.

- Monitoring for complications: regular screening for complications; *see* Viva Q3 above.
- Drug treatment: see table below.

TABLE 5.11 Various drug treatments available

Drug	Description
Biguanides, e.g. metformin	Metformin decreases liver glucose production and increases peripheral sensitisation of target tissues to insulin. It is the first-line agent in overweight patients (as it causes anorexia) and has been used in combination with sulphonylureas in those patients who are normal or underweight, or when a single agent has failed to control glucose levels. It can cause lactic acidosis and should be avoided in those with severe liver or renal failure. Hypoglycaemia does not occur as a side effect.
Sulphonylureas, e.g. glibenclamide or gliclazide	These drugs promote insulin secretion. They are preferred in T2DM patients who are normal or underweight. Weight gain and hypoglycaemia are common side effects.
Alpha-glucosidase inhibitor, e.g. acarbose	This inhibits intestinal alpha-glucosidases and thus prevent carbohydrate absorption by attenuating the conversion of complex sugars to simple sugars. This reduces post-prandial glucose peaks. It is used as a third-line agent in combination with two other drugs. It can cause GI side effects, especially bloating and diarrhoea.
Thiazolidinediones, e.g. pioglitazone	Pioglitazone activates peroxisome proliferators-activated receptor gamma (PPAR). These drugs increase insulin sensitivity. They are used in combination with metformin or sulphonylureas. Rosiglitazone has been withdrawn due to concerns regarding an increased risk of cardiac events. These are contraindicated in those with heart failure or liver disease.
Insulin	Synthetic human insulin (animal derivatives are also available) is widely available in developed countries and is administered as a subcutaneous injection. Versions are available as ultrashort-acting, short-acting, intermediate- or long-acting. They also come as mixed preparations. Regimes vary widely in clinical practice, and it often needs trial and error to find one regime that suits the individual patient; however, 8 units of an intermediate-acting insulin given 30 minutes before breakfast and the evening meal is a perfectly reasonable starting point.

For management of the diabetic emergency, *see* Chapter 11.

The HbA1c can be used as a form of assessment of the overall level of glycaemic control. A value of 4%–7% suggests good blood glucose control over the lifespan of the Hb molecule, which is approximately 6 weeks. It therefore gives an indication of the level of control in the preceding 6 weeks.

Honours response

History Case 2: Phaeochromocytoma

Instructions: Take a history from this 50-year-old man who has presented with palpitations and headaches.

Key features to look for

History of presenting complaint
- ❑ increased anxiety, panic, tremors and palpitations
- ❑ increased sweating, nausea and vomiting
- ❑ fainting due to postural BP drop

❑ nausea and vomiting, altered bowel habit
❑ weight loss

These symptoms may be exacerbated by local pressure over the adrenal glands, increased stress (physical or emotional) and medications, e.g. beta blockers/IV contrast.

Family history
❑ can be part of a syndrome: MEN2a/b, Von Hippel–Lindau, neurofibromatosis

Completion

Phaeochromocytomas are rare tumours of adrenalin-secreting chromaffin cells. Clinical signs include hypertension which may be intermittent or constant, tachycardia, postural hypotension, fever and flushing.

Viva questions

Q1 How would you investigate this patient?

Difficult question

- **Urinary catecholamines:** collected over 24 hours
- **CT/MRI imaging of adrenal glands:** gives a bright signal on T_2-weighted MRI imaging
- **MIBG scan:** useful in finding extra-adrenal disease

Q2 What treatment options are available?

Difficult question

- alpha and beta blockade
- surgical resection of tumour
- chemotherapy if disseminated disease

Beta blockers if given alone are dangerous in the management of phaeochromocytoma, as there can be an alpha-adrenergic crisis from unopposed alpha-adrenergic stimulation.

The 'rule of 10' in phaeochromocytoma helps in remembering its key features:
- 10% are familial
- 10% are bilateral
- 10% occur outside of the adrenal glands
- 10% are malignant

CHAPTER 6

Gastroenterology, renal & haematology

6.1 EXAMINATION OF THE GASTROINTESTINAL SYSTEM

The gastrointestinal system is a core examination system and will be a certainty in finals. Although a lot of the pathology in the abdomen will be surgical (see our companion text), the emphasis in medical finals will be on recognising hepatomegaly and splenomegaly on clinical examination, and the most common cases will be either ascites or a patient with chronic liver disease. Occasionally, a renal transplant patient may be seen. Haematological malignancies like lymphoma and chronic myeloid leukaemia are unlikely to appear due to the sensitive nature of their diagnosis; however, you should still be able to state this as a differential for your hepatosplenomegaly and know some of the common haematological malignancies well.

Below, we describe a basic schema for you to follow. Note that there is great similarity between the surgical examination and medical examination, with some subtle differences.

Clinical examination

Introduction

As for any clinical encounter (*see* Chapter 1, Section 3); specifically for this case:

❑ **Expose patient adequately:** The patient needs to have their chest and abdomen fully exposed. Ideally, from nipples to knees, but in practice, from xiphisternum to the pubis is acceptable. Offer a chaperone as necessary.

❑ **Position patient appropriately:** The patient needs to be in a supine position, head resting on one pillow and their arms by their side; the level of the bed needs to be at an appropriate height to make the examination comfortable for the examiner from a kneeling position.

Inspection

❑ **Perform a general inspection from the end of the bed**

■ **Paraphernalia:** Look around the bed for peripheral stigmata of disease, such as dialysis machines, any sick bowls, IV drips and drugs. Is there a box to measure the patient's blood sugar? Is there a PCA or any other medications around? Comment on each of these to the examiner.

■ **Patient's demeanour:** Does the patient look ill, uncomfortable or in obvious pain? Do they look pale or jaundiced, cachectic (weight loss is a feature of carcinoma as well as IBD and malabsorption)?

- **Degree of illness:** Does the patient look well or septic? Are they peripherally shut down, is there pallor or are they clammy? In a peritonitic state, the patient will classically look pale with sunken eyes and have a greyish tinge to their face. (It will however be very unlikely that a sick, unstable or septic patient will be put forward for the examination.)
- **Weight loss:** Is there evidence of weight loss or wasting? An individual considered to be cachectic (severe weight loss) will normally have an underlying malignancy, although it can also be a feature of alcoholism, TB and is also seen in heart failure and advanced COPD. Keep in mind that weight loss or wasting can also occur secondary to malabsorption.
- **Dehydration:** Does the patient appear to be dehydrated? Closer examination of the patient's skin turgor and mucous membranes will assist in deciding this.
- **Respiration:** Assess their respiratory rate and pattern: if the patient is peritonitic, they may take rapid shallow breaths.
- **Jaundice:** Does the patient look jaundiced? This is seen as a yellow discolouration to the skin and sclera resulting from an excess of bilirubin, which can be unconjugated or conjugated. Jaundice becomes clinically detectable at levels greater than 30 mmol/L; this may indicate liver disease or biliary tract obstruction.
- **Skin changes:**
  - Look for purpura, which is an indication of impaired clotting.
  - Look for spider naevi. More than five above the nipple line in a superior vena caval distribution are pathognomonic of liver disease.
  - Caput medusa – these are distended veins radiating away from the umbilicus secondary to severe portal hypertension. In obstruction of the inferior vena cava, blood flows superiorly in the dilated epigastric veins present on the abdominal wall.
- ❑ **Examine the hands**
  - **Temperature:** Feel for temperature: are they warm or cold and clammy?
  - **Nail changes:**
    - **Digital clubbing:** present in malabsorptive conditions such as coeliac disease, IBD. Also present in cirrhosis and chronic liver disease. Clinically seen as a loss of the angle between the nail and the nail bed, the so-called diamond sign (*see* Chapter 9 Case 8)
    - **Leukonychia:** due to hypoalbuminaemia seen in chronic liver disease
    - **Koilonychia:** spoon-shaped nails seen in iron-deficiency anaemia (*see* Chapter 9, Nail signs).
  - **Hand abnormalities:**
    - **Palmar erythema:** indicative of a hyperdynamic circulation, redness of the palms sparing the centre; seen in liver failure, pregnancy, thyrotoxicosis and rheumatoid arthritis
    - **Dupuytren's contracture:** thickening of the palmar fascia, seen in alcoholic liver disease
    - **Pale palmar skin creases:** a sign of anaemia
    - **Pyoderma gangrenosum:** may be present on the dorsum of the hand in inflammatory bowel disease, although rare in the upper extremity, it is relatively more common over the shins

— **Scratch marks:** due to excessive pruritis from excessive bile-salt deposition

— **Tattoos:** can be a risk factor for contraction of hepatitis

— **Arteriovenous fistulae:** in renal dialysis patients; look to see if there are puncture marks from recent use; they are typically situated anywhere between the wrist and upper arm.

■ **Tremor:** Examine for a flapping tremor, seen in hepatic encephalopathy. A similar tremor can also be seen in respiratory failure and other metabolic encephalopathies. To examine for this, ask the patient to extend their arms out in front of them and cock their wrists back; now look for flapping movement of the hand at the wrist. Though not part of the abdominal examination as such, this will be a good thing to do as part of the complete examination if there are other signs of liver disease.

■ **Assess the pulse:** Palpate the patient's radial pulse and assess for 15 seconds, then multiply by four to get the rate. Are they tachycardic? Suggestive of pain, sepsis, dehydration, the presence of a fever or may be a feature of alcohol withdrawal. Bradycardia in a patient with other stigmata of chronic liver disease may suggest that they are on a beta blocker for portal hypertension. Ask the examiner for the patient's temperature.

❑ **Examine the face, neck and chest**

■ **Eye signs:**

— Kayser–Fleischer rings are present in Wilson's disease and appear around the cornea as a yellow/brown ring. Naked-eye examination may fail to detect this, and a slit-lamp examination is the best way to look for it.

— Pale conjunctiva are indicative of anaemia. To assess this, pull down the lower eyelid of one eye after warning the patient what you are about to do. This does not confirm the patient has anaemia, as only a haemoglobin measurement can do that.

— Look for evidence of jaundice in the sclera (ideally in natural daylight). Jaundice typically becomes noticeable in the eye at levels over 30.

— Look for xanthelasma, which appear as yellow plaques around the eyelids. These are seen in hypercholesterolaemia, dyslipidaemia associated with primary biliary cirrhosis and in chronic cases of biliary obstruction.

— A lemon-yellow tinge is often seen in the sclera of patients with pernicious anaemia.

— Scleritis or uveitis may been seen in association with IBD.

■ **Mouth signs:** Look in the mouth for dry mucous membranes, furring of the tongue as seen in dehydration, aphthous ulcers in Crohn's disease, angular stomatitis in iron-deficiency anaemia and an enlarged red beefy tongue as seen in anaemia (vitamin B_{12} deficiency). Note if the patient's breath smells ketotic (described as a sweet pear-like smell), or does their breath smell of alcohol? Advanced liver-disease patients may have a musty or ammoniacal odour called fetor hepaticus.

■ **Assess for lymphadenopathy:** Briefly palpate for lymph nodes in the neck triangles; in particular, palpate for the presence of a lymph node in the left supraclavicular fossa. When present, this is known as Troisiers' sign and is called a Virchow's node. The thoracic duct, which receives lymph drainage from the abdomen and the left side of the thorax, drains into the left supraclavicular lymph node area. It is enlarged as a result of metastatic deposit from a malignancy anywhere in this region, although classically it is attributed to a gastric malignancy.

AUTHOR'S TOP TIP

Make it obvious that you are palpating for this node. We suggest you hold the patient's head in slight flexion with one hand and feel with the fingers of the other hand, so that you're showing the examiner exactly where you are palpating in the left supraclavicular fossa.

- **Chest wall signs:** Look for gynaecomastia and spider naevi in the superior vena caval distribution above the nipple line. Both are present in chronic liver disease. There is general paucity of hair, but particularly in the male patient look in the axilla for loss of axillary hair. Along with gynaecomastia, these are both signs of increased circulating oestrogen which may be seen in liver failure and obesity. Spironolactone, often prescribed to chronic liver disease patients with fluid overload, can cause gynaecomastia (often painful). True gynaecomastia will have not only hypertrophy of the pectoral fat pad but also a palpable enlarged breast disc under the areolar skin.

❑ **Closer inspection of abdomen**
You should, if able to, kneel down on the right side of the patient to the level of their abdomen.
- **Abdominal contour:** Is it flat, scaphoid or distended?
  — **Scaphoid:** seen in starvation, malnutrition
  — **Distension:** aetiology easiest remembered as the 5 Fs: fluid, fat, flatus, faeces and foetus.
- **Scars:** Describe their location. Remember that scars have the potential to cause adhesions which can cause intestinal obstruction. Laparoscopic scars may be difficult to see. Always check for an incisional hernia at this point.

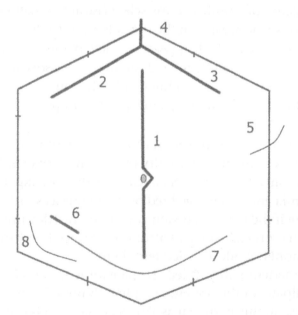

FIGURE 6.1 Common surgical scars

- **Abdominal wall hernia:** Describe its location; it could be a paraumbilical hernia or incisional hernia occurring at sites of old scars. Look for divarication of the recti; this is caused by weakening of the abdominal muscles causing separation of the rectus abdominis muscles. It is commonly seen in multiparous women and the elderly due to poor musculature. This can be accentuated in the exam by asking the patient to lift their head off the couch and touch their chest wall with their chin or to lift their legs straight up from the examining couch without bending their knees. We suggest you use the latter method, as in our experience this makes any abnormalities easier to see.

- **Presence of stoma:** Describe its location, and start considering what type you think it may be.

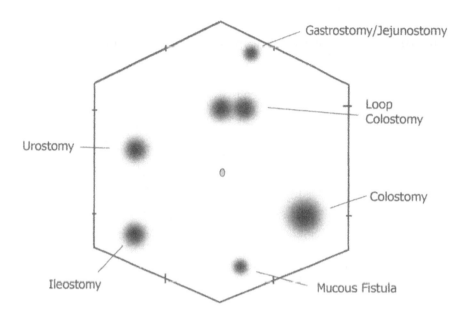

FIGURE 6.2 Abdominal stomas

- **Skin changes:** Look for bruising; striae, which generally occur as a result of rupture of the reticular dermis; silver striae, which signify significant changes in weight; bluish striae, which are present in hypercortisolism; prominent veins – these are present in obstruction of the inferior vena cava or portal hypertension. Discolouration/bruising may also be found in patients with coagulopathy associated with chronic liver disease. They may also be associated with haemoperitoneum secondary to haemorrhagic pancreatitis or ruptured ectopic pregnancy (Cullen's sign – bluish discolouration around the umbilicus; Grey Turner's sign – bluish discolouration at the flanks); unlikely to be present in patient used during the exam.
- **Abnormal movement:** Peristalsis (visible in intestinal obstruction), abdominal respiration (this is absent in peritonitis) or transmitted pulsation from the aorta in the epigastric region.
- **Masses:** If large, these may be visible, in which case describe their location, shape and size.
- **Presence of drains:** You may see indwelling catheters, such as those used for peritoneal dialysis or for draining ascites.
- **Cough test:** Ask the patient to cough. This will be extremely painful in the presence of peritonitis, and the patient may even refuse to do this as a result.

Palpation

Remember the nine regions of the abdominal wall whenever you are examining the abdomen.

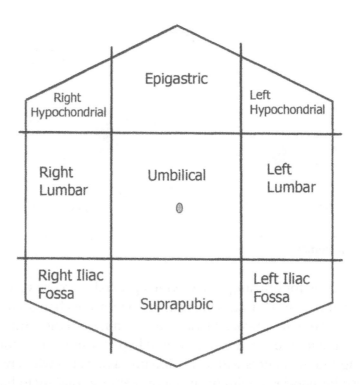

FIGURE 6.3 The nine abdominal wall regions

❑ **Light and deep palpation**
- To palpate, use your four fingers flexing at the MCP joints.
- Palpate systematically around the abdomen in all nine regions, begin with light palpation, then repeat the process with deeper palpation.
- On palpation, note:
  — **Soft/hard:** If the abdomen is rigid all over and 'board-like' due to involuntary contraction of abdominal muscles, this is a strong indication of peritonitis. The patient will also be lying very still.
  — **Guarding:** Tensing of the abdominal wall muscles as you apply pressure, in response to underlying peritoneal inflammation. Guarding can be voluntary or involuntary.

— **Rebound tenderness:** As you examine the patient, swiftly remove your palpating hand from the patient's abdomen: the patient experiences pain as the inflamed peritoneum is forced into contact with the underlying inflamed organ. A kinder way to examine for this is using percussion to elicit tenderness. This sign is seen in peritonitis; a board-like rigid abdomen is a characteristic feature. The abdomen will not move with respiration, and the patient will be lying very still.

❑ **Palpate the liver**

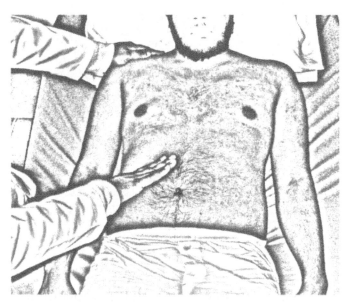

FIGURE 6.4 Liver palpation

- Place the dorsal edge of the index finger on the abdominal wall, starting at the right iliac fossa, and palpate deeply; if pain allows, gradually moving up towards the right hypochondrium so you end up parallel to where you expect the liver edge to be.
- To feel for the liver edge, ask the patient to take in a deep breath whilst you are pressing inwards and upwards with your hand. As the patient is at maximal inspiration, ease the inward pressure, and at this point you will feel the liver edge if it is palpable.
- The liver will normally be palpable just below the costal margin as it moves down a few centimetres on maximal inspiration. Follow the edge of the liver across the abdomen, working medially to the xiphisternum.
- If the liver is enlarged, then state how many finger breadths (or in centimetres if you can) below the costal margin it is palpable.
- If you diagnose hepatomegaly, ensure you actively examine for splenomegaly.

· EXAMINER'S TOP TIP

A common mistake, or rather omission, is to say that the liver is enlarged once it is palpable on abdominal examination without doing percussion over the intercostal spaces to find the actual liver span.

❑ **Palpate the spleen**

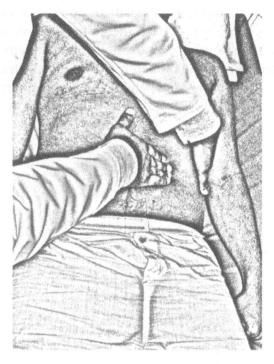

FIGURE 6.5 Spleen palpation

■ This time, working from the RIF towards the left hypochondrium, using the tips of your fingers, press inwards and upwards as the patient takes in a deep breath for you and work your way slowly up towards the left costal margin. In splenomegaly, you will feel the edge of the spleen before you reach this point.

■ If this fails to elicit a palpable spleen, you can ask the patient to slowly roll onto their right-hand side and repeat the above procedure to accentuate any splenomegaly. You can place your other hand on the patient's ribcage on the left to offer them support.

■ In a normal individual, the spleen is not palpable. In pathological states, it increases in size and is thus palpable below the left costal margin.

❑ **Ballot the kidneys**

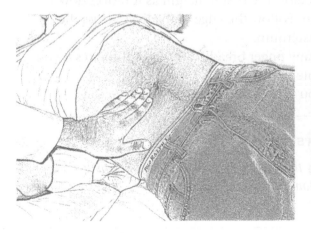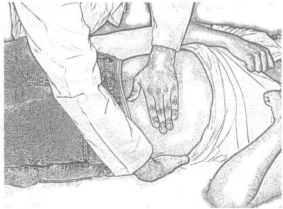

FIGURE 6.6A–B Balloting

- Here, you will be using two hands; begin with the right loin, place one hand under the loin and use the other hand to palpate over the right lumbar region. Instruct the patient to take deep breaths in and out and move your hands together to feel for an enlarged kidney, kidney masses or tenderness in the loin. Now repeat this on the other side with your hands in a position which you find comfortable.
- Normally, the lower pole of the right kidney is palpable; this is especially true in thin individuals. Enlargement of both kidneys is seen in polycystic kidney disease; unilateral enlargement may be seen in the presence of a tumour or hypertrophy.

❑ **Palpate other organs**
- **Examine for an abdominal aortic aneurysm:** This can be felt just to the left of and above the umbilicus, with your index and ring finger placed on either side. Remember, an aneurysm will be expansile as well as pulsatile. In a thin individual, you will normally be able to feel the transmitted pulsations of the aorta; this does not mean they have an aneurysm. If enlarged, try to measure the width using your finger breadths.
- **Focused visceral examination:** If necessary from the history, you can palpate for an enlarged bladder or other palpable masses arising from the pelvis. Use the same method to palpate, but this time starting at the umbilicus and moving inferiorly to the symphysis pubis. If the patient is jaundiced, you may wish to palpate for a gall bladder, which if found is always pathological according to Courvoisier's law.
  — **Examine any masses:** Note that if any mass is palpable, it needs to be described in terms of its position, size, surface, consistency and all the factors that you would normally use to describe a lump. State whether the edge is palpable or whether the mass is associated with an enlarged palpable organ; you must note whether it is pulsatile or tender.

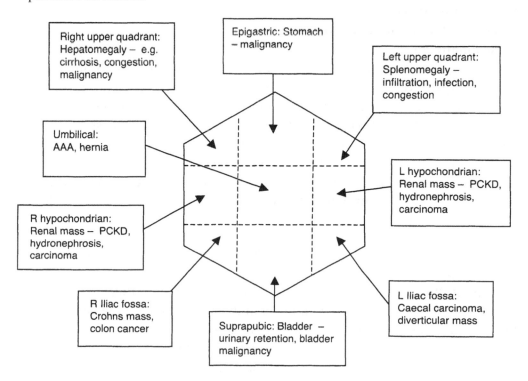

FIGURE 6.7 Causes of abdominal masses

— Interestingly, in cases of severe constipation, you will be able to palpate faeces in the large bowel, most commonly in the sigmoid colon. You will know these are faeces, as there are usually multiple masses which are easily indentable on examination.

AUTHOR'S TOP TIP

If you feel a lumpy area on the abdomen which is indentable, this may be caused by long-standing chronic constipation. But in order to distinguish this from a colonic malignancy which may feel similar, re-examine the patient once they have opened their bowels. If the lump disappears, then this is likely to be constipation and what you felt were hard stools.

AUTHOR'S TOP TIP

If you are describing an abdominal mass ensure you describe its: site, shape, size, dimensions, surface, edges, consistency, tenderness and any other associated features, such as overlying skin erythema (see our companion text for further details).

❑ **Percussion**
- This will allow you to determine the nature of any distension.
- This is performed by placing your index finger flat on the abdominal surface horizontally and tapping on this with the index finger of your other hand, listening for the sound it generates:
  — **Dull:** solid or liquid underneath
  — **Resonant:** air.
- You can also use percussion to demonstrate an enlarged intra-abdominal organ, such as an enlarged liver, spleen or bladder. Some candidates prefer to do this immediately after palpating each organ, rather than performing this as a separate routine.
- **Percussing the liver:** Percuss from the right nipple down to the costal margin or beyond until you hear a difference in sound, then percuss up from the right iliac fossa towards the costal margin, identifying where the percussion note changes.
- **Percussing the spleen:** Percuss from the right iliac fossa up to the left hypochondrium for the spleen, identifying where the percussion sound changes note, if it does.

❑ **Examine for ascites**

If the history is suggestive of ascites or there is fullness at the flanks, you can demonstrate the presence of ascites by:
- **Shifting dullness:** Percuss from the umbilicus laterally until there is a change in percussion note to dull. Keep your finger at this point, and ask the patient to roll onto the opposite side, so now your resting hand is at the apex of the patient's abdomen, and wait for about 30 seconds to allow the fluid to displace to the other side; then start to percuss again, listening for a change in percussion note from dull to resonant. If the spot you have marked now has a different percussion note, then this is positive

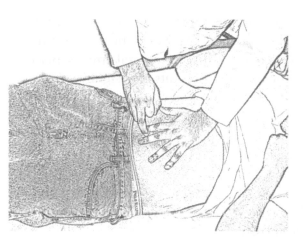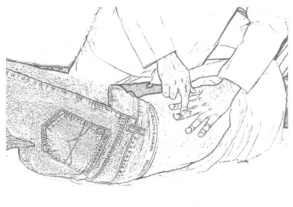

FIGURE 6.8A–B Shifting dullness

for the presence of ascites. Repeat this by asking the patient to lie on their back again and percuss back to the umbilicus and now towards the opposite flank.

- **Fluid thrill:** This requires some experience. With the patient lying on their back, place your left hand on the patient's flank; using the right hand flick at the right flank and feel for a fluid thrill/impulse at your left hand. This now needs to be repeated with the patient's hand placed in the midline of the abdomen, repeating the flick. Again, repeat this on the opposite flank. The presence of a thrill is a positive sign.

AUTHOR'S TOP TIP

We suggest you use the shifting dullness technique in finals, as a fluid thrill is difficult to perform unless the patient has massive abdominal distension due to ascites.

Auscultation

❏ **Listen for bowel sounds**
- Peristalsis of the bowel results in gas and fluid being passed through the bowel lumen; this produces bowel sounds. In a normal state, these are heard as intermittent low-pitched sounds. In pathological states, this changes.
- Place the diaphragm of your stethoscope over the abdomen and listen for bowel sounds. This can be repeated in three different locations, and if no bowel sounds are heard, you must continue listening for at least 3 minutes to be confident of this.
  - **absent sounds:** paralytic ileus, peritonitis, obstruction, mesenteric ischaemia/ infarction
  - **increased sounds:** diarrhoea, obstruction
  - **tinkling:** ileus, a later phase of obstruction.

❏ **Listen for bruits**
- **Abdominal aorta:** Listen over the aorta for abdominal bruits caused by turbulent blood flow; your stethoscope needs to be placed above the level of the umbilicus as the aorta bifurcates at the level of L4, which is approximately at the level of the umbilicus. Bruits are best heard in the epigastric region.

- **Renal artery:** Bruits may also be heard in renal artery stenosis, for which you place your stethoscope in the upper quadrants, although best heard over the epigastrium.
- **Iliac/femoral artery:** To listen for bruits related to the iliac or femoral arteries, place your stethoscope in the lower quadrants. The presence of bruits here signifies the potential presence of peripheral vascular disease.
- **Liver bruits**

Complete the examination

❑ **Further examination**
- *'To complete my exam, I would like to perform a digital rectal examination, dip the urine, examine the external genitalia and check the hernial orifices. In all female patients of childbearing age, I would request a urinary beta HCG'*

❑ **Thank the patient**

❑ **Wash your hands**

❑ **Present your findings**

Occasionally, you may be asked to perform the digital rectal examination on a prosthesis. Below, we suggest a schema to follow.

6.1.1 Digital rectal examination

The rectum is approximately 12 cm in length and constitutes the terminal part of the large bowel. The rectum can be divided into thirds.

- The upper 2/3 of the rectum is covered in peritoneum; in men, this peritoneum is in contact with the surface of the base of the bladder, whilst in women this peritoneum comprises the pouch of Douglas (the rectouterine pouch) and can contain loops of bowel.
- The structures just above the lower 1/3 section of rectum:

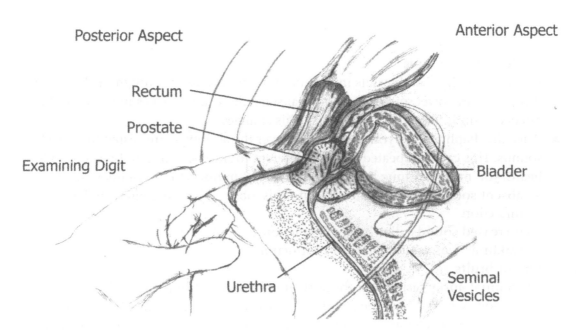

FIGURE 6.9 The rectum

— **Men:** working proximally lies the urethra, prostate, base of the bladder and seminal vesicles
— **Women:** the vagina and cervix (the very experienced may be able to palpate a retroverted uterus)

The rectum is continued as the anus, which is 3–4 cms in length and joins the perineum. The anus has two sets of sphincters: external (voluntary) and internal (involuntary) sphincter muscles.

Examination of the rectum can be very revealing and is an integral part of any abdominal examination. As a junior doctor, this task is usually delegated to you, so it is important you have a good grasp of the examination. Increasingly, this is being examined as a separate OSCE station in its own right. You will often be asked to examine a mannequin, with the most common finding being a smoothly enlarged prostate on a male mannequin. Therefore, spend some time in your clinical skills lab, as the pathological specimens will be very similar to the ones used in the actual exam. For variation, the station may have an actor for you to interact with, but the principles of examining any system are the same.

Clinical examination

Introduction
As for any clinical encounter (*see* Chapter 1, Section 3); specifically for this case:
❏ **Explain purpose, gain consent and ask for a chaperone.**
❏ **Build rapport:** It is important to get the patient to relax as much as possible, because if they don't this will make it very difficult for you to perform the examination.

Preparation
❏ **Collect your equipment**
  ▪ You will need to collect disposable gloves, lubricant and some wipes.
  ▪ And if indicated, a stool-sample tube.
❏ **Position patient appropriately**
  ▪ First, **ensure privacy** by drawing a curtain around you.
  ▪ Ask the patient to lie on their left-hand side facing away from you, i.e. the left lateral position, with their hips and knees flexed up to their chest wall and their buttocks at the edge of the examining couch.

Inspection
❏ **Inspect the perineum and anal margin**
  ▪ Part the cheeks with the fingers of one hand and inspect the perineum and anal margin, commenting on the presence of:
    — skin tags, pilonidal sinus
    — anal fissures (this would cause immense pain on initiation of DRE, so a suppository containing local anaesthetic should be used first, before conducting the examination)
    — anal fistulae
    — external haemorrhoids, external thrombosed piles, rectal prolapse
    — skin discolouration, eczema

Palpation

❑ **Examine the anal canal**
  ▪ Warn the patient that you are about to start the intrusive part of the examination.
  ▪ Lubricate the index finger of the other hand and press this against the posterior anal margin (at the 6 o'clock position).
  ▪ Then slip the lubricated finger into the anal canal following the curve of the coccyx and sacrum upwards and backwards, feel for any obvious masses (if found, describe as you would any lump).

❑ **Examine the anterior rectal wall**
  ▪ Rotate your finger 180 degrees by pronating at the wrist and noting the consistency of the rectal wall as you rotate your finger; you are now at the 12 o'clock position. Complete the examination of the rectum by examining the entire circumference, all 360 degrees.
  ▪ Anteriorly will be the prostate in the male, and the cervix and a retroverted uterus if present in the female. Whilst examining, note the presence of:
    — **lumps/masses:** a carcinoma will be palpable as an irregular mass; there may be faeces present in constipation which will be indentable on examination
    — **tenderness:** this may be present in cases of pelvic appendicitis; in women, comment on whether you can elicit any tenderness whilst palpating the cervix anteriorly, which may indicate the presence of endometriosis in the pouch of Douglas
    — **haemorrhoids:** only palpable when thrombosed
    — **ballooning of the rectal cavity:** present in proximal obstructions to the rectum.

❑ **Examine the prostate**
  Remember that the normal prostate measures approximately 3.5 cm in width and will protrude approximately 1 cm into the lumen. The normal consistency is rubbery with a smooth surface and a palpable sulcus between the two lobes.
  ▪ **Surface:** Is the surface irregular, craggy, hard or are there any palpable lumps all suggesting carcinoma of the prostate gland? May feel like a protuberant nodule in some cases.
  ▪ **Size:** Is the gland generally enlarged? Can you feel a palpable sulcus? Obliteration suggests gross enlargement secondary to a malignancy. If the enlargement is symmetrical, this suggests prostatic hypertrophy.
  ▪ **Tenderness:** If there is any tenderness on palpation of the prostate, this suggests prostatitis.

❑ **Assess for anal tone**
  ▪ You can ask the patient to bear down on your finger now, to assess the anal tone if appropriate.
  ▪ This is useful in cases of faecal incontinence or neurological disease. This procedure also helps assess any lesions in the upper rectum missed by the examining finger, which moves caudally.

❑ **Inspect the examining finger**
  ▪ Remove your finger; note the presence of faeces, blood or mucus on the examining finger.

Complete the examination

❑ **Thank the patient**

- Wipe the examining surface of the patient, cover them up with a sheet and leave them in privacy to dress.

❑ **Wash your hands**

❑ **Further examination**

- *'To complete my exam, I would like to examine the abdomen and send off a stool sample for faecal occult blood.'*

A stool sample for testing is often sent in combination with the DRE to help with the diagnosis of anaemia or GI bleeding.

Viva questions

Q1 What are the causes of an enlarged spleen?

- The causes of splenomegaly can be divided according to its size:

TABLE 6.1 Causes of splenomegaly according to size

Massive (> 8 cm)	Moderate (4–8 cm)	Small (< 4 cm)
Chronic myeloid leukaemia	Myelo- and lymphoproliferative disorders	EBV infection
Myelofibrosis		Infective endocarditis
Malaria	Gauchers	Haemolytic anaemia
Leishmaniasis (visceral)	Amyloid	
Kala-azar		

Average response

- Or more commonly, it is classified according to causative agent:

TABLE 6.2 Causes of splenomegaly according to aetiological sieve

Classification	Aetiology
Infective	**Bacterial:** typhoid, brucella, TB, endocarditis
	Viral: hepatitis, EBV, glandular fever
	Protozoan: malaria, leishmaniasis
Myeloproliferative	CML, PCR, myelofibrosis
Lymphoproliferative	CLL, lymphoma
Haemolytic anaemia	Sickle cell, thalassaemia, hereditary spherocytosis, autoimmune haemolytic anaemia, cold haemagglutinin disease
Portal hypertension	Congestive cardiac failure
	Liver cirrhosis, portal vein thrombosis
Storage disorders	Andersen's disease, Gaucher's disease, amyloidosis
Collagen diseases	SLE, Felty's syndrome
Others	Splenic metastasis

Good response

Q2   What are the causes of a Dupuytren's contracture?
- familial, usually affecting Caucasians of northern European descent
- idiopathic
- associated with alcoholic liver disease, epilepsy, smoking, diabetes, manual labour with vibrating tools

Q3   What are the causes of jaundice?
- Jaundice refers to the yellow skin tone caused by the build-up of excessive bilirubin in the bloodstream. Bilirubin is formed during the breakdown of haem products.
- The causes can be divided into:

TABLE 6.3 Causes of jaundice

Classification	Causes
Prehepatic	Congenital hyperbilirubinaemia, e.g. Gilbert's syndrome, Crigler–Najjar
	Haemolysis which can be:
	• **Infective:** malaria, parvovirus, *E. coli*, haemolytic uraemic syndrome
	• **Drugs:** antimalarials, dapscine
	• **Inherited:** G6PD deficiency (especially when exposed to certain drugs), sickle cell
Intrahepatic	**Congenital:** Dubin–Johnson (failure of hepatic excretion), Wilson's disease (copper accumulation)
	Infective: hepatitis A, B and C; CMV, EBV
	Drugs: anti-TB medication (rifampcin, isoniazid), valproate, phenothiazines (chlorpromazine), halothane, paracetamol overdose, alcohol
	Cirrhosis: most commonly caused by alcohol, amongst other causes
	Hepatic congestion: CCF, portal vein thrombosis
	Cancer: primary hepatic or metastasis to the liver
Post-hepatic or cholestatic	**Gallstones**
	Pancreatic cancer causing obstruction

Q4   What are the causes of hepatomegaly?
- The causes of hepatomegaly can be classified in two main ways.
- Either as in the presence or absence of jaundice:

TABLE 6.4 Causes of hepatomegaly

Without jaundice	With jaundice
CCF, cirrhosis, lymphoma	Hepatitis
Carcinoma (primary or secondary)	Biliary tract obstruction, cholangitis
Polycystic disease	Liver cirrhosis
	Carcinoma (primary or secondary)

Average response

TABLE 6.5 Causes of hepatomegaly using aetiological sieve

Classification	Causes
Cirrhosis	**Alcohol** (most common)
	Genetic: hereditary haemochromatosis, alpha-1-antitrypsin deficiency
Carcinoma/infiltrative	Secondary metastatic cancer, primary hepatocellular carcinoma
	Myeloproliferative disorder
	Amyloidosis
Congestive	Congestive cardiac failure; right heart failure
Congenital	Polycystic disease
	Glycogen storage diseases
Immune	Primary biliary cirrhosis, primary sclerosing cholangitis, autoimmune hepatitis
Infection	Acute hepatitis A, B and C
	EBV, CMV, HIV
	Pyogenic liver abscess, amoebic liver abscess
	Hydatid cyst

Good response

AUTHOR'S TOP TIP

For finals, we would suggest you use the aetiological sieve as this demonstrates your breadth and depth of knowledge.

Q5 A bruit is heard on auscultation over the liver. What does this indicate?
- This may indicate the presence of an AV malformation, active hepatitis, or a tumour.
- A venous hum may be heard in portal hypertension.

Q6 What are the causes of hepatosplenomegaly?

TABLE 6.6 Causes of hepatosplenomegaly

Classification	Causes
Infective	Glandular fever
	Brucellosis, leptospirosis
Haematological	**Myeloproliferative disorders:** chronic lymphocytic leukaemia
	Lymphoproliferative disorders: chronic myeloid leukaemia, polycythaemia rubra vera
Infiltrative	Amyloidosis, sarcoidosis
Cirrhosis	Liver cirrhosis

AUTHOR'S TOP TIP

If you ever feel hepatomegaly in the exam, make sure you actively seek out splenomegaly and vice versa. You may miss an important diagnosis!

Q7   What are the causes of an enlarged kidney?
  ▪ polycystic kidney disease
  ▪ hydronephrosis
  ▪ perinephric abscess
  ▪ carcinoma

Q8   How would you differentiate between a spleen and a kidney on examination?
  ▪ The spleen is not ballotable.
  ▪ You cannot get above the spleen.
  ▪ The spleen moves diagonally with respiration, not vertically.
  ▪ The kidneys are resonant to percussion normally (due to overlying bowel).
  ▪ The spleen has a palpable notch.
  ▪ The spleen enlarges towards the right iliac fossa.
  ▪ The kidney has a palpable upper border, whereas top border of spleen is under ribs.

It is important you are able to distinguish between the three organs likely to be palpated in the exam:

TABLE 6.7 Organomegaly

Variable	*Liver*	*Spleen*	*Kidney*
Site	Right hypochondrium; can extend into epigastrium if very large	Left hypochondrium	Left or right flank (if very large, may involve the ipsilateral hypochondria)
Palpation	Can't get above it	Can't get above it	Can get above it
Moves with respiration	Yes	Yes, down towards RIF on inspiration	Yes, moves vertically down on inspiration
Ballotable	No	No	Yes
Percussion	Dull	Dull	Usually resonant due to overlying bowel
Special features	Can be associated with splenomegaly	Palpable notch; enlarges towards the umbilicus/RIF	If bilateral, consider polycystic kidney disease

Q9 How would you distinguish between Hodgkin's and non–Hodgkin's lymphoma?

TABLE 6.8 Lymphoma

Feature	Hodgkin's lymphoma	Non–Hodgkin's lymphoma
Pathology	Reed–Sternberg cells (mirror image) nuclei seen	No Reed–Sternberg cells seen
		Most of B-cell lineage
		Covers a much more diverse group of conditions, e.g. MALT, follicular, Burkitt's
Symptoms	**B symptoms (systemic):** night sweats (drenching), fever ($> 38°C$), anorexia, weight loss ($> 10\%$ in 6 months), pruritis	Night sweats, fever and weight loss (although less common than in Hodgkin's)
	Alcohol-induced lymph node pain	Symptoms of mediastinal enlargement and resultant compression on bronchus or SVC
	Symptoms of mediastinal enlargement and resultant compression on bronchus or SVC	
Signs	Lymph node enlargement (cervical, axillary or inguinal)	Lymph node enlargement
	Hepatosplenomegaly	Extranodal enlargement, e.g. skin, bone, lung
		Pancytopenia due to bone marrow involvement
Diagnosis	B symptoms suggest more extensive disease	Lymph node biopsy
	Blood test: increased LDH indicates increased cell turnover	CT/MRI imaging
	CT or MRI imaging	Bone marrow aspiration used for staging
	Lymph node biopsy is optimal, usually guided by initial imaging, otherwise image-guided needle biopsy can be used	
Treatment	Chemotherapy +/- peripheral stem cell transplant	**Low-grade disease:** hard to treat, often widespread at presentation
		High-grade disease: more aggressive disease, but potentially more treatable
		Chemotherapy +/- localised radiotherapy

Honours response

Q10 Do you know of any staging systems used in lymphoma?

Honours question

- The Ann Arbor system is used to stage lymphoma:

TABLE 6.9 Ann Arbor system

Stage	Description
Stage I	Single lymph node region
Stage II	Two or more nodal regions on the same side of the diaphragm
Stage III	Involving lymph nodes on both sides of diaphragm
Stage IV	Spread beyond lymph nodes, e.g. liver/spleen

Case 1: Renal transplant

Instructions: This 55-year-old Asian woman has a palpable soft tissue mass in her RIF. Please examine the gastrointestinal system.

Key features to look for

Inspection

☐ **Hands/arms**

▪ **AV fistulae:** Check to see if recent use (puncture), feel for turbulent flow and listen for bruit; these can be anywhere from the wrist to upper forearm, so look carefully. These may be tied off once they have had their transplant, and so you may see a scar instead.

– **Skin changes:** Viral skin, warts and squamous cell carcinomas of the skin are common for patients on immunosuppression such as ciclosporin.

☐ **Face/neck**

▪ **JVP:** raised if fluid overloaded

▪ **Scars:** IJV or subclavian scars from old tunnelled lines and central lines used for dialysis; a parathyroidectomy scar

▪ **Eyes:** conjunctival pallor due to anaemia

▪ **Mouth:** gum hypertrophy due to ciclosporin use

▪ **Face:** an overall Cushingoid appearance due to chronic steroid use, hirsutism

– **Hearing aids:** in patients with Alport's syndrome or Wegener's granulomatosis.

☐ **Chest/body**

▪ **Surgical scars**

– **peritoneal dialysis catheter scars:** small scars on the abdominal wall from previous dialysis

– **renal transplant scar:** an L-shaped scar usually in the right iliac fossa

– **nephrectomy scars:** a posterior-lateral scar in the loin suggesting nephrectomy, possibly of a renal carcinoma or in polycystic kidney disease (PCKD).

Palpation/percussion

Transplanted kidneys

☐ often sit low in the abdomen, and if patient is not properly exposed, you will miss them

☐ firm, non-tender, slightly mobile masses, dull to percussion

---

AUTHOR'S TOP TIP

Transplanted kidneys that are rejecting can become tender; remember to ask about pain before you palpate!

Polycystic kidneys

☐ These may still be present as well as transplanted kidneys.

☐ These are usually bilateral flank masses which are felt as firm, irregular and cystic.

☐ They can be massive in size and tender if recent infection or rupture of cyst.

AUTHOR'S TOP TIP

Remember the rules for differentiating kidneys from the spleen. See previous Viva Q8.

Complete the examination

❑ **Further examination**
   ■ *'To complete my exam, I would like to assess the BP and check the blood sugar.'*
❑ **Thank the patient**
❑ **Wash your hands**
❑ **Present your findings**

Viva questions

Q1 What pertinent features in the history would you like to know?
   ■ **Indication for transplant:** What was the cause of their end-stage renal failure? This can be:
      — **Diabetic nephropathy** and **hypertensive nephropathy** are the most common.
      — **Polycystic kidney disease.**
      — **Glomerulonephritis:** This can be the membranous, progressive, focal segmental, lupus or membranoproliferative forms.
      — **Interstitial nephritis**, which can be due to:
         • drug reactions: NSAIDs, penicillins
         • immunological: lupus, vasculitides such as Wegener's, Sjögren's syndrome
         • infections: viral such as hep B, CMV, HIV; bacterial, parasitic such as *Leishmania*, toxoplasmosis infections
         • heavy metals: lead, cadmium.
   ■ **Family history/past history:** Polycystic disease is inherited, via either AD or AR, with AD being much more common. Alport's syndrome is associated with sensorineural deafness.
   ■ **Drug history:** A history of drug induced renal failure; patients are usually on long-term immunosuppression.

Q2 How would you investigate this patient?
   ■ **MSU:** haematuria, proteinuria
   ■ **Bloods:** raised urea and creatinine if impaired graft function with hyperkalaemia, hyperphosphataemia and acidosis
   ■ **ECG:** RAD, right atrial and ventricular hypertrophy, RBBB; chronic renal failure patients often have a longstanding hyperkalaemia and may not show ECG changes that you would normally see in a patient with acute hyperkalaemia
   ■ **CXR:** may show signs of pulmonary oedema if fluid overloaded or central lines in situ

- **USS:** used in the assessment of PCKD and can demonstrate small atrophic kidneys in chronic renal failure

Q3 What is the mainstay of treatment in this patient?
- Renal transplant patients are often on many medications for various reasons. Immunosuppression is a key part of their treatment regime.
- Immunosuppression is on the whole used to prevent T-cell alloimmune response to donor kidney.

TABLE 6.10 Immunosuppressive drugs in renal transplant

Drug	Action
Steroids	Reduce inflammation, capillary permeability and polymorph activity
	Side effects include unstable BM control, thinning of skin, easy bruising
Azathioprine	Inhibits lymphocyte proliferation
Mycophenolate	Inhibits lymphocyte proliferation
Ciclosporin	Calcineurin inhibitor, reduces IL-2 production in active T cells
	Side effects include: gum hypertrophy, hirsutism
Tacrolimus	Calcineurin inhibitor, reduces IL-2 production in active T cells
Basiliximab	Blocks IL-2 on T cells
Alemtuzumab	Anti-CD-52 induces lympholysis

Q4 What is their overall prognosis?

Difficult question

- Live donor grafts and cadaveric grafts can both be used; 1-year survival rates are slightly better for live donor grafts, with both being > 75% in developed countries.
- The greater the HLA match, the better the survival, with best outcomes seen from identical-twin grafts.
- Grafts are expected to last 10–20 years, with live donor grafts surviving almost double the length of cadaveric grafts.
- Cardiovascular disease is the main cause of mortality in renal failure patients, with hypertension being another common problem. Atheromatous disease is increased compared to the general population.
- Malignancy is another problem for those on long-term immunosuppression. Typical malignancies in renal transplant patients include SCC and to a lesser extent BCC of the skin, lymphoma and anogenital cancer.

Q5 Are there any contraindications to renal transplantation from a recipient's perspective?
- active infection
- cancer
- severe heart disease or medically unfit for surgery

There are many factors that need to be considered before a donor can be considered suitable to donate a kidney; this is particularly the case for non-heart-beating donors (i.e. cadaveric donors), including cause of death and certain medical problems. This is not necessary for finals level.

Q6 What do you know of adult polycystic kidney disease?
- It is an autosomal dominant disorder (although can be autosomal recessive) which results in renal failure, large polycystic kidneys, hypertension, haematuria and urosepsis.
- There are associated cysts in other organs, e.g. liver, pancreas and spleen.
- Patients may complain of loin pain due to infected or bleeding cysts.
- Patients are also predisposed to valvular lesions, especially mitral regurgitation.
- There is an association with intracranial aneurysms; thus berry aneurysm may initially present as a subarachnoid haemorrhage following an intense headache.

Q7 What are the stages of renal failure?

Difficult question

Renal failure is classified according to the patient's glomerular filtration rate (GFR) in mL/min/1.73m²; this is normally > 90 in healthy individuals.

TABLE 6.11 GFR in renal failure

Stage	Description
Early renal failure	GFR < 90
Moderate renal failure	GFR < 60
Severe renal failure	GFR < 30
End-stage renal failure	GFR < 15

Q8 What types of renal replacement therapy do you know of for end-stage renal failure patients?
- Generally, these can be either haemodialysis or peritoneal dialysis.
- There are various subsets within each, and these are beyond the scope of this revision guide.
- In peritoneal dialysis, a surgically placed catheter is inserted into the peritoneum that acts as a membrane through which dialysis can occur.
- The benefit is that patients can dialyse in the comfort of their home, and so it provides a level of independence.
- Haemodialysis requires venous access; this can be in the form of a temporary double-lumen central line, commonly called a vascath, inserted into any central vein, or a permanent surgically created anastomosis between an artery and vein, the so-called arteriovenous fistula (AvF). This requires several weeks to mature before use.
- Patients can spend up to 3 times a week in hospital being dialysed and so become long-term patients well known to the hospital.
- Haemodialysis requires specific prescriptions for the dialysate contents and the duration of dialysis as well as frequency.

AUTHOR'S TOP TIP

Never cannulate an AvF in a renal patient. This may seem obvious, but we can assure you this still happens every so often in actual clinical practice. Also, you should never cannulate anything proximal to the wrist in a renal patient unless it's a dire emergency, as this area will serve as sites for potential fistula creation in the future.

Common complications associated with haemodialysis are difficult venous access, line sepsis and accumulation of beta-2 microglobulin leading to amyloidosis. There are massive fluid shifts associated with haemodialysis and consequently haemodynamic instability.

Q9   What are the complications of renal transplants?
- **Immediate:** surgical complications, e.g. infection, leaking ureters, stenosis of the transplanted renal artery or ureters, amongst many other complications
- **Long term**
  — **Drug side effects:** patients will be on numerous drugs, and these all have side effects, e.g. ciclosporin-induced hirsutism
  — **Immunosuppression:** side effects associated with chronic steroid use, such as Cushing's syndrome, bone necrosis; risks from immunosuppressive drugs including increased risk of opportunistic infections such as *Pneumocystis carinii*, malignancy such as skin cancer, post-transplant lymphoproliferative disorder, particularly lymphoma and leukaemia
- **Organ rejection**
  — **Hyperacute rejection:** occurs within hours of the surgery and is due to antibodies already present in the recipient's blood
  — **Acute rejection:** occurs in the first few days and is due to cytotoxic mediated immunity against the graft
  — **Late rejection:** occurs in the subsequent period and is due to graft antibodies, with T cells from the recipient interacting with the HLA tissues of the graft, with resultant complement cascade activation; especially important is the production of interleukin 2

It is important that the donor's and recipient's immune systems are similar enough so as to avoid rejection. There are various features which are taken into account to ensure a match. First-degree family members tend to match the closest, and of course genetically identical twins are the ideal match. All recipients and donors require detailed immunological matching to avoid graft failure. This involves, amongst other factors, blood-group crossmatching, HLA typing and lymphocytotoxic crossmatching. Despite this, due to the impressive capabilities of the immunosuppressive agents available today, there can be a degree of mismatching between non-related live donors and recipients, but this level of knowledge is beyond the scope of this revision guide, and for finals purposes it is enough to know that such transplants can occur and are successful, provided certain criteria are met and the post-operative course is meticulously managed.

Patients who have had repeated blood transfusions for anaemia may be susceptible to HLA sensitisation and therefore limited in their match potential. Therefore, anaemia should be tolerated in renal patients as much as possible to avoid blood transfusions. Pregnancy may also sensitise the patient to HLA antigens.

Case 2: Chronic liver disease

Instructions: This 45-year-old man presents with abdominal swelling and a background of heavy alcohol intake. Please examine the gastrointestinal system.

Key features to look for

Inspection

❏ **General features**
- jaundice
- confusion in acute liver decompensation (unlikely to be seen in finals)
- lack of body hair
- tattoos and track marks, suggestive of viral hepatitis
- muscle wasting
- slate-grey pigmentation seen in haemochromatosis

❏ **Hands/arms**
- **nail signs:** digital clubbing, leuconychia, koilonychia
- **liver flap (asterixis):** flap seen in encephalopathy; do not confuse with a tremor that can also be seen in acute withdrawal from alcohol (occurring ~12–72 hours after last drink)
- **palm:** Dupuytren's contracture (thickening of the palmar fascia), palmar erythema
- **skin changes:** purpuric bruising due to deranged clotting and multiple falls from alcohol, scratch marks from pruritis

❏ **Face/neck**
- icteric sclera (seen before skin colour changes)
- parotid enlargement, suggestive of alcoholic liver disease
- anaemia, Kayser–Fleischer rings in Wilson's disease

❏ **Chest/body**
- spider naevi
- gynaecomastia

❏ **Abdomen**
- caput medusae
- generalised swelling with **shifting dullness**, the swelling may be tense with **eversion** of the umbilicus; this is most likely to be ascites
- hepatomegaly and/or splenomegaly; these may be difficult to palpate due to the ascites (dipping your hands into the abdomen may help palpation)
- may be a venous hum over the liver
- testicular atrophy

Complete the examination

❏ **Further examination**
- *'To complete my exam, I would like to assess for signs of encephalopathy.'*

❏ **Thank the patient**

❑ **Wash your hands**
❑ **Present your findings**

Viva questions

Q1 What are the causes of ascites?
- The causes of ascites can be divided into transudates and exudates depending on the protein concentration of the ascites:

TABLE 6.12 Causes of ascites

Classification	Causes
Transudate (< 30 g/L protein concentration)	Cardiac failure, nephrotic syndrome, hypoalbuminaemia secondary to malnutrition, cirrhosis, Budd–Chiari syndrome, myxoedema
Exudate (> 30 g/L protein concentration)	Pancreatitis, TB, peritonitis, malignancy, e.g. gastric, ovarian and liver

Ascites is thought to occur due to sodium and water retention as a result of vasodilatory stimulation of the renin angiotensin aldosterone system. The majority of cases of ascites seen in finals will be due to chronic liver disease.

Currently, the best way to classify ascites is to calculate the serum-ascites albumin gradient (SAAG). This is done by subtracting the numerical value of the ascitic fluid albumin level from the serum albumin level measured concurrently. If the difference is greater than or equal to 11, then it is called a high-SAAG ascites and for all practical purposes is due to portal hypertension. Other causes of high SAAG are CCF and nephrotic syndrome. If the difference is less than 11, it is called low-SAAG ascites and can be due to malignancy, tuberculosis and pancreatitis, amongst others.

Q2 How would you manage ascites?
- Identify and treat the underlying cause if possible.
- Specifically for ascites, this will depend upon whether the ascites is an exudate or transudate:

TABLE 6.13 Treatment of ascites

Classification	Treatment
Transudate	**Low-salt diet:** < 80 mmol per day
	Diuretic therapy: spironolactone (an aldosterone antagonist), frusemide
	Therapeutic paracentesis: for tense ascites with protein replacement (typically 100 mL of 20% human albumin solution for every 2–3 L ascites drained)
Exudate	Paracentesis without protein replacement

Good response

If the patient has alcoholic liver disease, as the majority of cases do, also mention alcohol cessation programmes and vitamin B replacement.

Q3 What are the commonest causes of cirrhosis?
- ❑ The most common cause is alcohol-induced and chronic viral hepatitis (hepatitis B and C).
- ❑ Other causes include non-alcoholic steatohepatitis (NASH), autoimmune hepatitis, idiopathic, drug induced, congestive cardiac failure leading to congestive hepatopathy, haemochromatosis, Wilson's disease and alpha-1-antitrypsin deficiency, among others.

Cirrhosis of the liver is a term used to describe certain histopathological changes that occur due to a number of causes (mentioned above). These changes inevitably involve cell necrosis, inflammation, fibrosis and nodular regeneration of the liver.

Q4 What are the causes of abdominal swelling?
- fluid
- fetus
- faeces
- fat
- flatus
- fibroids

AUTHOR'S TOP TIP

These are commonly referred to as the six Fs.

Q5 What investigations would you request?
- **Bloods**
  - **LFTs:** raised ALT/AST/ALP/GGT, as liver synthetic function declines; raised bilirubin, low albumin
  - **Clotting:** prolonged prothrombin time due to impaired synthetic function of coagulation factors and prothrombin depletion
  - **FBC:** low platelets is a sign of secondary hypersplenism
  - **Raised alpha-fetoprotein** is an indicator of hepatocellular carcinoma (HCC)
- **CXR:** can have dilated cardiomyopathy
- **USS:** hepatomegaly, fatty infiltration, cirrhosis, Doppler may show signs of portal hypertension and signs of reverse portal flow
- **Ascitic tap:** *see* Viva Q6 below

AUTHOR'S TOP TIP

Remember that serum albumin, bilirubin and prothrombin time are more accurate indicators of liver function as opposed to liver enzymes. Indeed, these are features in addition to the presence of ascites and encephalopathy used to measure severity and prognosis in liver failure.

Q6   What tests would you request for an ascitic tap?
- **Macroscopic appearance:** this helps identify possible causes.
  - Straw-coloured is the usual colour.
  - Bloody suggests malignancy.
  - Coloured chyle suggests pancreatitis.
  - Turbid suggests TB.
- Send fluid for cell count and differential, Gram stain, cytology and culture, protein, albumin and amylase levels; serum albumin and ascitic albumin levels to calculate SAAG.
- Always inoculate the fluid into blood culture bottles at the bedside rather than sending it in a white-topped sterile container to the lab for the technician to inoculate into culture bottles for culture, as this vastly increases the chance of getting a positive culture and reduces false-negative results.

AUTHOR'S TOP TIP

If the patient has ascites, it is important you consider spontaneous bacterial peritonitis if they are acutely unwell.

Spontaneous bacterial peritonitis is treated with broad-spectrum antibiotics until sensitivities are available from ascitic tap. Note that the ascitic tap itself is a risk factor for infection.

Q7   What blood test results would suggest alcoholic liver disease as a cause?
- **FBC:** MCV is raised, i.e. macrocytosis
- **LFT:** raised gamma-glutamyl transferase (gamma GT) as a result of enzymatic induction

However, neither of these nor any other biochemical test can give any confirmatory clue. Even a liver biopsy may fail to establish a definitive diagnostic aetiological cause by the time cirrhosis has developed. Features of NASH and alcoholic steatohepatitis can often be very difficult to differentiate with certainty.

Q8   Clinically, how can you differentiate between caput medusae and IVC obstruction?

Difficult question

- In IVC obstruction, the venous flow is cephalad from the groin.
- Whereas in caput medusae, the veins radiate from the umbilicus.
- So by obstructing any of these veins with your fingers and noting the pattern by which they refill, you can tell whether the vein fills from below or from the umbilicus.

Q9   What is portal hypertension?
- Normal portal pressure is < 10 mmHg.
- When the portal vein is obstructed, portosystemic shunting occurs whereby

collateral veins are formed which carry blood to the main venous systems of the body; these collaterals are called varices.

- **Aetiology:** the most common cause worldwide is post-viral hepatitis, and in the UK it is alcoholic liver cirrhosis, but in general these can be divided into hepatic, prehepatic or post-hepatic:
  - **prehepatic causes** – portal vein thrombosis
  - **hepatic causes** – liver cirrhosis, veno-occlusive disease of liver; a degree of portal hypertension occurs in any case of acute hepatitis causing swelling of hepatocytes and is particularly common in acute alcoholic hepatitis
  - **post-hepatic causes** – constrictive pericarditis, Budd–Chiari syndrome
- **Signs of portal hypertension:** splenomegaly (and hypersplenism), caput medusae, oesophageal or rectal varices and a venous hum over the liver, recanalisation of umbilical vein in the ligamentum teres hepatis.

Honours response

Q10 What are the features of hepatic encephalopathy (HE)?
- low affect, irritability and insomnia (grade I HE), confusion, problem with memory, slurred speech, drowsiness, progressing to coma or decerebrate posturing (grade IV HE)
- asterixis (liver flap) is present in grades I–III HE but is absent in grade IV HE
- reflexes: hyperreflexia (although reflexes can be diminished)
- hippus (seen in grade IV HE), alternating constriction and dilatation of pupils

Acutely decompensated liver disease is a state which includes features of hepatic encephalopathy with acute-onset jaundice, ascites or portal hypertension.

Honours response

6.2 HISTORIES IN THE GASTROINTESTINAL SYSTEM

Abdominal pain tends to be the most common symptom associated with the gastrointestinal system. However, this is more likely to be covered in surgical finals, as abdominal pain in clinical practice is referred to surgeons. There are still, however, many presenting complaints that could appear in medical finals. *See* Chapter 2 for the general history-taking schema described. Here, we focus on specific points related to the gastrointestinal system.

History Case 1: Inflammatory bowel disease

Instructions: This 19-year-old boy has presented with diarrhoea, PR bleeding and weight loss. Please take a focused clinical history.

Key features to look for

TABLE 6.14 Features in the history of IBD

Type	Pertinent features in history
Ulcerative colitis	Diarrhoea with blood and mucus
	Abdominal pain
	Increased stool frequency
	Non-smoking
	Acute presentation/exacerbation: fever, anorexia, malaise, urgency, tenesmus
Crohn's disease	Diarrhoea
	Abdominal pain
	Weight loss
	Smoking
	Acute presentation/exacerbation: fever, anorexia, malaise

Completion

You should elicit a history of altered bowel habit (*see* Short Case 2 below), and consider colorectal cancer and infective causes of this patient's symptoms.

Ulcerative colitis is defined as inflammation of the large bowel, usually confluent in nature extending proximally; it can extend into the small bowel with backwash ileitis. Inflammation is usually superficial. Crohn's disease affects the bowel from the mouth to anus, but is often not confluent with 'skip' lesions; commonly seen in the terminal ileum. There is a significant family history of IBD with a tenfold increased risk in a first-degree relative.

Viva questions

Q1 What are the pathological features of inflammatory bowel disease?

TABLE 6.15 Pathological features of IBD

Diagnosis	Pathology
Ulcerative colitis	Superficial ulceration, i.e. mucosa/submucosa
	Crypt abscesses
	Inflammatory cell infiltration
	Confined to large bowel
	Almost always affects rectum
	Decreased incidence in smokers

(*continued*)

Diagnosis	Pathology
Crohn's disease	Transmural ulceration
	Granulomata (non-caseating)
	Skip lesions with normal mucosa in between
	Lymphoid aggregates and neutrophil infiltrates
	Fissures and abscess formation
	Increased incidence in smokers

Q2 What are the extraintestinal signs associated with IBD?

Honours question

- erythema nodosum
- pyoderma gangrenosum
- renal stones (urate stones in ulcerative colitis and oxalate in Crohn's)
- fatty liver, gallstones in Crohn's, primary sclerosing cholangitis
- arthritis and inflammation of other organs, e.g. eyes (anterior uveitis)
- clubbing

Q3 How would you investigate this patient?

Difficult question

- **Bloods:** raised ESR, CRP, WBC; low Hb and albumin
- **Stool cultures**
- sigmoidoscopy, capsule endoscopy, endoscopy; colonoscopic surveillance for bowel cancer begins 10 years post-diagnosis, as the incidence increases from this point in ulcerative colitis
- **Barium study:** in ulcerative colitis, there will be loss of haustrations and a shortened colon; in Crohn's, the study will demonstrate cobblestone mucosa with rosethorn ulcers, strictures and skip lesions

Q4 What treatment options are available?

Difficult question

- Management depends on the diagnosis (ulcerative colitis versus Crohn's), disease activity, site of disease and the presence of any complications.

TABLE 6.16 Treatment options in IBD

Type	Treatment measures
Ulcerative colitis	**Medical**
	Steroids: given as oral, enemas (for proctitis), or IV if acute/severe
	5-ASA compounds, e.g. mesalazine PO/PR; may be needed lifelong to maintain remission
	Sulfasalazine, infliximab (antibody therapy)

(continued)

Type	Treatment measures
Ulcerative colitis (*cont.*)	**Surgical** **Colectomy:** this is curative; there is higher mortality if carried out as an emergency. Surgery is indicated if: ● failure to respond to medical therapy ● bowel perforation or toxic dilatation ● haemorrhage
Crohn's disease	**Medical** **Steroids:** given orally, IV if acute and severe **5-ASA compounds**, e.g. mesalazine, although less beneficial than in UC **Azathioprine, sulfasalazine, methotrexate, elemental diet, infliximab** **Smoking cessation** **Surgical** Most will need at least one operation in their life. Surgery is not curative. Indicated if: ● failure to respond to medical therapy ● strictures, perforation ● fistulae, abscesses

Q5 What are the possible complications of IBD?

Difficult question

- **Ulcerative colitis:** toxic megacolon, increased risk of bowel cancer, anaemia
- **Crohn's disease:** fistulae, slightly increased risk of bowel cancer, abscess formation, B_{12} and iron deficiency due to terminal ileum involvement
- **Treatment side effects:** azathioprine can cause bone marrow suppression; patients are often on corticosteroids, which has many well known side effects

History Case 2: Alcoholic liver disease

Instructions: This 45-year-old man presents with abdominal swelling with a background of heavy alcohol intake. Please take a focused clinical history.

Key features to look for

❑ **History of presenting complaint**
- **Jaundice:** frequency, severity
- **Increased abdominal swelling**
- **History of GI bleeding:** has it ever happened before? If so, how frequently? Have they ever had an endoscopy? If so, when was their last one and what did it show? Ask specifically about varices
- **Spontaneous bruising:** sign of liver function impairment
- **Alcohol use:** how much alcohol do they drink? Ask what they drink on a daily basis and specify it in terms of wine, spirits, lager and any other drinks
- **Weight loss:** increased risk of hepatocellular carcinoma (HCC) if cirrhosis present
- **Co-morbidities:** presence of hep B/C can accelerate cirrhosis and is associated with higher rates of HCC

☐ **Social history**
  ■ **Recreational drug use:** patients who abuse alcohol often abuse other medications; IV drug use
☐ **Drug history**
  ■ **Beta blockers:** e.g. propranolol for varices and portal hypertension
  ■ **PPI:** for GI bleeding
  ■ Are they usually on vitamin B and thiamine replacement?

Completion

Perhaps the most important questions to ask in this history are the CAGE questions to help determine whether your patient is at risk of alcohol abuse. *See* Viva Q1 below.

Viva questions

Q1   What are the CAGE questions?

TABLE 6.17 CAGE questionnaire

CAGE criteria
C – Have you ever felt you should **C**ut down on your drinking?
A – Have you ever felt **A**nnoyed by people asking about your drinking?
G – Do you feel **G**uilty about your level of drinking?
E – Do you have an **E**ye-opener drink in the morning?

Answering two or more with a 'yes' is deemed clinically significant and puts patients at risk of alcohol abuse and alcoholism.

6.2.1 History short cases

The following are other symptoms that may appear in finals.

Short Case 1: Jaundice

Key features to look for

TABLE 6.18 Jaundice

Diagnosis	Pertinent features in history
Hepatitis	**Travel history:** recent travel history may suggest hep A/E
	High-risk behaviour: intravenous drug use, tattoos (hep B/C/D), sexual contacts
	History: associated abdominal pain, myalgia, malaise, anorexia
Cirrhosis	**Alcohol intake:** remember that other conditions can proceed to cirrhosis, not only alcohol

(continued)

Diagnosis	Pertinent features in history
Gallstones	**Classical history:** right upper quadrant pain, pain exacerbated by eating especially fatty foods, indigestion, dyspepsia
	Risk factors: female, obese (fat), forties (age); remember that many people have asymptomatic gallstones that may be found incidentally on ultrasound or associated with mildly deranged LFTs
Malignancy	Weight loss, anorexia, abdominal pain, anaemia (especially if large bowel malignancy with secondaries)
Pancreatic cancer	Weight loss, can be otherwise asymptomatic until quite late in the disease, epigastric pain radiating to the back

Completion

For further information on jaundice, see our companion text, *The Ultimate Guide to Passing Surgical Clinical Finals.*

Short Case 2: Change in bowel habit

Key features to look for

❑ **Duration and frequency of defecation:** how this has changed over time, an important sign in bowel cancer

❑ **Stool consistency:** change from solid to fluid stools or vice versa

❑ **Household contacts:** are there any others affected similarly? If family members or a travelling group also affected, consider infective causes

❑ **Mucus:** presence can be a sign of cancer or IBD

❑ **Tenesmus:** this is highly suggestive of rectal carcinoma, but can also occur in such conditions as ulcerative colitis and prolapsed haemorrhoids

❑ **Pain on defecation:** this is linked to rectal carcinoma, anal fissures and thrombosed haemorrhoids

❑ **Weight loss:** always think of cancer, IBD, coeliac disease and other conditions causing malabsorption or increased loss of nutrients from the gut, e.g. infective diarrhoea

❑ **Dysphagia:** often upper GI malignancy, strictures, rings and webs of the oesophagus as well as gastric outflow obstruction

❑ **Nausea/vomiting:** can relate to obstruction, subacute obstruction or constitutional symptoms of disease. The higher the level of obstruction, the more likely they are to present with vomiting versus diarrhoea and vice versa if a lower-level blockage

❑ **Family history:** it is important to ask about family history, as there are links to FAP, HNPCC, bowel cancer, IBD

❑ **Social history:** red-meat diet, barbequed food – links to bowel cancer, smoking – reduces UC symptoms, worsens CD

Completion

The most likely cases to appear in finals would be either bowel cancer or inflammatory bowel disease.

Short Case 3: Rectal bleeding

Key features to look for
❑ **Colour of blood:**

TABLE 6.19 Rectal bleeding

Colour	Description
Fresh red	Suggests bleeding from rectum or anus, e.g. haemorrhoids, rectal cancer, large bowel cancer, diverticular disease
Dark red/clotted	Suggests bleeding from large bowel, e.g. carcinoma, diverticular disease
Altered/black	Upper gastrointestinal tract, e.g. gastric cancer, peptic or duodenal ulcer

❑ **Location of blood:** Enquire about where the blood is seen; blood seen in the toilet bowel or on wiping with paper suggests a low-level bleeding, e.g. the large bowel or locally in the rectum or anus. Blood mixed in with the stools suggests that bleeding is coming from the large bowel or higher.

Completion

Other causes include angiodysplasia, which can affect any area of the bowel and may need capsule endoscopy or angiography to determine the site of bleeding. Infective diarrhoea can lead to rectal bleeding due to salmonella or shigella; in these conditions, you would expect some other constitutional symptoms, such as anorexia and fever.

Short Case 4: Haematemesis

Key features to look for
❑ **Duration:** How long has this been going on for? Acutely after multiple retching attempts is suggestive of a Mallory–Weiss tear.
❑ **Features of blood:** What colour is the blood? Bright red? Clots of blood? Or is it black? The latter suggests that it has been sitting in the stomach for some time and has been broken down by the acid in the stomach.
❑ **Volume of blood:** Ask them to try to quantify the amount (this will be difficult for them), but you can help by asking if it was vomit streaked with some bright-red blood or if it was just blood they brought up, and if so, how much, e.g. half an egg cup full, a small cola bottle worth (330 ml)?
❑ **Frequency:** How often has this happened?
❑ **Malaena:** Do they have black tarry stools? Remember, this is very important to elicit, as the commonest cause of PR blood loss is an upper GI bleed. Note that it does not only have to be malaena, as a severe upper GI bleed will result in a brisk bright-red PR blood loss also.
❑ **Previous history:** Do they have a previous history of haematemesis? When was the last time they had haematemesis? Were they hospitalised? If so, what investigations or treatment did they receive? Were they given a diagnosis at the time?
❑ **Past medical history:** Do they have a history of dyspepsia, a known history of peptic ulcers; were they diagnosed on previous OGDs?

❏ **Social history:** Do they have a history of excessive alcohol intake?
❏ **Drug history:** Is the patient taking steroids or NSAIDs?

Completion

Common causes of haematemesis include:

TABLE 6.20 Causes of haematemesis

Aetiology of haematemesis
Mallory–Weiss tear
Gastric/duodenal ulceration
Gastritis
Oesophagitis
Gastric/oesophageal cancer

Neurology

Neurology is considered by many medical students and junior doctors to be the most difficult subject examined for in clinical finals. However, the key to unlocking this subject is to keep things simple and classify as much as possible, including your clinical examination itself. Detailed neuroanatomy is not required, nor are the finer aspects of neurology. Being able to conduct a slick cranial nerve and peripheral nerve examination will be more than enough to pass finals. There is only a finite amount of things you need to recognise and remember for finals, and we will cover these in this chapter.

7.1 CRANIAL NERVES

When it comes to the 12 cranial nerves, there is divided opinion on how best to describe them, whether numerically or by name. Students tend to stick to numerical descriptions as they are easier to remember; however, this is bad practice, as in postgraduate examinations names of cranial nerves tend to be preferred, and it makes it harder to correlate numbers with names quickly in your mind. We therefore recommend you learn the cranial nerves by their respective names and only refer to their numerical forms when grouping nerves together for memorisation purposes or for recall of certain conditions.

The 1st cranial nerve, the olfactory nerve, is tested in the exam by simply asking whether the patient has noticed any alterations in their sense of smell. There are formal methods of testing using smelling or scent bottles, but this is not normally required or expected in finals.

Often in finals, the eye component of the cranial nerves examination – that is, cranial nerves II, III, IV and VI – is examined separately under an 'eye examination'. This will be covered in Section 7.2, Neuro-ophthalmology.

Another major component of the cranial nerves is typically examined as part of a group of three nerves: the trigeminal, facial and vestibulocochlear nerves (CN V, VII and VIII). This is because pathology occasionally involves all three nerves due to their close proximity to one another – the so-called cerebellopontine angle.

The final component of the grouped nerves for examination comprises the 9th, 10th, 11th and 12th cranial nerves. These lower four cranial nerves are located in the medulla, and any lesions therefore tend to affect all four – the so-called bulbar palsy.

If you remember to examine the cranial nerves in the above four groups, it will help you to not only remember them and their names but also enable you to practice conducting a slick examination.

Traditionally, the nerves when numbered were written using Roman numerals; however, this is not an absolute rule, and many of us find it easier to number using simple numbers, as this avoids mistakes in communication between professionals, which is more likely if using Roman symbols.

TABLE 7.1 Cranial nerves

Cranial nerve groups	Description
CN I	Olfactory
CN II, III, IV, VI	Ophthalmology: optic, oculomotor, trochlear and abducens
CN V, VII, VIII	Trigeminal, facial and vestibulocochlear
CN IX, X, XI, XII	Bulbar: glossopharyngeal, vagus, hypoglossal and accessory

7.2 NEURO-OPHTHALMOLOGY

This tests cranial nerves II, III, IV and VI. It's best you group these cranial nerves together and perform an eye examination as a whole.

❑ **General**
  ■ Start by looking at the face and eyes in general; note any abnormality of head or eyes. This includes any facial droop or CN palsies.
  ■ Look for any signs of basal or squamous cell carcinoma on the face or eyelids.

❑ **Eyelids and lashes**
  ■ Eyelid droop (CN III palsy, congenital, or due to Horner's (sympathetic paralysis), lid retraction (hyperthyroidism).
  ■ Look to see if the lid is turned in (entropion) or out (ectropion). Entropion is usually congenital or age-related, but can occur secondary to infection or trauma (spastic form). Due to the inversion of the eyelashes, you get redness and irritation of the eye with excessive lacrimation. Ectropion usually affects the lower lid, with signs of corneal exposure, lacrimation, scarring of the conjunctiva and eventually vision loss. Ectropion is commonly involutional and rarely congenital. Styes (hordeolum) are an acute focal infection, usually staphylococcal involving the glands of Zeis or meibomian glands (external and internal hordeola respectively) at the base of the eyelash.

❑ **Eye**
  ■ Look at the general condition of the eyeball: any obvious gross scarring, cataracts or artificial eyes.
  ■ Look for any signs of proptosis: abnormal protrusion (sometimes interchangeably used with exophthalmos when underlying cause is endocrine). Proptosis is caused by increased volume in the fixed-volume orbital cavity forcing the orbit forward; this can be due to inflammatory, infectious or vascular pathologies. In Graves' disease, there is an autoimmune reaction in the orbital tissues, which become infiltrated with inflammatory cells and matter, often with an associated myopathy of the optic muscles.
  ■ Look at the iris: colour, also look for Kayser–Fleischer rings (green, indicate copper deposit in Wilson's disease). Iritis is often present in systemic disease and in conditions such as ankylosing spondylitis, where there is pupilary constriction with a mudded iris.
  ■ Look at the conjunctiva, sclera and cornea: colour, discharge, haemorrhage, ulceration, scarring or any corneal arcus surrounding the cornea.

- Assess for the direct and consensual light reflex using a pen torch:
  — pupils constrict in bright light, infancy, old age, sleep
  — dilated in fear, excitement, poor light
  — accomodation reflex – pupils constrict when eyes converge
  — the pupil may be fixed and not respond to light in acute closed-angle glaucoma – associated with a headache.

TABLE 7.2 Miosis and mydriasis

Small Pupil (Miosis)	Description
Argyll Robertson	Due to syphilis, small irregular pupil that doesn't react to light but normal reaction to accommodation
Horner's Syndrome	Lesion of the sympathetic chain, associated with ptosis and anhydrosis (loss of sweating) on affected side, reacts normally to light and accomodation
Iritis	Poor reaction to light and accommodation
Large Pupil (Mydriasis)	*Description*
Homes-Adie	Congenital, pupil slow and incomplete reaction to light, accommodation is slow/normal, associated with loss of deep tendon reflexes
CN3 lesion	Interruption of parasympathetic chain, no reaction to light or accommodation, normal side still reacts consensually

❑ **Visual function**
- Acuity: use a Snellen chart at 6 m; allow the patient to wear their spectacles if normally worn.
- Visual acuity is recorded as the distance in metres from the chart over the number of the smallest line the patient can read.
- Each line of the Snellen chart has a number ascribed to it, e.g 60, 36, 24, 18, 12, 9, 6. This is the distance at which an individual with normal vision could read that line. 6/6 is normal visual acuity.
- In refractive errors such as myopia, vision is improved if looking through a pinhole; this will not improve vision in other causes of visual disturbance.
- Colour vision: Ishihara plates are most commonly used for this.

❑ **Visual field**
- Assess function of retina. Defects are described as peripheral or central and carried out by confrontation.
- Sit approximately 1–2 m in front of the patient. Test each eye separately. Ask the patient to cover the right eye with their right hand, you cover your left eye with your left hand (the opposing eye), ask the patient to look at your nose, and wriggling your fingers in from the side equidistant between you, ask them to let you know when they see your fingers wriggling. This should be roughly the same time you see the fingers wriggling. This test can also be carried out with a red Neurotip pin if you have one available. This is done from the upper and lower nasal and temporal quadrants. When assessing the temporal field, you can swap the hand you use to cover your own eye. Remember, this is a comparative study where you compare your visual field to that of the patient. Repeat with the opposite eye covered and map out any defects.
- Inattention can be elicited by asking the patient to open both their eyes whilst still sitting and facing you, assuming the peripheral visual fields are intact. Hold your

arms on out both sides of the patient so they are in their peripheral vision. Ask the patient to look at your nose and tell you which hand is moving. Carry out a random combination of L and R finger movement, assessing whether the patient can correctly identify the side of movement. In amongst these, you should move both hands together, as some patients may have selective inattention.

TABLE 7.3 Visual field lesions

Pathology	Aetiology	Left Eye	Right Eye
Arcuate scotoma	Glaucoma		
Central scotoma	Macular degeneration		
Unilateral deficit	Arterial occlusion, Branch retinal vein occlusion, Retinal detachment		
Superior deficit (quadrantinopia)	Right field deficit means left temporal lesion		
Inferior deficit (quadrantinopia)	Right field deficit means Left parietal lesion		
Homonomous hemianopia	Right field deficit means Left optic radiation or visual cortex		
Bitemporal hemianopia	Pituitary lesion at optic chiasm		
Loss of vision in one eye	Optic nerve lesion, Complicated lesion of chiasm		

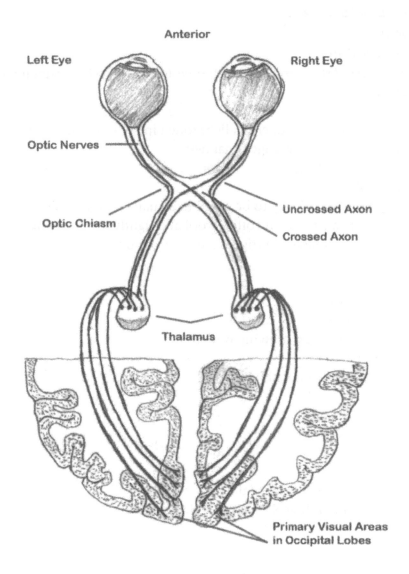

FIGURE 7.1 Optic chiasm

❑ **Ocular movements**
- Ask the patient to keep their head still and only move their eyes; if you find they are moving their head, you might want to put two fingers on their chin to hold them in the neutral position after warning them.
- Move your index finger laterally left and right and then up and down, assessing for visual movements of the eyeball: look for any abnormalities, including a squint and nystagmus. Some use an H pattern to assess for eye movements, but it is up to you whichever you find more comfortable

---

AUTHOR'S TOP TIP

There is a normal physiological nystagmus if you move your hands too laterally or too quickly on assessment of eye gait.

7.3 CRANIAL NERVES 5, 7 & 8

Trigeminal nerve

❏ Check motor function
  ■ **Assess masseters:** Ask patient to clench their teeth and feel the strength of the muscles around the jaw.
❏ Check sensation
  ■ With the patients eyes closed, check light touch in the ophthalmic, maxillary and mandibular divisions of the trigeminal nerve.
  ■ Ensure you assess both sides.
❏ Assess corneal reflex
  ■ In the OSCE, you are unlikely to be asked to actually perform this.
  ■ This is done by using a wisp of cotton wool and lightly touching the cornea.
  ■ Its absence is an early sign of a trigeminal nerve lesion.

Facial nerve

❏ Check for facial asymmetry
❏ Assess motor function
  ■ **Test buccinators through blowing out cheeks**
    — Raise eyebrows.
    — Close eyes as tight as possible.
    — Show the teeth.

Viva questions

Q1   What are the branches of the facial nerve?
  ■ There are five major branches: temporal, zygomatic, buccal, marginal mandibular and cervical

---

AUTHOR'S TOP TIP

The famous mnemonic 'Two Zulus buggered my cat', helps one to remember the branches.

Knowledge of the course the facial nerve traverses is beyond the scope of this study guide. It is enough to mention to the examiner that such knowledge is useful in determining the site of a facial nerve lesion, as lesions at various places lead to characteristic features, e.g. lesions distal to the stapedius branch results in hyperacusis, as the stapedius cushions noise.

The facial nerve is mainly motor in function; however, one of its major branches, the chorda tympani, carries taste from the anterior two thirds of the tongue. This branch arises during the facial nerve's course through the facial canal of the petrous temporal bone, and so damage to the temporal bone from, e.g. Bell's palsy, may lead to loss of taste in the anterior two thirds of the tongue.

Q2   What are the causes of facial cranial nerve palsy?

Difficult question

TABLE 7.4 Causes of facial nerve palsy

Aetiology	Description
Bell's palsy	This is idiopathic, but can be viral.
	Typically, facial weakness is the only sign.
Infective	**Ramsay–Hunt syndrome:** reactivation of herpes zoster in the geniculate ganglion leading to altered taste and vesicles in the external auditory meatus
	Lyme disease, TB
Brain lesions	**Brainstem:** tumours, multiple sclerosis, CVA
	Cerebellopontine angle: meningioma, acoustic neuromas
Others	**ENT:** otitis media, cholesteatoma, parotid tumours
	Trauma: traumatic head injury to base of skull, barotrauma during diving
	Others: diabetes, Guillain–Barré syndrome

Note that by default a facial nerve lesion is a lower motor neuron lesion. The most common cause of an upper motor neuron lesion of the facial nerve is a stroke (*see* below).

Case 1: Facial nerve palsy – Bell's palsy

Instructions: Please examine the 7th cranial nerve of this 46-year-old man who has a facial droop.

Key features to look for
- [ ] **Unilateral** facial paralysis; facial droop
- [ ] **Bell's phenomenon:** on attempted closure of eye, the eyeball rolls up; weak orbicularis oculi muscles resulting in difficulty in closing eyes
- [ ] **Inability to raise eyebrow:** weakness of frontalis muscle
- [ ] **Inability to frown**
- [ ] **Smooth nasolabial fold**

Complete the examination
- [ ] **Thank the patient**
- [ ] **Wash your hands**
- [ ] **Present your findings**

As with any isolated cranial nerve exam, state to the examiner that you will examine the rest of the cranial nerves and peripheral nervous system. Particularly when examining the 7th cranial nerve, ensure you mention focusing on the 5th and 8th cranial nerves also. Specifically mention you will aim to localise the lesion by asking about any changes in hearing (hyperacusis), taste, impaired lacrimation and salivary secretion (*see* Viva Q1 above).

The incidence of Bell's palsy is 15 per 100 000, and the risk increases in pregnancy and diabetes. If the patient presents within 6 days, a course of steroids and aciclovir is indicated in addition to eye protection.

Viva questions

Q1 How would you distinguish between a UMN lesion and LMN facial weakness?

TABLE 7.5 Comparison of UMN and LMN facial nerve palsy

Facial Weakness	Description
Upper motor neuron	**Distribution:** lower part of face only, upper face spared
	Slight mouth droop
	Flattening of nasolabial fold
	Normal eye closure
	No wrinkling of forehead
	Affects contralateral side to lesion
Lower motor neuron	**Distribution:** upper and lower face affected
	Poor eye closure
	Weakness of forehead and mouth

AUTHOR'S TOP TIP

Remember that a facial nerve palsy is in fact a lower motor neuron lesion. Upper motor neuron lesions occur due to supranuclear lesions.

The reason for sparing of the upper facial muscles in a UMN lesion is that the upper facial nerve supply is bilaterally innervated by supranuclear pathways; whereas supranuclear innervation from the contralateral side supplies the lower face.

Vestibulocochlear nerve

It is important to remember that there are two components to the vestibulocochlear nerve: the cochlear aspect for hearing and vestibular in equilibrium. Hearing and detailed examination of the ear is a postgraduate topic. However, you would still be expected to perform a basic examination of the 8th cranial nerve.

❑ **Perform screening test:** Assess whether they can hear you rustling your fingers in either ear.
❑ **Perform Rinne's test**
   ■ This test compares bone conduction from air conduction.
   ■ **Bone conduction:** sound emanating from a vibrating 512-Hz tuning fork placed on mastoid process.
   ■ **Air conduction:** sound emanating from tuning fork heard via the external auditory canal.
   ■ Air conduction is normally better than bone conduction; this is called Rinne positive.
   ■ If bone conduction is better than air conduction, this is abnormal and can be due to a number of causes.
   ■ **Technique:**
      — Strike tuning fork and place directly over the mastoid process.
      — Ask the patient to indicate when they can no longer hear the sound.

— When indicated to that the sound has disappeared, remove tuning fork and place in the air close to the external auditory canal of the same side and ask if the sound is now audible.
— If yes, this indicates that air conduction is better than bone conduction, i.e. a positive Rinne's test, which is normal.
— If abnormal (i.e. bone conduction better), this may be due to conductive hearing loss as a result of wax or middle ear pathology (otosclerosis, effusions).
— Repeat on other side.
❑ **Perform Weber's test**
  ■ **Technique:**
    — Strike tuning fork and place over vertex of head
    — Sound should be audible in both ears equally; this is normal.
    — If there is a noticeable difference, this can be either:
      • **conductive hearing loss:** sound is louder in abnormal ear
      • **sensorineural hearing loss:** sound diminished in abnormal ear

Complete the examination
❑ **Further examination:** ask to perform a peripheral nerve exam
❑ **Thank the patient**
❑ **Wash your hands**
❑ **Present your findings**

Ideally, hearing should be assessed with formal audiometry. Vertigo is the illusion of movement, the causes of which can be classified into peripheral or central causes. Vestibular neuronitis or acute labyrinthitis is a common cause of peripheral vertigo in young, previously well patients post-URTI. Nystagmus is a sign suggestive of an 8th cranial nerve lesion.

7.4 CRANIAL NERVES 9, 10, 11 & 12
These cranial nerves when affected tend to occur together in clusters, as they are located in the medulla, or the bulb – hence the term 'bulbar palsy'. Isolated nerve lesions are rare. The following constitutes the clinical examination and findings in pathological states.

TABLE 7.6 Cranial nerves 9, 10, 11 & 12

Cranial nerve	Description
Glossopharyngeal nerve (CN IX)	**Examination:** gag reflex may be attempted (although not recommended, simply mention to the examiner)
Vagus nerve (CN X)	**Signs:** unilateral absence of reflex is pathological
	Examination: 'Open your mouth and say "Aah"'
	Signs: the uvula is pulled to the opposite side of the lesion
Accessory nerve (CN XI)	**Examination:** 'Shrug your shoulders'
	Signs: weakness of the trapezius
	Examination: tests ability to resist lateral neck movement. 'Turn your head to one side and stop me from pushing it back'
	Signs: weakness of sternomastoid

(continued)

Cranial nerve	Description
Hypoglossal nerve (CN XII)	**Examination:** *'Open your mouth, then stick your tongue out'* **Signs:** tongue fasciculations, wasting; deviation of the tongue to the side of the lesion

---

AUTHOR'S TOP TIP

Remember that when assessing the accessory nerve, it is the contralateral sternomastoid which rotates the head to the other side, i.e. the right sternomastoid turns the head to the left and vice versa.

Viva questions

Q1 What is the difference between bulbar palsy and pseudobulbar palsy?

Difficult question

TABLE 7.7 Difference between bulbar and pseudobulbar palsy

Lesion	Description
Bulbar palsy	**Incidence:** rare **Lesion:** LMN; site is the medulla **Aetiology:** most commonly motor neuron disease, myasthenia gravis, Guillain–Barré syndrome and rarely poliomyelitis **Clinical features:** dysarthria, dysphagia, nasal regurgitation; tongue wasting, weakness and fasciculations; normal affect; lower motor neuron lesion
Pseudobulbar palsy	**Incidence:** common **Lesion:** UMN; site is typically the internal capsule **Aetiology:** CVA, MS and motor neuron disease **Clinical features:** dysarthria, dysphagia, nasal regurgitation; exaggerated jaw jerk; small and spastic tongue with no fasciculations; affect is emotionally labile; upper motor neuron lesion

Such patients are at high risk of aspiration pneumonia due to difficulty in swallowing. They would therefore need speech and language therapy (SALT) with video fluoroscopy if required.

7.5   PERIPHERAL NERVOUS SYSTEM

Examining the peripheral nerves will help delineate whether a patient is suffering from an upper motor neuron (UMN) or lower motor neuron (LMN) lesion. This examination can be divided into examination of the upper limbs and lower limbs.

Upper limbs

❑ Inspection
  ▪ Look for any muscle wasting, fasciculations or abnormal movements, tremor or posture.

❑ Tone

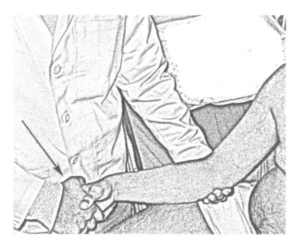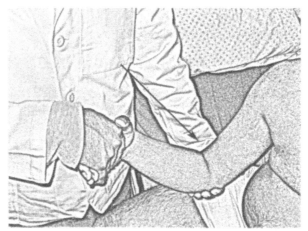

FIGURE 7.2A–B Assess upper limb tone

  ▪ **Method:** Grasp the patient's arm, as if taking their hand for a handshake, and rotate their wrist, flex and extend their elbows and abduct and adduct their shoulders, assessing for the ease with which this can be conducted.
  ▪ **Increased tone:** This is when these actions become more difficult to do, appearing to the candidate as increased resistance to the aforementioned passive manoeuvres.
    — The 'clasp-knife spasticity' suggests pyramidal disease, as seen in upper motor neuron lesions, and can be elicited by passively flexing and extending the patient's elbow rapidly.
    — 'Cogwheel rigidity', a feature of extrapyramidal disease, can be elicited by slowly pronating and supinating the patient's wrist.
  ▪ **Hypotonia:** If the passive movements appear extremely floppy or easy and effortless to perform, then this suggests decreased tone, as seen in LMN lesions.

❑ Power
  ▪ Assess power in all upper limb muscle groups; however, in the exam it is not practical to do so. It is therefore advisable to chose specific muscle groups to examine to save time; *see* below.
  ▪ It is easiest to avoid long-winded instructions to the patient; simply demonstrate what you would like them to do, then provide resistance and ask them to either push down, up, away or towards you (depending upon the muscle action involved).
  ▪ This keeps things short and makes your examination look slick.

Shoulder

*AB*duction	*AD*duction
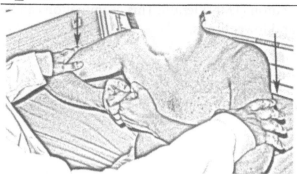	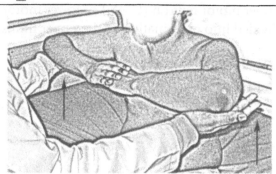

FIGURE 7.3 Shoulder abduction

FIGURE 7.4 Shoulder adduction

- **Nerve root:** C5
- **Muscle:** supraspinatus and deltoid

- **Nerve root:** multiple, mainly C7
- **Muscle:** pectoralis major, latissimus dorsi

Elbow

Flexion	*Extension*
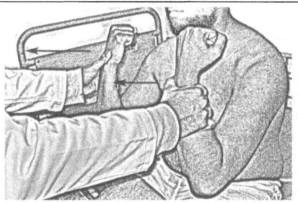	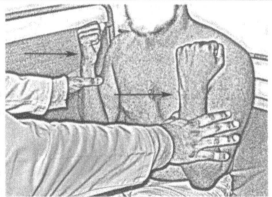

FIGURE 7.5 Elbow flexion

FIGURE 7.6 Elbow extension

- **Nerve root:** C5, C6
- **Muscle:** biceps, brachioradialis

- **Nerve root:** C7
- **Muscle:** triceps

Wrist

Flexion	*Extension*
• **Nerve root:** C7, C8	• **Nerve root:** C7
• **Muscle:** wrist flexors	• **Muscle:** wrist extensors

Fingers *Abduction & Adduction*
- **Nerve root:** T1
- **Muscle:** interossei
- Grade overall muscle power

TABLE 7.8 Medical Research Council (MRC) muscle strength scale

MRC Grade	Description
0	No visible movements
1	Flicker of movement on active contraction
2	Active movement with gravity eliminated
3	Active movement against gravity, but not resistance
4	Active movement against gravity and resistance, but not normal strength
5	Normal

❏ Coordination
- **Finger–nose test**

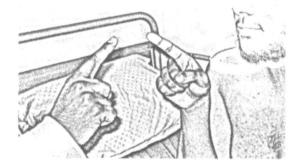 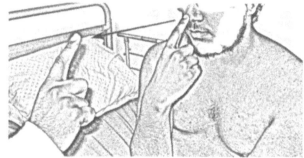

FIGURE 7.7A–B Finger-nose test

— Ask the patient to alternately touch their nose and thence your finger rapidly.
— Repeat on the other side.
— Difficulty with past pointing and intention tremor suggests cerebellar disease (*see* case 1 section 7.5, p. 183).
- **Dysdiadochokinesis**
  — Ask patient to place their hands over each other and to pronate and supinate the top hand as fast as possible; repeat on the other side.
  — Difficulty in doing so suggests cerebellar disease.

You may also test fine finger movements by asking the patient to oppose their thumb with each of their digits and repeat on the other side, performing this as rapidly as possible.

❏ **Reflexes**
These can be either normal, reduced, hyperreflexic or equivocal. Do not get too bogged down with grading systems for reflexes, as these are highly subjective among examiners.

■ **Check supinator reflex (C5, C6)**

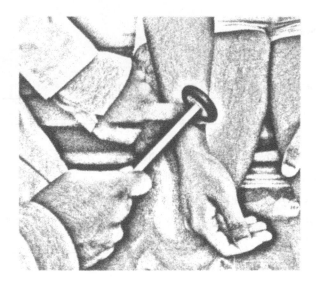

FIGURE 7.8 Supinator reflex

— Place your finger over the wrist and strike with the hammer. You are looking for contraction of the brachioradialis muscles (resulting in finger and elbow flexion)

■ **Check bicep reflex (C5, C6)**

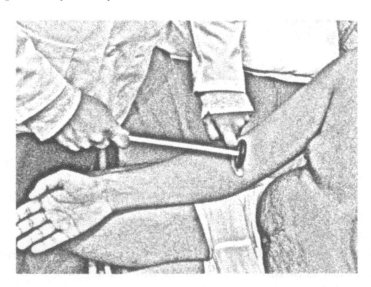

FIGURE 7.9 Bicep reflex

— Place your finger over the bicep tendon and strike with the hammer. You are looking for contraction of the bicep muscle.
— Repeat on the other side.
■ **Check triceps reflex (C7)**
— Keeping the elbow in flexion, strike the tricep tendon, looking for contraction of the tricep muscle.
— Repeat on opposite side.

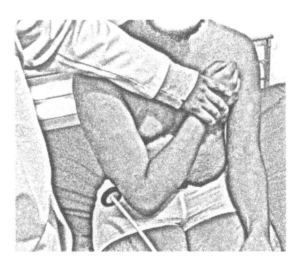

FIGURE 7.10 Tricep reflex

AUTHOR'S TOP TIP

Despite the use of the word 'strike' when referring to eliciting tendon reflexes, it is suggested you allow the tendon hammer to fall with its own weight as opposed to actively striking the tendon. This makes your examination look smoother and is more comfortable to the patient.

If you are finding it difficult to elicit a reflex, firstly ensure the muscle group involved is kept as relaxed as possible. Otherwise, you may try to reinforce the reflex by asking the patient to clench their teeth just before you test the reflex.

❏ **Assess sensation**
This involves assessing several different sensory modalities. For each, ensure the patient has a point of reference and thus an understanding of the sensation expected by firstly demonstrating the test on their sternum before you start. It is advisable to keep their eyes closed during assessment to improve accuracy.
❏ **Assess light touch**
  ■ Using cotton wool or your finger tips, lightly touch the patient in each dermatome bilaterally.
  ■ Do not use a stroking motion.
❏ **Assess pinprick**
  ■ Using a neurological pin, standardise the sensation initially by testing against the patient's sternum, ensuring they appreciate the difference between what is sharp and what is dull.

In the exam, do not accept anything less than a neuro pin. You should certainly never use venepuncture needles.
❏ **Assess temperature**
  ■ Ideally, this is performed using ethyl chloride spray, which is cold spray; however, using the 'cold' sensation of the tuning fork is acceptable.

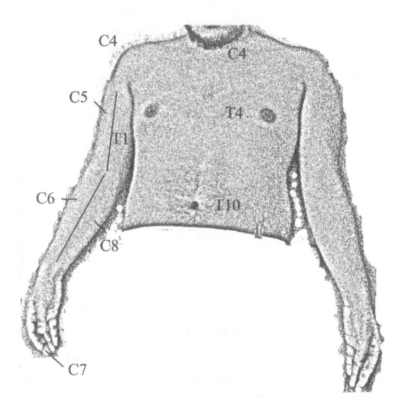

FIGURE 7.11 Upper limb dermatomes

- Again assess in a dermatomal pattern bilaterally.
- Temperature sensation is an assessment of the spinothalamic tracts.
❏ **Assess proprioception**

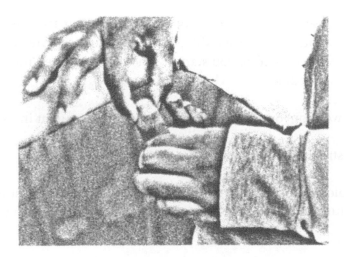

FIGURE 7.12 Proprioception

- To assess dorsal columns integrity with joint position sense, stabilise the PIP joints and flex and extend the finger at the DIP joint, firstly demonstrating to the patient that flexion is 'down' and extension is 'up'.

- Repeat this with the patient's eyes closed and ask them to describe whether their finger is being moved 'up' or 'down'.
❑ **Assess vibration**
  - Select a 128-Hz tuning fork and strike the prongs such that the fork is vibrating; place this over the sternum to demonstrate the test to the patient and then place over any bony prominence in the upper limb, ideally starting distally and moving proximally.
  - Compare both sides.
  - Vibrations assess the integrity of the dorsal columns.

Lower limbs
❑ **Inspection**
  - Look for any muscle wasting, fasciculations or abnormal movements, tremor or posture.
❑ **Tone**
  - With the patient supine, gently roll the legs by externally and internally rotating each leg at the hip. Then grasp onto the back of each knee and gently lift the leg off the examining couch at the knee joint whilst observing the ankle to see if it remains in contact with the bed or not. If it does, then the leg is flaccid; if the heel lifts off the bed, then this suggests spasticity, i.e. increased tone.
  - Assessing tone in the lower limbs is best learnt by watching someone do this.

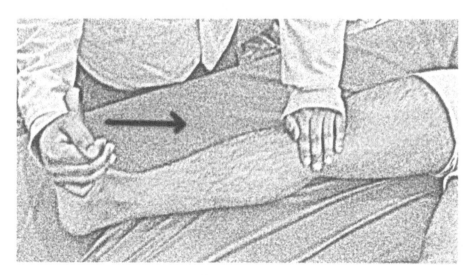

FIGURE 7.13 Ankle clonus

  - **Assess for ankle clonus:** Keeping the knee slightly flexed with the foot relaxed, suddenly jerk the foot (dorsiflexion) and hold it there, looking for sustained contractions of the ankle joint
❑ **Power**
  - With the patient supine, assess power in specific lower limb muscle groups and grade as per the MRC scale.

Hip

Flexion	Extension

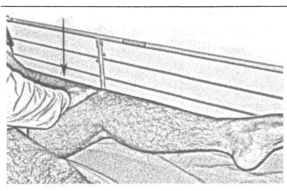 |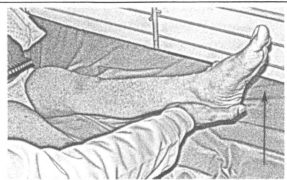

FIGURE 7.14 Hip flexion

FIGURE 7.15 Hip extension

- **Nerve root:** L1, L2
- **Muscle:** iliopsoas; ask patient to keep their leg straight, and then raise against resistance

- **Nerve root:** L5, S1
- **Muscle:** gluteus maximus

Knee

Flexion	Extension

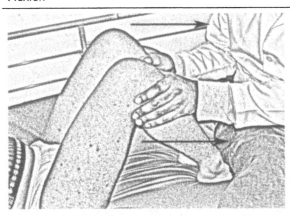 |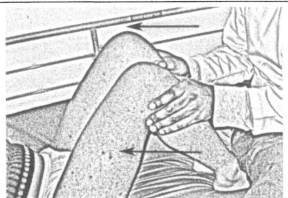

FIGURE 7.16 Knee flexion

FIGURE 7.17 Knee extension

- **Nerve root:** L5, S1
- **Muscle:** hamstrings

- **Nerve root:** L3, L4
- **Muscle:** quadriceps

Ankle

Dorsiflexion	Plantar flexion

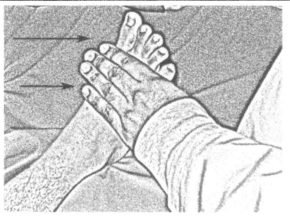

FIGURE 7.18 Dorsiflexion

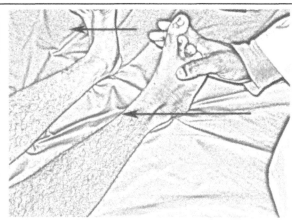

FIGURE 7.19 Plantar flexion

- **Nerve root:** L4, L5
- **Muscle:** tibialis anterior

- **Nerve root:** S1
- **Muscle:** calf muscles

❑ Coordination

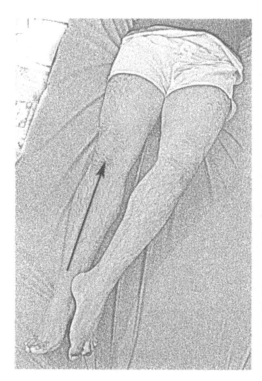

FIGURE 7.20A–B Heel–shin coordination

- **Heel–shin test:** Ask patient to run their heel down the contralateral shin and repeat as fast as possible, repeating on the other side. You are looking for any difficulty in performing this or tremors.

❑ **Sensation**
  ■ Assess light touch, pinprick, temperature, vibration and proprioception.

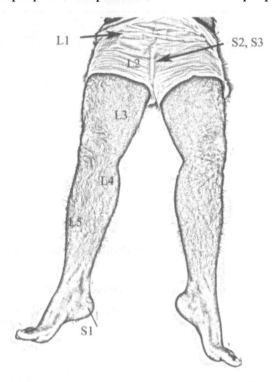

FIGURE 7.21 Lower limb dermatomes

  ■ As for the upper limbs, perform a similar sensory examination of the individual lower limb dermatomes.
❑ **Reflexes**
  ■ Check knee reflex (L3, L4)

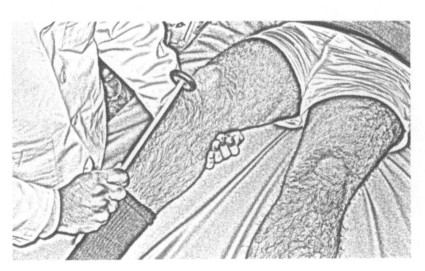

FIGURE 7.22 Knee reflex

- Hold the patient's leg, support with the knee flexed at 15 degrees, ensure the quadriceps are relaxed.
- Using the tendon hammer, strike the patella tendon.
- You are looking for knee extension and quadricep-muscle contraction.
- Repeat on the other side.

❑ **Check ankle reflex (L5, S1)**

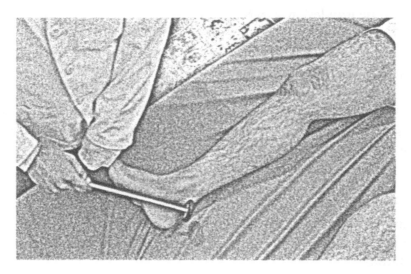

FIGURE 7.23 Ankle reflex

- With the knee in slight flexion and the leg externally rotated, ask the patient to let their leg go floppy.
- Hold onto the forefoot and dorsiflex the ankle slightly; strike the Achilles tendon with the tendon hammer.
- You are looking for plantar flexion of the ankle and contraction of the calf muscle.

Babinski response

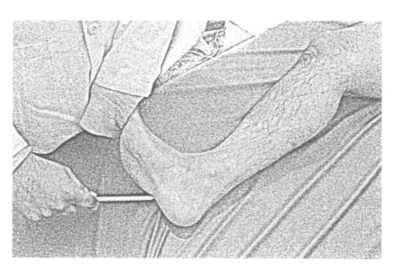

FIGURE 7.24 Babinski response

- Warn the patient this may be uncomfortable.
- Scrape along the plantar aspect of the foot with the sharp end of the tendon hammer.
- Begin at the lateral border of the heel, moving up along the sole of the foot to the big toe, following around like a curve.
- You are looking for plantar flexion of the toes, which is normal.
- An abnormal response is dorsiflexion of the toes, sometimes called an 'extensor plantar response' or simply described as 'upgoing plantars' which would indicate an upper motor neuron lesion (UMN).

There are many ways to elicit this. We have seen car keys and even a fingernail, amongst many others. Use what you find most comfortable.

❑ **Assess gait**
  - You are looking for characteristic gait patterns, such as the shuffling gait with loss of arm swing in Parkinsonism, or the inability to tandem walk in cerebellar disease.
  - Assess for a sensory ataxia using Romberg's test, which is positive if the patient is more unsteady with their eyes closed.

Complete the examination

❑ **Further examination:** ask to perform a cranial nerve exam
❑ **Thank the patient**
❑ **Wash your hands**
❑ **Present your findings**

AUTHOR'S TOP TIP

It is important you remember to ask the patient about any pain they may have before performing any of the above manoeuvres.

Viva questions

Q1 What are reflexes?
  - These are monosynaptic responses to muscle-fibre stretch, mediated via the spinal cord with inhibitory input from higher neurons.

In a UMN lesion, there is less inhibitory input from higher neurons, and so reflexes are increased, resulting in hyperreflexia. In LMN lesions, the reflexes are reduced or absent.

Q2 What is the pattern of signs elicited in a UMN lesion versus an LMN lesion?

TABLE 7.9 UMN vs LMN lesion

	UMN	*LMN*
Tone	Increased tone or spasticity Clonus may be present	Hypotonia
Power	Weakness mainly in arm extensors and leg flexors Drift of the outstretched arms	Weakness (symmetrical and distal)
Reflexes	Hyper-reflexia Babinski response positive	Loss of reflexes
Inspection	No muscle wasting or fasciculations	Muscle wasting, with or without fasciculations
Lesion location	Contralateral side	Ipsilateral side
Differentials	Stroke, MS	Radiculopathy, peripheral neuropathy, mononeuropathies

7.5 CEREBELLAR SYSTEM, SPINAL CORD AND PERIPHERAL NERVES

This section will primarily cover the cerebellum and the extrapyramidal system, as only certain conditions tend to crop up in finals cases. The cerebellum and extrapyramidal system coordinate movement, and so disorders of these systems may cause incoordination. Due to the nature of the aforementioned conditions, signs and symptoms, it is difficult to ask you to concentrate on a single examination system, and so usually a vague instruction is given at the doorway. This is what tends to alarm candidates, as they feel uncertain of what is expected of them upon entering the OSCE station. More recently, there has been a move away from this format with more focused instructions, such as to examine the upper limb peripheral nervous system, whereby you might elicit the cogwheel rigidity seen in Parkinson's disease. Occasionally, you may be asked to examine the patient's gait or assess coordination. The diagnosis is not the important aspect of the OSCE, as in most cases the diagnosis will be given to you or will be obvious from the outset. It is how you examine the patient's signs and symptoms, paying particular attention to those which are characteristic of the given disease, that will gain you those extra marks.

Examination of peripheral nerve palsies and injuries have been covered in our companion textbook, as they tend to be managed surgically.

Case 1: Cerebellar disease

Instructions: Please examine the coordination of this 36-year-old man who has been increasingly unsteady on his feet with slurred speech.

Key features to look for

- ❑ **Dysdiadochokinesis**
- ❑ Limb **Ataxia and hypotonia**
- ❑ **Horizontal Nystagmus;** fast component towards the side of the lesion
- ❑ **Intention** tremor with past pointing
- ❑ **Staccato** or slurred speech (usually with bilateral lesions)
- ❑ **Heel** shin ataxia

❏ Wide-based, unsteady ataxic gait (patient falls to the side of the lesion)

AUTHOR'S TOP TIP

A helpful mnemonic for the above is DANISH.

AUTHOR'S TOP TIP

To assess whether the tremor is an action tremor, rule out any muscle activation by taking the patient's arms into your own and while supporting their arms a truly cerebellar tremor will disappear.

Complete the examination

❏ **Thank the patient**
❏ **Wash your hands**
❏ **Present your findings**

The lateral lobes of the cerebellum are each responsible for movement coordination of the ipsilateral limb. Therefore, signs on the left indicate disease of the left lateral lobe. The cerebellar midline vermis maintains midline or axial balance and posture. Lesions of the cerebellar vermis may therefore cause a trunkal ataxia, whereby patients are unable to sit or stand up.

Viva questions

Q1   What are the causes of cerebellar disease?
  ■ space-occupying lesions, e.g. tumours, abscess, bleed
  ■ multiple sclerosis
  ■ chronic alcohol abuse
  ■ anti-epileptic drugs

Case 2: Parkinson's disease

Instructions: Please examine this 46-year-old man who is being seen in clinic with suspected Parkinson's disease.

Key features to look for

Inspection
❏ **Tremor:** unilateral, pill-rolling of hand; a 4- to 7-Hz resting tremor

❑ **Bradykinesia:** lack of facial expression, drooling of saliva, difficulty in initiating movement and performing rapid alternating movements (touching each finger with their thumb)

❑ **Gait:** slow starting, shuffling gait with lack of arm swing and difficulty in turning; patient keeps gaze on floor with body leaning forward as they walk (festinant gait), poor balance and postural instability

Palpation/tone

❑ **Rigidity:** increased tone in opposing muscle groups causing lead piping at the elbow and cogwheel rigidity at the wrist

Some candidates like to perform the glabellar tap test, which in a normal individual causes patients to cease blinking, whereas in Parkinson's disease it causes patients to continue blinking.

Complete the examination

❑ **Further examination**

- *'To complete my exam, I would like to assess the patient's speech and handwriting.'*

There is a slowing down of speech, dysphonia and lack of gestures seen in early Parkinson's disease. Micrographia is also a feature of Parkinson's.

❑ **Thank the patient**
❑ **Wash your hands**
❑ **Present your findings**

This is an important clinical triad to demonstrate with an emphasis on the asymmetry of signs, with initial involvement of the upper limbs and fluctuations in symptom severity. There are many differential diagnoses, including dementia, multisystem atrophy, progressive supranuclear palsy, benign essential tremor and other causes of extrapyramidal signs and symptoms.

The extrapyramidal system is a term used to describe the basal ganglia and its connections, especially those to do with movement. The extrapyramidal system is charged with modulation and initiation of movement.

Viva questions

Q1 What is Parkinson's disease?
- This is a progressive neurodegenerative disorder characterised by Lewy bodies, neuronal loss and degeneration of the substantia nigra.
- Diagnosis is clinical, although some patients undergo trials of the dopamine precursor levodopa (L-dopa) or an apomorphine challenge. Others have PET or MRI scanning to exclude other diagnoses.

There are many causes of true Parkinsonism, the most common aetiology being idiopathic. It can also be drug induced. Patients may have periods of increased symptomatology; these are called 'on' states where there is levodopa-induced dyskinaesia or 'off' state periods where there is absence of movement. There may be coexisting depression. Treatment is dopamine replacement with levodopa, dopamine agonists such as ropinirole, cabergoline, bromocriptine and a peripheral dopa-decarboxylase inhibitor (Sinemet). Anticholinergic drugs such as selegiline are useful for tremors.

Case 3: Myasthenia gravis

Instructions: Please examine this 46-year-old man who is being seen in clinic with weakness induced by activity.

Key features to look for

Inspection
- ❑ **Thymectomy scar:** midline thoracotomy
- ❑ **Demonstrable fatiguability**
- ❑ **Speech:** dysarthria, poor swallowing (due to weak bulbar muscles)
- ❑ **Eyes:** ophthalmoplegia (weak extraocular muscles), ptosis, diploplia

To test for fatiguability, ask patient to gaze upwards for a few minutes; patients with myasthenia gravis will display worsening ptosis.

Palpation
- ❑ **Muscle power:** limb weakness

Complete the examination
- ❑ **Further examination**
  - ▪ *'To complete my exam, I would like to assess for signs of other autoimmune diseases.'*
- ❑ **Thank the patient**
- ❑ **Wash your hands**
- ❑ **Present your findings**

Many patients initially present with diploplia, characteristically worse when tired. Diagnosis is generally clinical, although the Tensilon test may be performed, whereby edrophonium, a short-acting anticholinesterase, is given to the patient, causing a rapid improvement in symptoms. EMG is useful in demonstrating fatiguability, with diminished amplitude of evoked responses with repetitive stimulation. Most patients have demonstrable antibodies to acetylcholine receptors, although some may not. There is an association with thymomas and thymic hyperplasia; patients may have had these surgically removed.

Viva questions

Q1 What is myasthenia gravis?
- This is an autoimmune disorder affecting the neuromuscular junction, whereby antibodies block the action of post-synaptic acetylcholine receptors.

This should be distinguished from Lambert–Eaton syndrome (LES), which also causes fatiguability. Unlike myasthenia gravis, the ocular and bulbar muscles are not affected; ptosis therefore is not a feature. The EMG characteristically shows improvement with repetition, as opposed to myasthenia gravis.

Q2 How would you treat myasthenia gravis?

Difficult question

- **Medical:** cholinesterase inhibitors, imunosuppressants and corticosteroids
- **Surgical:** thymectomy for thymomas

Patients are at risk of myasthenia crises if there is a coexisting infection, although some crises are drug induced.

Case 4: Multiple sclerosis

Instructions: Please examine this 28-year-old woman who is being seen in clinic with suspected MS.

Key features to look for

Inspection

❑ **Upper motor neuron (UMN) signs:**
- weakness, increased tone, and clonus bilaterally
- hyperreflexia and an extensor plantar response

❑ **Neuro-ophthalmology**
- internuclear ophthalmoplegia
- optic nerve damage

❑ **Cerebellar signs:** ataxia, dysarthria

❑ **Cranial nerve palsy:** facial nerve

❑ **Sensation:** altered in a variable fashion, altered temperature sensation, trigeminal neuralgia; Lhermitte's phenomenon, whereby electric shock sensation down arms/legs on neck flexion

Complete the examination

❑ **Further examination**

❑ **Thank the patient**

❑ **Wash your hands**

❑ **Present your findings**

AUTHOR'S TOP TIP

If you suspect the patient has multiple sclerosis, even though the patient is likely to be already aware of this diagnosis, it is best to state 'demyelinating' disease rather than multiple sclerosis when coming up with your differentials. Indeed, your diagnosis of MS may be wrong and cause undue stress to the patient. However, due to the sensitive nature of the disease, it is unlikely an actual case will be seen in finals.

An important differential based on the clinical signs is a spinal cord lesion, such as a tumour or trauma causing a spastic paraparesis; if all four limbs are involved, i.e. a quadraparesis, ensure you examine for a sensory level.

The most common cause of the above signs is, however, multiple sclerosis. There are many other clinical features of multiple sclerosis, which can be found on examination. Some patients may present with isolated symptoms. However, the diagnosis of MS is clinical and is demonstrated by multiple lesions in time and space. Diagnosis can be made on history, examination and MRI findings; CSF results also aid diagnosis.

Viva questions

Q1   What is MS?
- This neurological disorder of unknown cause results in multiple areas of plaques of demyelination in the brain and spinal cord, disseminated in time and space.
- Characteristically begins in early adulthood; the clinical course can be either progressive or relapsing-remitting.
- There is a female preponderance.

Poor prognosis is seen in male patients, older age of onset, motor symptoms, high number of relapses and incomplete remissions in between relapses, amongst others.

Q2   How would you investigate this patient?
- **MRI brain & spinal cord:** this is the first-line investigation and reveals plaques or multiple white matter lesions; particularly in the brainstem and periventricular areas
- **Electrophysiology:** prolonged visual evoked potentials
- **CSF examination:** raised protein; raised white cell count; electrophoresis demonstrates oligoclonal bands

Patients will require a multidisciplinary team management approach to treatment. The focus of treatment is to prevent disability and its progression. High-dose steroids may aid recovery and promote remission during an acute relapse; they do not, however, affect long-term prognosis. Beta-interferon has been shown to delay progression of disability, reduce relapse rates and reduce disease activity. Urinary catheterisation for those with bladder involvement (neurogenic bladder dysfunction), physical and occupational therapy to help aid mobility and limit disability; muscle relaxants such as baclofen for painful spasticity. All patients should be referred to patient and family self-help groups.

7.6 THE NEUROLOGICAL HISTORY

There are only a limited number of possible cases that could appear in finals under neurology. Those that tend to appear in undergraduate examinations are covered below.

History Case 1: Headache

Instructions: This 27-year-old woman presents with headache. Please take a focused clinical history.

Key features to look for

❑ **Pain history**
- **Site:** is the pain occipital or frontal?; unilateral or bilateral?; migraine pain is classical unilateral; over the superficial temporal arteries in temporal arteritis; retro-orbital pain in cluster headaches, and eye pain in glaucoma
- **Onset:** is this acute or chronic (over days or weeks)?; is there a specific time of day, e.g. first thing when they wake up?; has the pattern changed over time?; a sudden-onset headache may be due to a ruptured berry aneurysm causing a subarachnoid haemorrhage (SAH); headaches occurring over several minutes and lasting hours are seen in migraines; progressive severe headaches over days to weeks may suggest raised intracranial pressure from either a tumour or chronic bleed; meningitis may take hours to days to develop
- **Character:** is it a dull ache; or tight band-like pain in tension headaches; pressure, thunder clap or bursting pain in sudden raised intracranial pressure; throbbing pain in migraines?
- **Radiation:** does the pain spread from the front to around the head; any neck pain?
- **Aggravating factors:** does the headache come on after exertion, sexual intercourse, certain foods?, e.g. cheese in migraines, coughing/sneezing; bending over or other posture-related headaches are typical of raised intracranial pressure, work related, menstruation
- **Timing:** frequency of headaches: are they episodic/cyclical or constant; how is the patient in between attacks? Symptom-free in between attacks is a feature of migraines. Duration of symptoms, e.g. several hours up to 3 days can be seen in migraines; headache occurring at the same time each day for a few weeks is characteristic of cluster headaches; headaches worse in the morning are a classical symptom of raised intracranial pressure
- **Relieving factors:** staying in a quiet and darkened room, for example, may help in migraines
- **Scale:** the worst headache ever in a patient's life should prompt you to consider SAH

❑ **Associated symptoms**
- **Nausea & vomiting:** can be a feature of migraine or space-occupying lesions
- **Photophobia:** may be seen in subarachnoid haemorrhage, migraine or meningitis, glaucoma

- **Neck stiffness:** a sign of meningism; can be seen in SAH, meningitis
- **Aura:** presence of an aura suggests migraines; visual symptoms, e.g. spots, flashing lights; remember visual disturbances could be a sign of giant cell arteritis; reversible unilateral paraesthesia of hands or face
- **Visual disturbances:** these can occur in glaucoma, e.g. haloes; unilateral visual loss in temporal arteritis
- **Fever:** consider meningitis
- **Rash:** meningitis should be considered and actively treated as such
- **Jaw claudication:** consider temporal arteritis
- **Seizures:** consider an intracranial space-occupying lesion
❑ **Past medical & family history:** known history of migraines, prior investigations or treatments for headaches; family history of headaches
❑ **Drug history:** the OCP can precipitate migraines; drug side effects causing headaches, e.g. GTN
❑ **Social history:** cluster headaches are associated with male smokers

Completion

AUTHOR'S TOP TIP

Headache can be considered like any other 'pain'-based history; use SOCRATES as your framework.

Headaches can be classified into either primary or secondary headaches. Primary headaches include migraines, tension headache and cluster headaches. Secondary headaches incorporate a wide range of causes, including trauma, vascular disorders, e.g. SAH; trigeminal neuralgia, alcohol withdrawal–associated, amongst others. The key in the OSCE is to ensure you do not miss out a serious diagnosis, such as SAH, meningitis or a space-occupying lesion.

Viva questions

Q1 How would you investigate the patient with headache?
Firstly, perform a clinical examination, specifically focusing on peripheral and cranial nerve exams. Thereafter, your investigations will be tailored to your history, examination findings and differential diagnosis. However, in general, the following may be useful:
- **Bloods:** ESR raised in temporal arteritis, raised WCC in meningitis or cerebral abscess; renal failure as a cause of hypertensive headaches; blood cultures in meningitis
- **BM:** remember, the patient may have headaches due to hypoglycaemia
- **CT head:** there are various national guidelines for deciding which patient requires a CT; however, we suggest you use your clinical judgement in the OSCE; suggesting this in the exam is safer than not doing a CT head

- **MRI head:** this is normally done until after specialist referral to neurologists, who then request this
- **Lumbar puncture:** this is indicated if you suspect meningitis, as it will help distinguish the type of meningitis; if you suspect SAH, you must also send CSF off for xanthochromia

Good response

History Case 2: Seizures

Instructions: This 32-year-old man presents with seizures. His partner is waiting outside the room. Please take a focused clinical history.

Key features to look for

❏ **History of seizure event**
- **Frequency:** how many seizures have occurred in a certain space of time, how frequently do they tend to occur and has this changed?
- **Duration:** a few minutes or longer than 5 minutes?
- **Tongue biting:** this is very suggestive of epilepsy; patients may say their tongue or mouth feels sore
- **Incontinence:** not necessarily a feature of epilepsy itself
- **Presence of an aura:** this could manifest as a strange feeling in the gut, unusual smells or a feeling of déjà vu phenomenon; the presence of an aura suggests partial seizures, particularly temporal lobe epilepsy
- **Aggravating features:** strobe or flashing lights from, e.g. club lights, television screens; illicit drug or alcohol abuse, menstruation
- **Post-seizure injury:** were any injuries sustained?; more likely in tonic clonic
- **Pre- and post-seizure symptomatology (from patient):** presence of prodromal symptoms, which may occur hours to days prior; it is not actually part of the seizure; did they feel extremely tired and drowsy in the post-ictal state?

❏ **Witness account:** this will help fill in any gaps the patient may not recall
- A description of what was observed by the witness before, during and after the seizure
  - **Pre-seizure:** what events led up to the seizure?; was the patient exposed to strobe lighting in a dance club?
  - **During-seizure:** were they tonic-clonic, mouth frothing, incontinent?; was there a loss of consciousness or not?; duration of seizure
  - **Post-ictal state:** was there a slow recovery?; remember that a post-ictal state is very suggestive of epilepsy

❏ **Past medical history:** known to have epilepsy, prior history of traumatic head injury, known stroke, space-occupying lesion or meningitis

❏ **Family history:** epilepsy can occur in families

> **AUTHOR'S TOP TIP**
>
> *Information from a witness is essential in making a diagnosis of seizures, as your patient will often have no recollection of the events.*

Sometimes in the OSCE, examiners will purposely inform you that the patient has attended clinic with a family member or friend. It is always important not to ignore these invaluable sources of information. In actual clinical practice, you would welcome such information when the patient is unable to provide this. With the patient's permission, you may ask if they witnessed the event and you can ask for their description of events.

Completion

Although almost all patients have some form of neuroimaging performed, the accurate clinical history is crucial to diagnosing seizures. Remember that a normal EEG does not exclude epilepsy. Antiepileptic drugs are not usually commenced after a single episode of seizures unless there is some structural lesion identified on MRI.

There are many causes of seizures (too many to cover in this study guide), and these should be considered in your differentials, e.g. metabolic causes such as hyper- and hypoglycaemia, hyper- and hyponatraemia, hypoxaemia, renal failure causing uraemia and liver failure, amongst many others, including structural and infective aetiologies.

Once diagnosed, patients are advised to avoid operating any heavy machinery, driving, unsupervised swimming and to be especially careful when showering or coming into contact with hot water, as burns are not uncommon. Of particular concern is the pregnant patient and the teratogenicity of antiepileptic drugs balanced against the risk of uncontrolled seizures affecting mother and baby. Driving restrictions and the criteria required for reinstating of driving licences, whether for personal use or commercial purposes, are not required for finals.

Viva questions

Q1   What are seizures?
  - These are transient, abnormal events occurring due to spontaneous paroxysmal electrical activity in cerebral neurons.

Epilepsy is a condition whereby there is a continuing tendency for recurrent seizures; it occurs in 1%–2% of the UK population and so is fairly common. Status epilepticus is a medical emergency in which seizures occur consecutively without recovery in between. *See* Chapter 11.

Q2   How are seizures classified?
  - Seizures can be either partial or generalised.

TABLE 7.10 Seizure classification

Class	Description
Partial	Partial seizures arise from focal cortical lesions suggesting structural disease, e.g. the temporal lobe. They can be:
	Complex: loss of consciousness
	Simple: no loss of consciousness
	They can also progress from partial into secondary generalised seizures.
Generalised	Generalised seizures arise from bilateral cortical discharges. They can be:
	Tonic-clonic: once known as grand mal seizures; sudden stiff (tonic) limbs with jerks (clonic)
	Myoclonic: single or multiple jerking limbs
	Atonic: sudden loss of posture, flaccid
	Absence: brief sudden pauses; previously called petit mal

Q3   What antiepileptic drugs do you know of?

Difficult question

TABLE 7.11 Antiepileptic drugs

Drug	Description
Phenytoin	Due to its toxicity, it is not used as first-line treatment for either generalised or partial seizures.
	Toxicity can lead to dysarthria, ataxia, gum hypertrophy, depression, nystagmus, etc.
Carbamazepine	Is first-line for partial seizures, but can be used for generalised. Side effects: diplopia, rash, fluid retention, hyponatraemia and blood dyscrasias, amongst others.
Sodium valproate	First-line agent for generalised seizures; second-line for partial seizures. Side effects: liver failure, tremor, sedation, weight gain, etc.
Lamotrigine	Can be used in partial seizures; second-line agent in generalised. Rash is a common side effect.
Levetiracetam (Keppra)	This novel drug with minimal side effects is now being favoured by many neurologists for secondary generalised seizures.

CHAPTER 8

Ophthalmology

8.1 EXAMINATION OF THE EYE

Fundoscopy tends to provoke anxiety amongst finalists, mostly because many have not had the level of experience in examining an eye as they have for example examining the abdomen. There is really no way around this and it will probably remain so for the rest of your careers, unless you happen to go into ophthalmology. We suggest you therefore take the opportunity to examine every single patient's eyes that you clerk. This will give you the chance to appreciate what is normal and the various normal idiosyncrasies between patients. For example, darker-skinned patients tend to have darker-coloured retinas than their Caucasian counterparts; this is normal.

You must also remember that when examining the eyes, fundoscopy is not the only part of the examination, which involves examining the cranial nerves as well. For purposes of clarity, the initial assessment of the eye, that is, the visual fields – acuity, ocular movements and reflexes – will not be repeated in this chapter. (*See* Chapter 7, Neuro-ophthalmology, for further details.)

Spending a few afternoons in eye clinic is also a useful place to learn this skill; however you must remember that most patients get examined under slit-lamp examination anyway. We suggest that the easiest method to gain more experience in fundoscopy is to simply identify all patients who are either hypertensive or diabetic and examine their eyes on the wards. This will give you an opportunity to practice holding the ophthalmoscope with your non-dominant hand and looking with your non-dominant eye, as it is harder than it looks and practice certainly makes perfect. It is usually obvious to an examiner if the candidate hasn't examined using the ophthalmoscope, so make sure you are adept at executing this.

More often than not, most cases you will see in finals will be retinal pictures given to you to discuss, rather than an actual patient, as it is easier for both parties, although it is not unheard of for a patient to be brought into the exam for the sole purpose of fundoscopy. But as you can appreciate, being subjected to mydriatics and a bright light shining into their eyes for hours can be quite uncomfortable; therefore, we advise you to be extra-careful and kind to your patients in this regard. Remember, they give you marks too.

Clinical examination

Introduction

As for any clinical encounter (*see* Chapter 1, Section 3); specifically for this case:

❏ **Expose patient adequately**
❏ **Position patient appropriately:** position yourself such that you are level with the patient's line of sight, e.g. sitting on a chair opposite the patient.

See Chapter 7, Neuro-ophthalmology, for cranial nerve examination of the eyes.

Fundoscopy

❏ **Ensure optimal environment**
- **Dark room:** Ask for the lights to be switched off and the curtains drawn.
- **Pupillary dilatation:** Ask that the patient receive mydriatic dilating drops into their eyes to dilate their pupils. You can use tropicamide 0.5%, whose effects can last up to 8 hours and which is not to be used in patients with glaucoma, or 2.5% phenylephrine solution, which works within 15 minutes and lasts 2 hours. Consequently, you must warn the patient their eyesight may be blurred for a while afterwards and that they shouldn't drive or operate machinery until this has resolved. Any prolonged blurring or eye pain should be managed by seeking healthcare advice immediately. A simple way of causing pupillary dilatation is by asking the patient to fix their gaze on a distant object.
  — e.g. *'Can I get you to look at the corner of the ceiling and keep looking at that?'*
- **Ensure patient comfort:** Remember that you will be in close proximity to the patient during the examination, so warn the patient of this; also that you will be shining a fairly bright light into their eyes, which in itself may be uncomfortable. Sit the patient on a chair and ensure that they are comfortable. Ask the patient to focus on an object in the distance, remembering to remove both yours and the patient's glasses as this creates a physical distance barrier between yourself and the patient.
  — e.g. *'I will be shining a bright light into your eyes and coming up quite close to you. Is that OK?'*
- **Assess for refractive errors:** If the patient wears glasses, ask whether they are long- or short-sighted. The ophthalmoscope can accordingly correct for any refractive errors of either the patient or the candidate (if they too wear glasses). Remember the following:
  — **Ophthalmoscope dioptre number equals the sum of the observer's refractive error and the patient's refractive error.**
- **Correctly position observer**
  — Starting on the right side, stand about a metre away from the patient; stay level with the patient's eyes.
  — Hold the ophthalmoscope in your right hand, looking through your right eye to look into the patient's right eye.

AUTHOR'S TOP TIP

It is important you use your right hand to examine the right eye, looking through the ophthalmoscope with your right eye, likewise examining the left eye, with your left eye, with the ophthalmoscope held in your left hand. Some schools actually reserve marks for this very thing! Thus you must practice as much as possible with your non-dominant hand, as it can be tricky!

Specifically for the orientation of the eye, the terms 'medial' and 'lateral' are replaced by 'nasal' and 'temporal', respectively. The fundus can be thought of as a circle with two halves; the medial half is the nasal half and the lateral half is the temporal portion.

AUTHOR'S TOP TIP

Before you begin using the ophthalmoscope, ensure that the light source is turned on and is working optimally. You would be surprised how often the light switches are not turned on, especially during the stress of an examination. We suggest you take the time to use ophthalmoscopes found in clinics, particularly the ones attached to the walls as these are likely to be the ones used in the exam.

AUTHOR'S TOP TIP

As you approach the patient from either side, if you are using an ophthalmoscope which is attached to the wall, the wall extension lead tends to get in the way of the patient as it tries to recoil back into the wall unit. We suggest you pull the lead cord behind and around you so that if it does pull it pulls on you and not the patient.

❏ **Elicit the red reflex**
  ▪ From a distance shine the light from the ophthalmoscope into both eyes, checking to see if the eyes light up red; this is the red reflex. What you may see:
    — **Red reflex:** This is normal and indicates that the retina is firmly attached to the underlying choroid and that the various media in front of the retina are transparent and thus clear of any obvious pathology.
    — **White reflex:** This is due to opacity either in the lens, cornea, anterior or vitreous chambers. This is likely to be due to a cataract. In young children, a white reflex can be indicative of retinoblastoma.
    — **Opacity:** This will have a black outline.
    — **Absent or attenuated red reflex:** This will occur in any condition affecting transparency in the media anterior to the retina. This can be seen in retinal detachment, vitreous haemorrhage or classically a cataract or other lens opacity.

AUTHOR'S TOP TIP

It is important that you look 'through the ophthalmoscope' as you do so, or you won't see the red reflex normally!

❏ **Examine the anterior chamber, lens and vitreous**
  ▪ **Approach the patient**
    — This is best done from the temporal side of the patient at an angle so as not to obscure the patient's view.

— You may choose to hold the ipsilateral eyelid open with your fingers, simultaneously placing your hand on their head, thereby helping to stabilise your balance as you come closer to the patient.

— To make it easier, tilt your head sideways as you approach the patient's eyes.

■ **Adjust focal length progressively through chambers**

— **Dioptre settings:** Normally, there are numbers on the ophthalmoscope starting with zero, and on either side there are positive numbers clockwise and negative numbers anticlockwise. These numbers are dioptres (D) and they help adjust the focal length with which you are viewing and thus which section or chamber you are focusing on during fundoscopy. This is particularly important if you are examining a long-sighted individual, because setting your dioptre to zero will focus your view behind the eye; short-sighted patients will have a view focused on the vitreous.

— **Focus on individual chambers/sections:** Dial clockwise to set the lens to +10D (short focal length; yellow/green/white coloured numbers) and observe the eye from approximately 10 cm away; while at this point use this opportunity to examine the surface of the eye and the anterior chamber. As you move closer, progressively (remembering to warn the patient of this) dial anticlockwise, thereby increasing the focal length of the ophthalmoscope lens, allowing you to focus on each section progressively deeper into the eye starting from the anterior chamber, to the lens, vitreous and finally until you are able to view the optic fundus.

— **Purpose of focal length adjustment:** As you adjust the dial, you will be focusing progressively through the eye, allowing you to identify any floaters, posterior vitreous detachments and general degenerative changes of the vitreous body.

❑ **Examine the optic disc**

■ **Locate the optic disc**

— Your initial approach above should have you looking directly towards the centre of the back of the head, as this will in most cases get you looking directly at the optic disc; if not then position yourself 30 degrees from the temporal side of the patient.

— Otherwise, identify a vessel, focus on this visible vessel and follow this back towards the optic disc, which is a coin-like object seen in the middle of the retina and is essentially the head of the optic nerve.

■ **Focus onto the optic disc**

— The dioptre number required to focus on the optic disc gives an indication of the patient's refractive error, assuming your eyesight is normal.

TABLE 8.1 Dioptre settings

Sightedness	Fundoscopy settings
Myopia	Short-sightedness requires negative, or commonly called 'minus' or concave lenses, i.e. the dioptre setting will need to be negative so it has a longer focal length.
Hypermetropia	In long-sightedness positive or commonly called 'plus' or convex lenses are used, as the eyes are short and so the focal length required will be short also, and thus the dioptre setting will be more positive.

Note that if the patient is wearing their glasses, assuming their glasses are optimally set, zeroing the dioptre setting on the ophthalmoscope will focus your view onto the retina.

- Examine the optic disc
  - **Describe the margin:** Normally, the temporal margin is well demarcated compared to the nasal margin, and there may be an area of pigmentation on the temporal side. This is also normal.
  - **Assess the colour:** This is variable but can be pink or white; the more vascular the more pink it is, and so elderly patients may have very pale discs. A very pale disc would suggest optic atrophy due to MS or chronic glaucoma.
  - **Assess the central cup:** Normally, the central cup is paler in comparison to the rest of the optic disc, with central vessels appearing to converge there. Measure cup size relative to disc radius; the diameter should be < 50% of the disc. 'Cupping' is the term used to describe an excavated appearance and is suggestive of glaucoma.

Remember that the optic disc contains no photoreceptors and is thus termed the 'blind spot'.
- ❏ **Examine the quadrants**
  - Identify the four major vessels (branches of the retinal artery), one going into each quadrant.
  - Then systematically examine all four quadrants, identifying any abnormalities in the quadrants as well as the major branch itself, for the presence of narrowing, tortuosity, arteriovenous (AV) nipping and vessel transparency.
  - Abnormalities should be described as if you were looking at a clock face with the disc at the centre, e.g. haemorrhage at the 3 o'clock position one disc diameter from the disc.

Abnormalities are measured according to the disc diameter as a reference for distance and size.
- ❏ **Examine the macula**
  - **Locate the macula**
    - It can be difficult to locate but is generally temporal, i.e. lateral to the optic disc.
    - It is a pale-yellow area against a much darker surrounding retina, found two disc diameters from the optic disc.
    - It is easiest found by asking the patient to look directly at the light.
    - Pathology of the macula therefore can lead to central scotomas.

The macula contains many densely packed photoreceptors with an important and much paler central area, the fovea, giving rise to central vision.

Complete the examination
- ❏ **Further examination**
  - *'To complete my exam, I would like to perform a slit-lamp examination.'*

Slit-lamp examination allows a more detailed examination of the fundus and enables measurement of intraocular pressure.
- ❏ **Thank the patient**
- ❏ **Wash your hands**
- ❏ **Present your findings**

TABLE 8.2 Fundoscopic abnormalities

Abnormality	Description
Hard exudates	**Morphology:** these are well-defined yellow/white deposits in the retina due to lipoproteins leaking from leaky blood vessels. They are arranged in circinate rings but can appear star-shaped at the macula. The ring centre may appear more white/yellow due to lipoprotein leakage. They appear more bright and crisp than cotton-wool spots
	Pathology: seen in diabetes and hypertension
Soft exudates	**Morphology:** these look like cotton wool deposited on the retina. They tend to deposit in regions of retinal infarction due to ischaemia; consequently, associated features of retinal ischaemia such as new vessel formation and haemorrhage may also be seen
	Pathology: they occur due to axonal nerve fibre swelling
Retinal haemorrhages	**Morphology:** superficial retinal haemorrhages appear **flame-shaped** because the blood tracks along the horizontally arranged nerve fibres and adopts this pattern; deep haemorrhages look similar to microaneurysms, of which they both appear like dark-red dots or blots
	Pathology: hypertension and diabetic retinopathy
Vitreous haemorrhages	**Morphology:** abnormal or absent red reflex, with an absent or distorted fundus view; they can be diffuse or localised in clumps, appearing like floaters
Cotton-wool spots	**Morphology:** deposits of cotton-wool-like lesions, that look similar to soft exudates
	Pathology: these occur due to arteriolar occlusion indicating regions of retinal ischaemia
Neovascularisation	**Morphology:** this new vessel (veins) formation appears haphazard in appearance, like worms running off of veins; these are fragile and more likely to bleed
	Pathology: occurs due to angiogenic factor stimulation from occlusive ischaemia
Microaneurysms	**Morphology:** these are weakened vessel walls that bulge and therefore appear as red dots; they may be scattered throughout the fundus
	Pathology: occlusion of capillaries
Arteriovenous (AV) nipping	**Morphology:** this happens when thick-walled arterioles cross over venules and lead to compression of the vessel at this crossing, referred to as AV nipping; silver wiring refers to thickened arteriolar walls in arteriosclerosis which appear like a silver wire; this is an unreliable sign
	Pathology: sign of arteriosclerosis and is seen in hypertensive retinopathy

Viva questions

Q1   How can you tell which eye you are examining if only given a picture of a retina?
- Assuming you are holding the picture the right way up, the optic disc is usually more nasal.
- If the optic disc appears on the right in the picture (not your right), then the image is of the left eye and vice versa.

Q2   How would you recognise a glass eye?
- Usually, this is self evident, as the eye does not move with head movement or have a red reflex; newer prostheses are however very lifelike.

■ The question should be 'Why does the patient have a glass eye in the first place?', and the most likely answer apart from eye trauma would be malignant melanoma.

Q3 What is optic atrophy?

Difficult question

■ **Optic atrophy** is a condition characterised by a pale disc with sharp margins, although occasionally this may be diffuse, reduced vision with a central scotoma and an afferent pupillary defect (*see* Chapter 7, Neuro-ophthalmology). It is one of the features of optic nerve damage. There may be signs of cerebellar disease
■ **Aetiology:** demyelinating disease (commonest cause in UK), ischaemic neuritis from a vasculitis or atherosclerosis, compression from a tumour or aneurysm, retinitis pigmentosa, trauma to optic nerve, glaucoma, Paget's disease, methanol, lead or arsenic poisoning, neurodegeneration in vitamin B_1 and B_{12} deficiencies, amongst many others, including TB and sarcoidosis infiltration

Q4 How would you recognise age-related macular degeneration?

Difficult question

■ **History:** elderly patients who have progressive deterioration of central vision
■ **Examination findings:** reduced visual acuity, loss of central vision, clusters of drusen (pale-yellow spots) throughout the macula, areas of retinal hyper- or hypopigmentation and choroidal neovascularisation

It is also the most common reason for a person to be registered blind in the UK. As such, your patient may have a white walking aid. Treatment is with photocoagulation and photodynamic therapy, with regular screening for neovascularisation.

Case 1: Central retinal artery occlusion

Instructions: Please examine this patient who presented with sudden painless loss of vision.

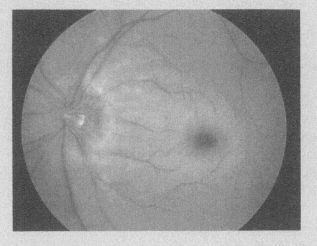

FIGURE 8.1 Central retinal artery occlusion

Key features to look for

❑ **Fundoscopy**
- pale appearance of retina in general
- there is a **cherry-red** spot at the fovea (of the macula)
- thin arterioles; there may be a cholesterol plaque
- Some neovascularisation

Complete the examination

- *'To complete my exam, I would like to examine for temporal arteritis, AF and ask about a history of previous CVA or MI.'*

❑ **Thank the patient**
❑ **Wash your hands**
❑ **Present your findings**

This type of patient would classically present to A&E complaining of sudden painless loss of vision and will require urgent ophthalmic referral to try and decrease intraocular pressure. Treatment is of the underlying cause and in those with a history of thromboembolism management would involve risk factor modification and/or appropriate anticoagulation.

Viva questions

Q1 How would you differentiate artery occlusion from central vein occlusion?

Difficult Question

TABLE 8.3 Artery occlusion versus vein occlusion

Condition	Description
Central retinal artery occlusion	**History:** There is sudden, painless vision loss. Past history of MI or temporal arteritis. Risk factors for AF. Cholesterol emboli as a possible cause post-percutaneous coronary intervention (PCI); may be seen as a shiny plaque in the arterioles. Patient may complain of amaurosis fugax.
	Fundoscopy findings: Pale opaque and swollen retina with development of cherry-red spots at macula. Optic disc swells then atrophies. If a branch is occluded by microemboli, you may get a visual field defect corresponding to the sector it supplies. The central retinal artery has upper and lower branches which supply the upper half and lower half respectively, divided by an imaginary horizontal line. Branch occlusion visual defects will therefore follow this pattern.
Central retinal vein occlusion	**History:** Visual loss is variable, but in general some vision is retained. Patients may complain of headaches from the raised intraocular pressure. History of glaucoma, diabetes, hypertension, vasculitis, atherosclerosis and polycythaemia or multiple myeloma.
	Fundoscopy findings: This is described as a stormy sunset appearance with swelling of the optic disc, retinal vein dilatation, large flame haemorrhages and cotton-wool spots all over the retina. These features may be restricted to a single quadrant in branch occlusion.

Case 2: Hypertensive retinopathy

Instructions: Please examine this gentleman who presents with a BP of 205/125.

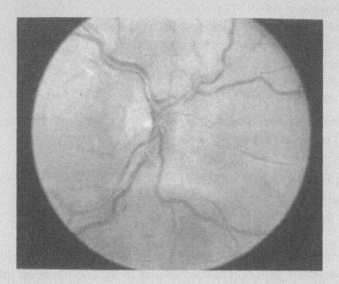

FIGURE 8.2 Hypertensive retinopathy

Key features to look for

❑ **Fundoscopy**
- AV nipping, thickened arteriolar walls appearing like 'silver wiring'
- arteriolar narrowing leading to cotton wool spots and flame shaped haemorrhages
- leakage of hard exudates due to leaking from vessels; leakage causing retinal oedema
- a macular star may be seen (a ring of exudates from the disc to the macula; star-like due to it following the line of retinal fibres around the macula)
- there may be optic disc swelling (papilloedema with its various features)
- features are bilateral

Complete the examination

- *'To complete my exam, I would like to examine the blood pressure and assess for other hypertensive end organ damage, particularly renal and cardiovascular complications.'*

❑ **Thank the patient**
❑ **Wash your hands**
❑ **Present your findings**

Hypertension causes changes to retinal microvasculature, with increased arteriosclerosis and closure of vessels leading to microinfarcts (cotton-wool spots and superficial haemorrhages). It is thought that intracranial hypertension secondary to systemic hypertension leads to the finding of papilloedema. In young patients without sclerotic changes to their vessels, there is arteriolar spasm and narrowing in response to hypertension; in the elderly, there are compensatory arterial changes seen, such as silver wiring and AV nipping.

Arteriosclerotic changes persist after blood pressure is lowered; however, some hypertensive retinopathy changes may resolve, such as cotton-wool spots, the macular star and papilloedema, though these may take weeks to months. Management would involve managing the hypertension and its underlying cause.

Viva questions

Q1   How would you grade hypertensive retinopathy?

TABLE 8.4 Hypertensive retinopathy stages

Grade	Description
Grade 1	Generalised arteriolar constriction (or narrowing/attenuation) causing: Silver wiring of vessels Vessel tortuosity
Grade 2	The above plus AV nipping
Grade 3	The above plus Cotton wool spots Flame and blot haemorrhages
Grade 4	The above plus Papilloedema

The prognoses of grades 3 and 4 are similar, irrespective of the presence of papilloedema; both represent malignant or the accelerated phase of hypertension, with a high incidence of severe end-organ damage and mortality. Accelerated hypertension is an acute increase in BP, higher than usual baseline hypertension resulting in vascular damage (flame haemorrhages, hard exudates) and optic disc swelling. End-organ damage may include renal failure, myocardial ischaemia and stroke.

Q2   What is the pathophysiology of papilloedema?
- Papilloedema can progress through various advanced stages.
- Papilloedema by definition is optic disc swelling as a result of raised ICP (which can appear within a few hours of this developing, but usually takes weeks or months to appear and is therefore usually a late sign of raised intracranial pressure).
- This raised CSF pressure is transmitted along the subarachnoid space of the optic nerve sheath, causing venous stasis, dilated tortuous veins and capillaries, leading to bilateral hyperaemic discs with blurred margins and loss of venous pulsations (this implies raised ICP).
- Once it progresses, retinal infarction leads to the development of cotton-wool spots and retinal haemorrhages from engorgement of retinal veins. This results in enlargement of the blind spot, which can be examined by assessing the visual fields. Following this, hard exudates appear on the disc.

■ Patients often have no visual disturbance.

■ The causes of papilloedema are any cause of raised intracranial pressure.

There are many other causes of optic disc swelling, of which papilloedema is the likely case in the exam. If you are asked to differentiate, note that the presence of spontaneous venous pulsation excludes papilloedema. Other causes of optic disc swelling include accelerated hypertension, pseudo-papilloedema, central retinal vein occlusion, hypercarbia and ischaemic optic neuropathy, amongst others.

Benign intracranial hypertension is a condition affecting young obese women on the oral contraceptive pill and steroids, who present with raised CSF pressures leading to headaches and papilloedema. Patients are managed by reducing the CSF pressure through therapeutic lumbar puncture with CSF siphoning.

Honours response

Q3   What are the clinical signs and symptoms of raised ICP?

■ early-morning headaches, which are worse on bending down, coughing or straining

■ nausea and vomiting

■ papilloedema

■ if severe:
— reduced levels of consciousness
— Cushing's triad – high systolic BP, low HR and wide pulse pressure

Good response

Case 3: Diabetic retinopathy

Instructions: Please review these images of a diabetic patient over the course of their disease.

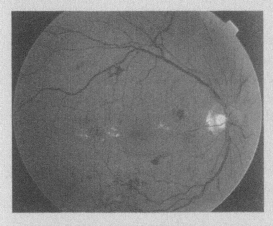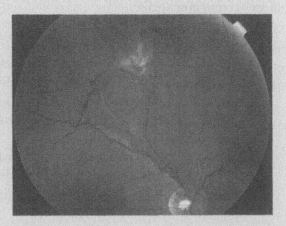

FIGURE 8.3A–B Diabetic retinopathy

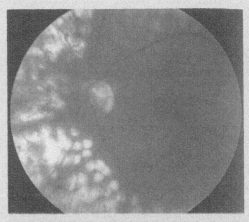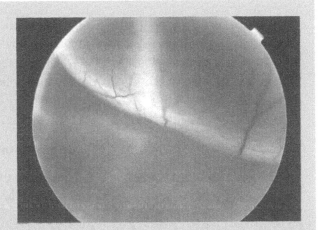

FIGURE 8.4A–B Diabetic retinopathy

Key features to look for
❏ **Non-proliferative**
- ■ **Background retinopathy (Figure 8.3A)**
  - — microaneurysms: small red **dots**; often the first clinical sign
  - — **blot** haemorrhages
  - — Leaking **hard exudates**

At this stage, good diabetic and blood pressure control is required to reduce progression. These signs don't affect visual acuity.
- ■ **Pre-proliferative retinopathy**
  - — the above features and:
    - • cotton-wool spots
    - • venous beading and dilatation of retinal veins
    - • larger blot haemorrhages
❏ **Proliferative (Figure 8.3B)**
- ■ the above features plus:
  - — neovascularisation
  - — preretinal or vitreous haemorrhage
  - — laser photocoagulation scarring may be seen (Figure 8.4A)
  - — retinal detachment due to new tissue production and scarring (Figure 8.4B)

AUTHOR'S TOP TIP

Pre-retinal haemorrhage can also occur in a subarachnoid haemorrhage. The appearance has been described as like a birds nest. It is also called a subhyaloid haemorrhage.

Complete the examination
❏ *'To complete my exam, I would like to examine for visual acuity and other diabetic eye complications.'* (*See* Viva Q2)

Diabetic retinopathy was historically classified into background, pre-proliferative and proliferative retinopathies; diabetic maculopathy and retinal detachment are also further classifications. Newer classification systems (used above) subdivide these into two main categories: proliferative and non-proliferative retinopathy. These are beyond the scope of this revision guide.

AUTHOR'S TOP TIP

The exact classification system is not too important for finals and simply being able to recognise the various degrees of changes that can be seen in progressive diabetic retinopathy is far more important, as well as differentiating from hypertensive retinopathy. The presence of microaneurysms distinguishes diabetic retinopathy from hypertensive retinopathy.

Diabetic eye disease occurs due to microvascular disease with endothelial cell wall damage, basement membrane thickening and loss of vascular pericytes which decreases structural integrity of the vessel wall.

Diabetes is a common cause of blindness; changes due to diabetes will be seen in type 1 diabetics after 10 years and the majority of type 2 diabetics who have had the disease for at least 15–20 years. It is far more common, however, in type 1 diabetics where almost all patients unfortunately develop retinopathy, despite optimal therapy.

The prevalence of diabetic retinopathy is 25%; prevention is therefore very important, and so routine screening of all diabetic patients annually via digital retinal photography has reduced vision loss in a significant number of diabetic patients. Another good preventative measure is tight glycaemic control, and so review patients' HbA1c regularly; however, be careful, as rapid correction of a poorly controlled diabetics glycaemic control may in fact worsen the retinopathy once present. A point to bear in mind is in those with background retinal changes, there can be a rapid development of proliferative retinopathy during pregnancy. The presence of renal failure and hypertension can also worsen retinopathy.

In some cases of diabetic retinopathy, laser photocoagulation may be required to prevent vision loss occurring. Most patients are, however, registered blind by middle age. By this stage, most patients would also have other complications, including other neuropathies as well as macrovascular complications such as MI or stroke.

Viva questions

Q1   What is diabetic maculopathy?
- This is a further stage of diabetic retinopathy whereby diabetic eye disease is seen within one disc diameter of the macula.
- Typically, the changes seen are of haemorrhages, exudates (circinate rings) and swelling within the macula.
- There is loss of vision, especially fine visual acuity.
- Maculopathy requires specialist referral to an ophthalmologist for consideration of focal laser therapy.

The macula is an important area of the eye containing the fovea, which has the highest concentration of cone cells, which allow for high levels of visual acuity; cone cells are also needed to see colours.

Good response

Q2   What other eye complications can occur in diabetics?

Difficult question

- increased risk of glaucoma and cataracts
- 6th cranial nerve palsy, amongst others
- increased risk of herpes zoster and conjunctivitis
- central retinal vein and artery occlusion

Q3   How would you treat diabetic retinopathy?
Aside from managing glycaemic control and screening (*see* Q4), treatment varies according to the stage of disease.

TABLE 8.5 Treatment of diabetic retinopathy

Disease stage	Management
Non-proliferative diabetic retinopathy	Mild disease, i.e. microaneurysms only, patients need annual screening and good diabetic control
(i.e. background & pre-proliferative)	More severe stages require specialist referral and prophylactic laser photocoagulation
Proliferative diabetic retinopathy	Laser photocoagulation therapy urgently
Vitreous haemorrhage	Surgical evacuation of vitreous blood. This has numerous complications including loss of eye.
Diabetic maculopathy	*See* Viva Q1 above.

Q4   What key features are very important for preventing diabetic retinopathy?

Difficult question

1. tight glycaemic control
2. tight blood pressure control (< 127/75 mmHg)
3. smoking cessation, due to smoking's prothrombotic and vascular damaging nature

Q5   How does laser photocoagulation therapy work?

Honours question

- The laser damages areas of the retina not involved with vision, the so-called ineloquent areas.
- Damage to ischaemic areas of the retina leads to inhibition of angiogenic factor production and thereby attenuating neovascularisation.
- It can also be used to treat oedema and microaneurysms as well as haemorrhages.

- There may be several thousand photocoagulation scars produced over a treatment course.
- Loss of peripheral vision is a known complication of treatment; however, the treatment aims to reduce the risk of severe debilitating vision loss.

Case 4: Retinitis pigmentosa

Instructions: Please examine this 30-year-old man who is complaining of difficulty seeing in the dark.

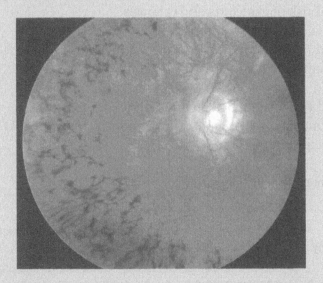

FIGURE 8.5 Retinitis pigmentosa

Key features to look for

❏ **Visual acuity**
- reduced

❏ **Visual fields**
- tunnel vision

❏ **Fundoscopy**
- web-like areas of hyperpigmentation which appear like pigmented bony spicules
- seen in the peripheries of the retina
- optic atrophy may be seen

Complete the examination

- *'To complete my exam, I would like to examine for poor colour vision using Ishihara plates and check to see if the patient has a white walking aid.'*

This is where you can demonstrate honours-level performance, by mentioning the white walking aids used by the registered blind.

❏ **Thank the patient**
❏ **Wash your hands**
❏ **Present your findings**

Retinitis pigmentosa is an inherited group of diseases resulting in progressive cases of blindness. The disorder can be inherited via autosomal dominance (AD), autosomal recessive (AR) or X-linked patterns, the latter two tending to be the more aggressive forms. This group of disorders affects the epithelium of the retinal pigment and the photoreceptors themselves. There is progressive apoptosis, traditionally affecting the rod cells to a greater extent than the cones. It is characterised by a triad of signs and symptoms (*see* Viva Q1).

Although the most common of the inherited retinal disorders, there is currently no medical treatment available which stops disease progression; however, aids are available to help augment night vision. Patients need regular follow-up as central visual field loss occurs late in disease and most patients are registered blind by middle age. Patients should be referred for genetic counselling.

Viva questions

Q1 What questions would you like to ask the patient?

Difficult question

Patients typically have a triad of signs and symptoms, so ask or actively seek findings along the lines of the following:

- **Tunnel vision:** progressive peripheral vision loss due to preferential cone loss; there may be cone involvement but this is variable with different forms of the disease
- **Night-time blindness:** due to loss of rods
- **Pigmented bony spicules:** features seen on ophthalmoscopy

There is often a family history of blindness due to the diseases' inheritance patterns, so this would be a potential question to ask the patient. Night-time blindness can be a complication of photocoagulation burns in those with diabetic eye disease; in fact, this is the most common non-inherited cause.

Q2 What are some of the conditions associated with retinitis pigmentosa?

Honours question

TABLE 8.6 Associations of retinitis pigmentosa

Association	Description
Refsum's disease	A disorder of phytanic acid metabolism inherited in an autosomal recessive pattern causing peripheral neuropathy, deafness, ichthyosis and cerebellar ataxia
Usher's disease	Autosomal recessive disorder with non-progressive sensorineural deafness
Kearns–Sayre syndrome	Mitochondrial inheritance disorder with ophthalmoplegia, heart block and ptosis
Abetalipoproteinaemia	Autosomal recessive disorder with neurological and muscular impairments. Commonly seen in Ashkenazi Jews.

AUTHOR'S TOP TIP

You would not be expected to know any of the above associations, and so being aware of just one will impress any examiner.

Q3 What does 'registered blind' mean?

Honours question

- The local authority in which the patient lives takes responsibility for registering persons who are blind.
- A voluntary application is made on behalf of the patient by an ophthalmologist.
- Eye disease criteria that need to be met for the requirements of registered blindness are complex; likewise with registration for partially sighted patients (and are beyond the scope of this revision guide). However, in general these are based on poor visual acuity and substantial visual field loss. Note that patients do not need to be completely unable to see to be registered.
- Registration offers the patient certain benefits, including tax allowances and various other concessions.
- Patients can be referred to the Royal National Institute for the Blind for any aids, including guide dogs.

AUTHOR'S TOP TIP

Remember, if you ever mention a term in finals make sure you know what it means. You may be questioned on it!

8.2 OPHTHALMOLOGY HISTORIES

Novices to ophthalmology may become overwhelmed by the level of knowledge and understanding required in this specialty to make an accurate diagnosis based upon history alone; it is very difficult to convince an examiner that you know how to take such a history if you've never had any experience of ophthalmological history-taking, as there are unique aspects to such a history, not least the terms used. However, having a basic understanding of commonly used terms will help ensure your referral to an ophthalmologist goes smoother. Whilst you would not be expected to have a special interest in ophthalmology for finals, you would be expected at the very least to know that eye signs and symptoms should be taken seriously, as the risk of visual loss is a significant cause of lifelong morbidity for the patient. Below, we describe commonly encountered short history cases you may come across.

TABLE 8.7 Ophthalmology terms

Term	Description
Floaters	These are vitreous opacities, which appear as small dark spots in the visual field
	Can be referred to as spots by patients
Haloes	A sign of acute glaucoma
	Can be referred to as spots by patients
Flashing lights	A sign of retinal detachment; can be seen in migraines
	Can be referred to as spots by patients

Visual disturbance or loss of vision can occur acutely or be gradual in onset. It is important to take a focused history trying to elicit whether there is pain, and whether visual loss is unilateral or affecting both eyes. Other features in the history that aid in diagnosis include: presence of double vision or blurred vision as opposed to loss of vision, visual loss confined to specific areas of the visual field, presence of floaters/flashing lights/haloes, or migraine-associated symptoms such as a visual aura. Chronically raised ICP classically leads to temporary loss of vision when bending over. Remember that neurophthalmological pathology (*see* Chapter 7) is also an important cause of vision loss. The following characteristic features help in coming up with a sensible differential diagnosis.

TABLE 8.8 Visual disturbance

Duration	Characteristic features & aetiology
Acute loss of vision	**Unilateral central vision loss:** optic neuritis
	Unilateral variable vision loss: retinal haemorrhage, detachment, central retinal artery or vein occlusion
Chronic loss of vision	**Unilateral or bilateral central vision loss:** cataracts, age-related macular degeneration
	Unilateral or bilateral peripheral vision loss: retinitis pigmentosa, retinal detachment, primary open-angle glaucoma

Probably the most common incidental eye-related finding you will see in clinical practice is a cataract. There are many causes, including steroid induced, trauma and hypoparathyroidism, amongst many others, however one of the most common is diabetes, and if you should find a cataract incidentally, always exclude this as a cause. It is age related and is therefore commonly seen in those over 65 years old. It is also one the most common causes of treatable blindness in the UK. Treatment is surgical, with either YAG laser or phacoemulsification.

History Case 1: Acute closed-angle glaucoma (ACAG)

Instructions: Please take a history from this 60-year-old lady who is complaining of new-onset acute right eye pain.

Key features to look for

- ❑ **Age:** tends to occur in middle age or later
- ❑ **Unilateral signs:** unilateral red eye should make you consider ACAG; bilateral disease is more suggestive of conjunctivitis

❏ **Red painful eye:** severe eye pain, described as 'deep boring pain'; vomiting can occur due to severe pain, there may be headache
❏ **Preceding symptoms:** blurry vision with haloes seen around objects, especially lights at night; these symptoms commonly precede acute attacks
❏ **Decreased vision**

Completion

Aqueous humor is produced in the eye by the ciliary body in the posterior chamber; it diffuses through the pupil into the anterior chamber and into the vascular system via the trabecular meshwork and Schlemm's canal. ACAG is caused by sudden closure of the drainage angle. Several anatomic variations predispose to ACAG:

❏ shallow anterior chambers
❏ thin iris
❏ thin ciliary body
❏ thicker lens which is anterior situated
❏ shorter eyeballs

Acute closed-angle glaucoma typically occurs in middle-aged and elderly patients who are long-sighted. Patients present with red eye, severe pain, decreased visual acuity, increased IOP, corneal oedema (steamy/hazy), a narrow anterior chamber and a fixed (unreactive) mid-dilated pupil; it is an emergency.

Viva questions

Q1 How would you investigate this patient?

Difficult question

- ask about precipitating events: dim light, medications (anticholinergics, sympathomimetics, e.g. dilating eye drops)
- intraocular pressure (IOP): raised to 60–70 mmHg, normal is 15–20 mmHg

Q2 What treatment options are available for this patient?
- analgesia
- acetazolamide: PO or IV reduces aqueous formation
- pilocarpine eye drops: to constrict the iris and open the channels for drainage
- beta-blocker eye drops
- laser or surgical peripheral iridotomy is usually performed 24–48 hours after IOP is medically controlled and is considered a definitive treatment for ACAG

Q3 What other causes of red eye do you know of?

Honours question

TABLE 8.9 Causes of the red eye

Aetiology	Description
Uveitis	Anterior uveitis usually presents acutely as an emergency and is more common than posterior uveitis. This is classically associated with HLA-B27 conditions such as Reiter's syndrome and anklyosing spondylitis. It is often idiopathic, but can also occur in Behçet's disease, IBD, SLE and RA. Uveitis causes an acutely painful and watery (excessive tearing) red eye with photophobia and blurred vision. Uveitis can also affect the posterior uvea. Posterior uveitis presents with **painless** impaired vision.
	Signs: pain, significant photophobia, decreased visual acuity, small pupils, and normal corneas and IOP
Scleritis	This is associated with vasculitis, sarcoidosis and rheumatoid disease, amongst others.
	Episcleritis, however, causes superficial redness with minimal pain. It is a self-limiting idiopathic condition, although it can be associated with rheumatoid arthritis.
Conjunctivitis	Usually, this is bilateral, and the conjunctiva is red, inflamed and hyperaemic. Can be infective in nature with an associated discharge, or have an allergic aetiology with associated lacrimation, itch and chemosis. Consider sexually transmitted diseases in young adults.
	Signs: minimal or no pain, minimal photophobia, but normal visual acuity, pupil size, cornea and IOP
Reiter's syndrome	This is a combination of arthritis, conjunctivitis and urethritis. It can present following infection with certain STDs such as gonorrhoea.
Subconjuctival haemorrhage	Can be caused by trauma or a sudden increase in intrathoracic pressure, e.g. coughing, Valsalva, hypertension and blood dyscrasias.
Keratitis	Inflammation of the cornea, commonly due to infections (HSV), trauma (particularly contact lens) or an immune reaction. Presents with blurring of vision, eye pain and a gritty feeling in the eyes.

Note that this is not an exhaustive list, and that trauma is also an important cause. The red eye is a common complaint for which you may be the first clinician assessing the patient, it is therefore important you do not miss serious causes of a red eye. If you are in doubt, tell the examiner that you will refer for a specialist opinion on the same day. In general, the presence of ciliary injection and pain is likely to be seen in serious causes of red eye as opposed to non-serious causes, such as episcleritis or conjunctivitis. A serious cause is usually seen as one where vision is threatened acutely.

History Case 2: Temporal arteritis

Instructions: Please examine this 60-year-old lady who is complaining of new-onset pain in her jaw on eating and intermittent disturbances to her vision.

Key features to look for

❏ **Age:** usually > 50 years old, but can be seen in the young
❏ **Headache**
❏ **Scalp tenderness:** often noticed when combing hair
❏ **Jaw claudication**
❏ **Visual disturbances:** amaurosis fugax/sudden blindness which occurs due to inflammation of temporal artery

❑ **Symptoms of PMR:** associated in around 25% of cases; large muscle group myalgias, e.g. shoulder, polyarthralgia, fever, malaise

Completion

On examination, you may find a pulsatile and tender temporal artery (scalp tenderness). It is an important diagnosis to consider in an elderly patient presenting with headache.

Viva questions

Q1   What investigations would you like to request?
- **Bloods:** raised ESR/CRP, low Hb, may have raised CK if concurrent PMR
- **Temporal artery biopsy:** is still the gold-standard investigation; demonstrates degeneration of the internal elastic lamina with inflammatory cell infiltrates and giant cells
- **Doppler US:** now being used to guide biopsy in order to gain greater yields

Q2   What treatment would you like to start on this patient?
- **Steroids:** to be started urgently; usually prednisolone 40–60 mg orally or IV hydrocortisone if ongoing optic involvement. Giant cell arteritis can lead to blindness, which is preventable with prompt steroid treatment once the diagnosis is suspected.

CHAPTER 9

Dermatology

9.1 INTRODUCTION

Dermatology is one of those specialties where during medical school if you blinked long enough you may have just missed it. Clinical attachments in dermatology are few and far between, and therefore, unsurprisingly, tend to be the Achilles heel of many medical students in finals. But no matter what your opinion is of the specialty, one thing is certain: you will see at least one case in finals. Although luckily, due to dermatology's short case nature, most of what you will see will be in the form of spot diagnoses, typically involving photographic images with a few quick-fire questions about management and differentials. For those unlucky enough to have a full station dedicated to this specialty, and consequently actual patients with lesions, you must take a standard approach as you would do for any other system examination, beginning with your introduction to the patient and examining the lesion as you would any other organ system. We have taken this latter approach, detailing the clinical examination and the possible viva questions that are not too infrequently seen in finals, as well as what would be expected of an honours student.

You must remember one key fact: the art of dermatology is about pattern recognition. It is this pattern rather than the actual phenotypic characteristics of the lesion that is paramount to diagnosis, as a psoriatic lesion can look different from one patient to another. It is therefore imperative you spend a great deal of time looking at images of the various skin conditions that could come up in finals. Clearly, it is not possible to include images of all the possible conditions you are likely to come across in finals in this study guide; we suggest therefore you spend some time in a dermatology clinic; most registrars and consultants would be more than welcoming. These are often walk-in clinics, so the variety of pathology you may see can be tremendous, ranging from the commonly seen acne and its various grades of severity to rare dermatological manifestations of clinically advanced systemic diseases. However, as we can appreciate, time is in short supply in the lead-up to finals, and so we recommend that a good dermatology atlas in colour would be well worth an investment.

A rather pessimistic colleague of ours once said that it doesn't really matter if you can't diagnose the lesion, his argument being that all patients get topical steroids anyway. This is not the manner with which you should present yourself in finals. Dermatology is a unique specialty, which you will undoubtedly come across and sometimes unexpectedly throughout your foundation years. No doubt a friend or family member will soon ask you if you wouldn't mind looking at this 'thing I have', only for you to be bemused by the lesion before you and simply diagnose a 'lesion' or worse yet, a 'mole'. The term 'mole' is vague and clinically not very helpful.

Although detailed management of skin conditions would not be expected of a final-year student, you must demonstrate to the examiner that you are able to describe a lesion succinctly and precisely over the phone such that the dermatologist on the other end can accurately diagnose your lesion; this is enough to pass finals. An important differential you must always consider is melanoma and/or other skin cancers. Examiners are keen to know that you will not dismiss such lesions and that you can recognise them. See our companion text, *The Ultimate Guide to Passing Surgical Clinical Finals*, for these lesions. As such, we will concentrate on the plethora of other skin conditions that can come up in medical finals.

For some of you, it is the first time you will come across these conditions; do not be overwhelmed by the detail in knowledge presented here, as it is unlikely that you will be expected to know the detail with which we discuss cases below. However, the fact you are aware of some of these and have a basic management plan will stand you in good stead and certainly make you stand out from the crowd. It is for this reason the majority of the viva questions would be considered difficult and/or at honours level. Remember, and we make no apologies for repeating this, simply being able to accurately describe the lesion and having one or two differentials would be enough to pass finals.

AUTHOR'S TOP TIP

Knowing the management of the conditions detailed here, as well as distinguishing features of the disease will be considered honours level.

Management in dermatology classically comprises conservative and medical measures, especially topical therapy, particularly emollients, followed by the addition of topical steroids to more 'systemic' therapies such as phototherapy and oral immunosuppressives. Occasionally, biopsies are performed in cases of doubt and managed according to a histological diagnosis. This is particularly the case in suspicious lesions, systemic diseases manifesting as skin lesions and of course in skin cancers.

Clinical examination

Introduction
As for any clinical encounter (*see* Chapter 1, Section 3).

Inspection
❑ **Describe general characteristics of lesion**
  ▪ **Site:** The site will help you in part decide the possible diagnoses; for example, is the lesion on a sun-exposed area, raising the possibility of a malignancy, or present on the palms and soles? Is there a special predilection for the flexor or extensor surfaces or is there sparing of certain areas?
  ▪ **Distribution:** Is it symmetrical (e.g. psoriasis, vitiligo), asymmetrical? On sun-exposed areas only? Bilateral lesions tend to be due to endogenous causes.
  ▪ **Size:** If a discrete lesion, estimate the size in centimetres.

- **Shape/surface appearance:** Whether round, oval or irregular.
- **Number:** Comment on the number of lesions present; is there a single lesion or multiple lesions? Or is the appearance more suggestive of a rash?
- **Extent of involvement:** Is the lesion localised, regionalised or is there widespread involvement? Is it disseminated?
- **Arrangement:** Comment also on the arrangement of the lesion, i.e. discrete, grouped, annular or linear.
- **Colour:** Describe colour of the overlying skin. Is it one discrete colour or is it variegated?

TABLE 9.1 Overlying skin colour

Colour	Possible pathology
Hypopigmentation/ paler skin	Loss of melanocytes
Red	Erythema – localised inflammation or infection
Yellow	Jaundice, xanthoma, xanthelasma
Orange	Hypercarotenemia – a benign condition following excess dietary intake of beta-carotene (a vitamin A precursor) found in orange/yellow vegetables and fruits. The skin discolouration is most obvious on the palms and soles
Purple	Kaposi's sarcoma and haemangioma, if violacious suggestive of lichen planus
Purple/grey	Ischaemic skin
Tanned	Haemochromatosis
Bluish or silverfish tinge to skin	Secondary to drug deposition, e.g. associated with amiodarone, minocycline
Black	Seen with melanocytic skin lesions such as naevi or melanoma. Also seen in infarcted skin or gangrene caused by arterial insufficiency
Blue	Mongolian spot/blue naevus
Discoloured fingernails	Green fingernails: infection by *Pseudomonas aeruginosa*
	White fingernails: hypoalbuminaemia, hereditary

- **Smell:** Sometimes, you can smell coal tar at the end of the bed, which should point you towards a diagnosis of psoriasis, although eczema is a differential.

Palpation

❑ **Describe the texture**
- This may be palpable or visible and helps in the diagnosis of the lesion, for example, in lichenification, where there is thickening of the skin following repeated rubbing, with skin markings becoming more obvious.
- Is the surface smooth, scaly, crusty or rough? Can you remove the crust or scales?
- On deeper palpation using the pulps of your thumb and index finger, is the lesion soft, firm or hard?

Lesion primary morphology

❑ **Describe characteristic morphology**
- This describes the physical changes in the skin and helps you describe the type of lesion.

■ This is a key part of your description of your physical examination findings and should include any of the following terminology:

TABLE 9.2 Terminology

Lesion	Morphology
Macule	Non-palpable lesions; usually < 10 mm in diameter, represented by a colour change on the skin, e.g. a freckle. If > 10 mm in diameter, then referred to as a patch
Papule	This is also < 10 mm in diameter, but this lesion is solid and palpable with distinct borders, e.g. a naevus, seborrhoeic and actinic keratosis
Plaques	Palpable lesions which are raised or depressed compared to the skin surface, these are > 10 mm in diameter, e.g. the plaque of psoriasis
Nodules	Solid raised lesion > 10 mm in diameter and extends to the dermis or subcutaneous tissue, e.g. lipoma, BCC
Vesicles	These are clear, fluid-filled lesions measuring < 10 mm in diameter. Seen in dermatitis herpetiformis
Bullae	Clear, fluid-filled blisters which are > 10 mm in diameter, e.g. seen following bites or burns and in pemphigus vulgaris and bullous pemphigoid
Pustules	Inflamed vesicles containing pus seen in bacterial infections, folliculitis; larger lesions are known as an abscess
Crust	Dry brown exudate
Scale	Dry skin fragments
Induration	Thickened area of the dermis and subcutaneous tissues
Annular	Ring-shaped lesions, e.g. erythema multiforme, fungal infections
Discoid	Round, oval or coin-like lesions, non-palpable, e.g. psoriasis, impetigo
Reticular	Net-like lesions, e.g. erythema ab igne
Lichenification	Skin thickening due to chronic inflammation
Excoriations	Linear erosions due to scratching. Erosions are areas of lost epidermis which heal without scarring
Petechiae	Small, non-blanching areas of haemorrhage in the skin, e.g. seen in vasculitis and meningitis
Purpura	This is a larger area of haemorrhage which may be palpable. Also known as ecchymosis or bruises
Urticaria (wheals/ hives)	This appears as pink raised lesions with a pale centre (wheal) secondary to localised oedema and can occur following drug hypersensitivity reactions or following local pressure, a reaction to temperature or sunlight, insect bites. This lesion is normally transient, lasting less than 24 hours. More severe forms can lead to angioedema
Ulcers	Here there is loss of some or all of the dermis with loss of the epidermis
Erosions	This is an area of skin that has lost its epidermal layer, seen commonly after trauma
Tumours	Solid mass of either the skin or subcutaneous tissue
Scars	Areas of the skin which have undergone fibrosis as a result of injury. This can sometimes become thickened and enlarged. For instance, a keloid scar is seen when the original scar has hypertrophied and extended beyond the initial scar margin

Lesion secondary morphology

❏ **Comment on lesion profile**
  ■ Is it flat-topped, dome-shaped, pedunculated, etc.?
❏ **Describe surface features**
  ■ Is there surface loss, i.e. loss of epidermis/dermis? Leading to erosions, ulcers or fissures?
  ■ Is there presence of an exudate on the lesion, e.g. blood or pus?
  ■ Is there crust on the surface where the exudate has dried up?

Complete the examination

  ■ Ensure you assess for any other conditions associated with your primary diagnosis, e.g. psoriatic arthropathy in psoriasis.
  ■ Assess the severity of the disease process (if possible), e.g. is there a flare-up?
  ■ Assess patient impact: discussing the psychosocial implications of skin disease offers to the examiner the understanding that you have spent time in a dermatology clinic and understand that there can be significant psychiatric comorbidity in severe skin disease.

It is not uncommon for examiners to ask if you would like to ask the patient any questions; aside from taking a quick dermatology history as for a short case, (*see* Section 3 below) it is important to assess the impact the disease process has on the patient.

EXAMINER'S TOP TIP

When the candidate mentioned he would consider referral to a psychiatrist for depression in this young woman with severely deforming skin disease, I was impressed he considered the patient as a whole and not a disease process. Well done.

Viva questions

Q1 How would you manage toxic epidermal necrolysis?
  ■ **Recognise urgency:** *'This is a medical emergency. I would resuscitate the patient, ensuring the patient's airway was patent and receiving supplemental oxygen, that his breathing was adequate and address the circulation by inserting two large bore cannulae, one into each antecubital fossa, and begin aggressive fluid resuscitation.'* (*See* Chapter 11 for overall format.)
  ■ **Initial resuscitation:** As above, and assess level of hypovolaemic shock.
  ■ **Emergency investigations:** No specific test required, but routine bloods for assessment of organ damage and/or required level of support, particularly U&Es for renal failure (due to hypovolaemia) and electrolyte disturbances. MC&S of urine, blood and skin. CXR if respiratory compromise seen. Skin biopsy enables accurate diagnosis and guides specific treatments and should be taken as early as possible.

- **Additional monitoring:** Temperature as hypothermia common. Assessment of fluid status with a CVP line.
- **Call for help:** *'After* discussion *with a senior colleague, I would like to consider the need for a specialist burns unit bed and specialist dermatology input.'*
- **Definitive treatment:** Stop the offending drug if identified and refer to burns unit or ITU for organ support as required (respiratory/renal) for wound care and sterile coverings by persons trained in burns units, as the barrier function of the skin is lost similarly to extensive burns patients. May require reverse isolation. Prevent hypothermia – ensure rewarming. Manage hypovolaemia and electrolyte disturbances. Adequate pain control and antibiotics as per microbiologist advice.

Although extremely rare (one per million incidence), mortality from TEN is 30%; therefore, it is crucial you recognise and manage the patient from the moment they attend hospital. This is a true dermatological emergency, commonly induced by drugs. Drugs which have been implicated include sulphonamides, allopurinol and penicillin, including some anticonvulsants. This mucocutaneous reaction results in widespread erythema, necrosis and detachment of the mucous membranes and epidermis. This results in exfoliation, which puts the patient at high risk of sepsis and septic shock due to the loss of protective skin barrier, which can be fatal. Respiratory failure and GI bleeding can occur with mucous membrane involvement. An important differential is Stevens–Johnson syndrome.

AUTHOR'S TOP TIP

If you mention drugs as a cause for anything in dermatology, especially antibiotics, be prepared to give at least one or two examples, as examiners will love to catch you out. Knowing the drug classes is more than enough for finals.

Dermatology is like any other specialty when it comes to emergencies. Remember all emergencies need to be managed according to ABCDs. In reality, treatment and assessment occur simultaneously. It is with this time-honoured approach to the sick patient that treatment is administered seamlessly. Do not forget to mention in your answer that early specialist referral to a burns unit as well as dermatology input are both vital components in your management plan. This shows you have spent time on a dermatology ward and are aware of the practicalities of managing such a sick patient.

AUTHOR'S TOP TIP

It is important that you do not lose your cool. Often, very able candidates falter when faced with an unfamiliar situation. Dermatology may seem alien to many of us and has the potential to catch everyone out, but if you think logically and structure your answers as you do for any medical specialty than you should sail through. Use your tried and tested strategies!

Q2 How would you manage dermatitis?

- Treat the cause if any, e.g. contact dermatitis due to patient's occupation or certain foods to be avoided. Advise to avoid frequent bathing and clothing that may cause abrasions to skin.
- **Topical:** adequate hydration of skin via emollients, bathing emollients, steroids, antibiotics if infected skin, antifungals and shampoos. Greasy ointments for dry scaly skin and water-based creams for crusted lesions. Steroid creams, ointments or lotions.
- **Oral:** antihistamines for pruritis, immunosuppressants in severe refractory cases.
- **Phototherapy:** PUVA light in refractory cases.

There are many forms of eczema, most commonly the atopic form followed by allergic contact dermatitis, a type IV hypersensitivity reaction where nickel is commonly implicated. Eczema and dermatitis are interchangeable terms. Typical features include itchy erythematous scaly patches, especially affecting the flexural areas, particularly the elbows, knees and neck. Scratching results in excoriation, lichenification and secondary bacterial infection if the skin is broken. Criteria for diagnosis include pruritus, the classical distribution on flexural surfaces in adults (extensor involvement in children) and a family history of atopy.

Q3 What are emollients?

Difficult question

- These are agents which smooth, hydrate and soothe dry, scaly skin.
- They are effective for short periods of time and thus require frequent application.
- They are commonly used in eczematous disorders and psoriasis, but can be used in any disorder causing dry skin whereby light emollients such as aqueous cream are preferred.
- Urea is the hydrating agent; occasionally topical corticosteroids are added to enhance penetration, e.g. E45, Dermol.
- In general, examples of emollients include aqueous cream, Diprobase and E45, among others.

AUTHOR'S TOP TIP

If you ever mention a drug or treatment in finals, be sure to know the mechanism of action of that drug, as the examiner is likely to question you on this. Although detailed pharmacology isn't expected for clinical medicine finals, as opposed to the pharmacology finals paper, you should still have prepared a quick verbal response to give the examiner should they ever question your general understanding of the drug you offer. In our experience, simply offering the class of the drug is more than enough to appease examiners and stop them from digging further into your knowledge!

Below are some medications you are likely to encounter in dermatology.

TABLE 9.3 Common drugs used in dermatology

Agent	Description
Calamine	An antipruritic agent; available as a lotion or cream. It is, however, often ineffective. Topical antihistamines are only marginally more effective. Insect bites are best treated with topical corticosteroids.
Daktacort	An example of a topical corticosteroid, with an added antifungal component. Many different agents are available, with various concentrations of hydrocortisone. Some contain antifungals, antimicrobials (Betnovate) or salicyclic acid. Topical steroids are used for inflammatory skin conditions such as eczema and insect bites, amongst others. It should be avoided in cases of skin infections.
Calcipotriol	Vitamin D analogue. Calcipotriol is an active form of vitamin D. Other examples include tacalcitol.
Coal tar	Crude coal tar has anti-inflammatory and anti-scaling properties. Used in chronic stable plaque psoriasis. Tar baths and shampoos are also available. Generally safe, but contact allergy and irritation can occur.
Dithranol	A hydroxyanthrone, anthracene derivative, used in chronic plaque psoriasis. Can cause staining, irritation and should be used with gloves. Burning sensation is a well known side effect.

The vehicle through which topical agents are given can affect the degree of hydration, drug penetration and has in itself a mild anti-inflammatory action. Lotions are preferred to creams/ ointments in hair-bearing areas and have a cooling effect. Ointments are greasy anhydrous water-insoluble preparations, suitable for dry chronic lesions. Creams are oil/water emulsions, which absorb well into skin. Creams are preferred by patients due to their cosmetically appealing nature; less greasy than ointments.

Case 1: Psoriasis

Instructions: Please examine this lesion.

Key features to look for
❑ There are multiple well-defined salmon-coloured plaques.
❑ Variable in size, with silver-coloured scaly surfaces.
❑ There is a preponderance on the extensor surfaces.

Complete the examination
❑ **Further examination**
- *'To complete my examination, I would like to assess the severity of disease by looking for the presence of psoriatic arthropathy, the extent of the lesions and whether there are any subtypes.'* (See Viva Q1.)
- *'I would also like to examine the nails for the characteristic pitting and onycholysis seen in psoriasis.'* (See Table 9.10.)

You may also wish to look at the scalp or behind the ears, as these tend to be coexisting sites of psoriasis. Severity in psoriasis is measured by the presence of psoriatic arthropathy, any psoriatic subtype (see Viva Q1) and the extent of plaques; there is also a formal Psoriatic Area

and Severity Index, which is beyond the scope of this revision guide. An important differential diagnosis would be dermatitis, which can look similar.
❑ **Thank the patient**
❑ **Wash your hands**
❑ **Present your findings**

Viva questions

Q1 What subtypes of psoriasis do you know of?

Honours question

TABLE 9.4 Clinical presentation of psoriasis

Presentation	Description
Nail signs	Thickening, with pitting and onycholysis, in 50%
Flexural psoriasis	Glazed smooth red lesions (erythema) commonly in the axilla and submammary regions, less scale-like lesions than other variants
	Uncommon
Erythrodermic psoriasis	Severe form with generalised erythema and scaling
	Can have significant morbidity & mortality through dehydration, fever and raised inflammatory markers
Guttate psoriasis	Numerous drop-like lesions
	Seen in adolescents commonly
	Can be due to infective causes such as streptococcal throat infection
Chronic stable plaque	These are well-demarcated, salmon-pinky-red, disc-like plaques
	Overlying silvery-white scale
	Classically affects scalp, elbows and knees
Pustular psoriasis	Erythema on soles of feet and palms of hand scattered with multiple small sterile pustules
	Can be generalised

Psoriasis is an inflammatory, proliferative disorder of the skin affecting 2% of the UK population. Its aetiology is idiopathic; however, we do know there is a genetic determination associated with various HLA genotypes, particularly HLA-B27. Some have a significant family history (30%), whilst in others it tends to appear in early adulthood following a psychosocial stressor such as trauma or pregnancy. It has been known to occur after abrupt withdrawal of steroids, exacerbated by drugs (lithium, beta blockers, indomethacin, antimalarials) and has been associated with infections, particularly HIV whereby previously existing psoriasis becomes refractory to treatment. There is overlap with rheumatological conditions such as spondyloarthropathies. On the whole, however, psoriasis tends to produce chronic stable plaques. Almost half demonstrate nail changes, and 7% can go on to develop psoriatic arthropathy, which can range from mild to severely deforming types and consequently physical limitations in activity.

Q2   What is the Koebner phenomenon?

Honours question

- Psoriasis demonstrates the Koebner phenomenon whereby lesions appear at the sites of minor trauma.
- This may even be the initial sign the patient has psoriasis.
- The Koebner phenomenon is sometimes referred to as the 'isomorphic response'.

Note that there are many other skin conditions that demonstrate the Koebner phenomenon, including vitiligo, bullous pemphigoid and lichen planus, amongst others.

Q3   What is Auspitz's sign?

Honours question

- This is when the silvery scaly covering of the psoriatic lesions can be readily removed by the examiner, revealing a vascular underlayer, with pinpoint bleeding.
- The scaly covering is keratin.
- Normal keratin is not produced, as the rapid epidermal turnover in psoriasis (nearly 10 × normal) prevents adequate differentiation of keratin.

AUTHOR'S TOP TIP

We advise you do not attempt to demonstrate Auspitz's sign! Simply mentioning this will win you plaudits.

Q4   How would you treat psoriasis?
     It is important to inform the patient that there is no cure for this disease and that treatment is indicated for symptom relief such as pain or physical limitations or cosmesis.

TABLE 9.5 Treatments for psoriasis

Therapy	Description
Topical (< 20% body affected)	**Emollients:** soft paraffin or aqueous cream
	Tar: coal tar is a safe and effective means of treating stable plaques
	Dithranol: this is the first-line treatment for stable plaques. A major drawback is that it can stain hair and plaques if applied longer than advised, therefore avoid the face. Burning can occur on flexure surfaces. Can be used in scalp psoriasis
	Vitamin D analogues: calcipotriol is used for mild to moderate stable plaques, but can cause hypercalcaemia in high doses
	Steroids: tachyphylaxis limits the use of topical steroids
	Ketarolytics: salicyclic acid can be used for scalp psoriasis, which is notoriously difficult to treat
	Topical combination steroid/antibiotic/antifungals are also available

(continued)

Therapy	Description
Systemic (oral/IV)	**Immunosupressants:** methotrexate (MTX) can be used for refractory cases where topical therapy has failed or in extensive severe psoriasis. It is also used for erythrodermic and pustular psoriatics. It is particularly helpful in cases of psoriatic arthropathy. Others include tacrolimus, ciclosporin and mycophenolate
	Systemic steroids
	Vitamin A derivatives and other retinoids
	Infliximab: this monoclonal antibody may be used for severe psoriasis
Phototherapy	**Ultraviolet B (PUVA-B):** phototherapy for guttate or widespread psoriasis. A narrow wavelength is used due to its longer disease remission rates and reduced incidence of burns. There is a risk of skin cancer and excessive skin ageing. PUVA is UVA and a psoralen. A psoralen is any naturally occurring compound used in the treatment of psoriasis; it augments the action of UVA

Honours response

There is an association with psoriasis and increased psychiatric comorbidity, particularly social phobia and major depressive disorder. As such, your answer should mention psychiatric evaluation in severely deforming skin disorders, the inclusion of which converts the previous answer into a gold-medal response.

Case 2: Alopecia areata

Instructions: Please examine this lesion.

Key features to look for

❑ A diffuse area of patchy hair loss (in normally hair-dense areas); this can be well defined.

❑ Absence of scarred hair follicles, i.e. the follicle is usually preserved in alopecia areata.

❑ There are 'exclamation mark' hairs (very short hairs that depigment as the tapering end approaches the scalp); this suggests active disease.

❑ Occasionally, fine downy depigmented regrowing hairs are seen.

Complete the examination

❑ **Further examination**

■ 'To complete my exam, I would like to assess the patient for other autoimmune disorders associated with alopecia.'

■ 'In particular, I would like to examine the nails for signs of nail pitting, ridging and thickening; the so-called sandpaper nail.'

There is an association with vitiligo and atopy.

❑ **Thank the patient**

❑ **Wash your hands**

❑ **Present your findings**

Do not confuse alopecia areata with alopecia totalis, which is loss of all scalp hair, and alopecia universalis, which is complete loss of hair from the entire body.

Viva questions

Q1 What are the treatment options available?
- **Topical:** steroids, dithranol, minoxidil, immunosuppressant such as diphencyprone (DPCP)
- **Oral:** systemic steroids
- Phototherapy

In general, treatment of a condition is divided up into conservative, medical and surgical measures. When discussing treatment options in dermatology, however, it is best to further classify your conservative and medical measures answer into topical, oral, systemic and/or phototherapy, if applicable.

Q2 What can cause alopecia?
- There are many causes of alopecia:
  - **Autoimmune:** associated with vitiligo
  - **Endocrine:** diabetes, thyroid disease (both hypo- and thyrotoxicosis), hypoparathyroidism, Addison's disease
  - **Drugs:** ciclosporin, cytotoxics, anticoagulants, anti-thyroid drugs (carbimazole, thiouracil), lithium, oral contraceptive pill
  - **Others:** androgenic baldness (male pattern), pregnancy induced, stress, Down's syndrome, nutritional deficiency (iron and zinc deficiency)
  - **Trichotillomania:** this is when patients pull out their own hair, sometimes unknowingly. Hair loss is typically unilateral, irregular and on the dominant hands' side

Note that when discussing alopecia this typically refers to the non-scarring type of alopecia, i.e. that is there is no destruction of hair follicles. The scarring form can occur in certain conditions, such as psoriasis, lupus, sarcoidosis, lichen planus and dermatitis, as well as burns. The scarring form is irreversible, whereas non-scarring alopecia may have some reversible causes.

The normal human hair follicle undergoes three phases of development, of which the resting phase (telogen) lasts up to 4 months and is typically the hair we normally find on hair brushes. Approximately 100 telogen hair follicles are lost each day normally; and at any one time the scalp contains 100 000 follicles.

Finasteride, a 5-alpha reductase inhibitor, can be used to treat male pattern baldness, whereby 70% of men can experience hair regrowth with continuous use. However, to sustain the effect, treatment would need to continue indefinitely, as discontinuation will result in hair loss.

Case 3: Acne vulgaris

Instructions: Please examine this lesion.

Key features to look for

❑ Skin appears greasy.
❑ With comedones (these may be open or closed comedones, commonly referred to as blackheads and occur due to keratin plugging of hair follicles), these are seen in

non-inflammatory cases; whiteheads may be seen (sebaceous glands that do not have a pore and are distended).

❏ Extensive scarring over the upper back (keloid scarring may be seen).

❏ Cysts may also be seen, containing sebum, i.e. inflammatory cases

❏ Sites of predilection: typically, these are areas of the body with the most abundant and largest sebaceous glands, i.e. the upper back, upper arms, face, neck and chest.

Complete the examination

❏ **Further examination**

  ■ *'To complete my exam, I would like to assess the severity of acne.'*

TABLE 9.6 Severity of acne

Severity	Features
Mild	**Morphology:** mostly comedones, which may be open or closed; some papules and pustules
	Distribution: mainly on the face
Moderate	**Morphology:** mostly inflammatory lesions, more papules and pustules than mild acne, there may be mild scarring
	Distribution: face, chest and back
Severe	**Morphology:** the above plus cysts, nodules, nodular abscesses and more extensive scarring
	Distribution: face, chest, or back

An important differential is acne rosacea; important distinguishing features are the lack of comedones and classical flushing that occurs after excess alcohol intake.

❏ **Thank the patient**

❏ **Wash your hands**

❏ **Present your findings**

Fundamentally, in acne there is increased sebum production (under androgenic and corticotrophin-releasing hormone regulation), with excessive sensitisation of sebaceous glands to androgens, rather than actual androgen excess. Abnormal follicular keratinisation leads to blockage of secretions and the formation of the classical lesion, the comedone.

Viva questions

Q1   Do you know if acne vulgaris is caused by bacteria?

                                                                          Difficult question

  ■ *Propionibacterium acnes* is the organism involved in acne vulgaris.
  ■ However, it is the colonisation and resultant growth of this organism in the pilosebaceous follicular unit which exacerbates the inflammatory response to follicular keratinisation and seborrhoea of the unit.

■ It does not actually cause acne vulgaris, rather the inflammatory response to this bacterium is what causes the lesions typical of acne.

This is almost a trick question, as on the face of it, the answer seems obvious, but do not get fooled, as it is your understanding of the organism's role in acne which is being tested, not the name of the bacterium.

Acne vulgaris is an inflammatory disorder of the pilosebaceous follicle, the causes of which are multifactorial, with genetic and hormonal factors playing a role in its development. A detailed understanding of this is not required, but simply knowing this and even correctly identifying the anaerobic organism involved will no doubt impress the examiner.

EXAMINER'S ANECDOTE

She was the first candidate to actually know and correctly pronounce the P. acnes *organism involved in acne vulgaris. She scored top marks!*

P. acnes is a normal skin commensal organism which, when follicles become blocked, flourishes in this new anaerobic environment. The importance of *P. acnes* comes to the forefront when in adolescent boys who exhibit a rare immune-mediated reaction to the organism resulting in necrotic lesions that can cause severe scarring. This is known as acne fulminans and requires admission to hospital for intravenous steroids.

Q2 What treatment options are available?
■ Options available are dependent on the severity of acne:

TABLE 9.7 Treatment for acne

Severity	Treatment
Mild	**Topical:** benzoyl peroxide, azelaic acid, topical antibiotics, e.g. clindamycin, topical retinoids
Moderate	**Oral antibiotics:** a 4–6 month course of antibiotics is first-line treatment for moderate acne, e.g. erythromycin, minocycline
	Synthetic oral retinoids: can be used in cases refractory to an antibiotic course
Severe	**Oral synthetic retinoids:** isotretinoin (Roaccutane) is the drug of choice in severe acne. It can also be used in less severe cases where there is scarring and/or associated psychiatric comorbidity. Given for a period of 4 months, up to 70% of patients have no further disease recurrence, whilst almost all patients demonstrate substantial improvement in symptoms. However, it must be prescribed by a specialist as it has many side effects, most notably teratogenicity, and so young women must take contraceptive precautions during and 1 month after course completion. LFTs will need monitoring as it can cause hepatitis. Other common side effects include headaches, myalgias and dry skin. There are reports of behavioural changes, with an increased risk of suicidal ideation. Patients will need informed consent before beginning a course

General features and aims of treatment include:
■ **Hygiene:** soap washing limited to not more than twice daily; avoid saunas or other methods causing steaming of skin

- **Manage excess sebum production:** reduce sebum production with oestrogens, anti-androgens
- **Decrease *P. acnes* activity:** benzoyl peroxide, retinoic acid, antibiotics (oral or topical)
- **Decrease inflammatory response:** topical/oral steroids
  — **Surgical management:** dermabrasion, laser resurfacing, chemical peeling

Honours response

If a course of oral antibiotics is given, these must be the same as the topical antibiotics, in order to avoid development of bacterial multidrug resistance.

Note that despite anecdotal evidence of the associations of various food items, most notoriously chocolate, with acne, studies have shown dietary restriction has no role in disease treatment.

Acne is common and the majority of patients seen in clinic will be complaining of this. The emphasis of your management and an important concept which you should get across to the examiners should be to prevent scar formation as the negative psychological impact it can have on such a young patient population cannot be underestimated. It is prudent, therefore, that you are aware of the various treatment options available, even the more invasive forms for severe disease states.

Case 4: Neurofibromatosis

Instructions: Please examine this lesion.

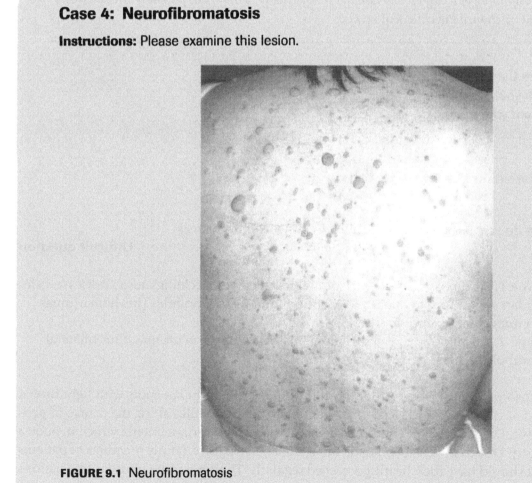

FIGURE 9.1 Neurofibromatosis

Key features to look for

❑ multiple, almost widespread, well-defined pedunculated lesions (subcutaneous nodules), occurring anywhere along peripheral nerves (neurofibroma)
❑ axillary/inguinal freckling
❑ at least six café au lait spots (brown macules)

Complete the examination

❑ **Further examination**

■ *'To complete my examination, I would like to examine visual acuity, hearing, the spine for scoliosis and check the blood pressure for possible hypertension.'*

You may also mention hypertension due to renal artery stenosis or phaeochromocytoma and the presence of Lisch nodules seen in 90% of patients (visualised on slit-lamp examination) and a feature of type 1 neurofibromatosis.

AUTHOR'S TOP TIP

If asked by the examiner if you would like to ask the patient any questions, aside from the above associated features, ask if there is a family history, as this demonstrates your understanding of its autosomal dominant inheritance. Thus if one parent is affected, there is a 50% chance the child will be also.

❑ **Thank the patient**
❑ **Wash your hands**
❑ **Present your findings**

Viva questions

Q1   What do you know of the two subtypes of neurofibromatosis?

Difficult question

■ **Type 1:** chromosome 17 association; also called von Recklinghausen's disease, café au lait spots more frequent (> 5), optic gliomas, Lisch nodules (iris hamartomas; an important diagnostic criteria)
■ **Type 2:** chromosome 22 association; bilateral acoustic neuromas, thus bilateral vestibulocochlear nerve palsies

It is an autosomal dominant disorder. Typically, there are café au lait spots with light brown macules > 1–2 cm in diameter. There may be subcutaneous nodules along the course of peripheral nerves. Diagnosis is on clinical evidence and based on certain criteria which include a family history. Due to the risk of bilateral 8th cranial nerve palsies, family members of patients with type 2 should have their hearing screened regularly. There are some unusual associations with this condition, aside from the aforementioned, which you are not required to know.

However, if asked as part of an honours question, some well-known associations include epilepsy, retinal hamartomas and learning disabilities. Most patients are asymptomatic and so require no treatment, although if painful some neurofibromas can be removed.

Case 5: Vitiligo

Instructions: Please examine this lesion.

Key features to look for

❏ symmetrically distributed patchy areas of hypopigmentation
❏ there may be hyperpigmented borders

Complete the examination

❏ **Further examination**
  ■ *'To complete my examination, I would like to examine the scalp for alopecia.'*
❏ **Thank the patient**
❏ **Wash your hands**
❏ **Present your findings**

Patients may complain of itchiness in the sunlight. In vitiligo, there is progressive autoimmune destruction of melanocytes. There is an association with other autoimmune diseases such as Addison's disease, alopecia areata, pernicious anaemia, Graves' disease and diabetes, amongst others.

Viva questions

Q1   How would you manage vitiligo?

Difficult Question

It is difficult to manage this condition, and treatment is on the whole unsatisfactory. Specific treatment depends on extent of involvement; however, in general:
  ■ **Topical:** cosmetic camouflage for disfiguring patches, steroids, sunscreen
  ■ **Phototherapy:** long-wavelength PUVA

A furanocoumarin derivative, methoxsalen has been used topically to enhance the effect of UV light, and/or given orally in more extensive vitiligo in combination with UV light therapy.

Case 6: Erythema multiforme

Instructions: Please examine this lesion.

Key features to look for

❏ well-defined concentric lesions, occurring anywhere on the body
❏ with a central pale oedematous area, which makes the lesion look like a 'target'
❏ surrounding erythema, which can be maculopapular, with or without blisters

Complete the examination

❑ **Further examination**
- *'To complete my examination, I would like to examine the mouth and eyes, in case this could be Stevens–Johnson syndrome.'*

❑ **Thank the patient**

❑ **Wash your hands**

❑ **Present your findings**

Viva questions

Q1 What are the causes of erythema multiforme?

Difficult question

- There are many causes of erythema multiforme, and they can be divided into:
  — Drug reactions: sulphonamides, penicillin, antimalarials, barbiturates
  — Infective causes: *Mycoplasma*, HIV, glandular fever and herpes simplex
  — Other: lupus, Wegener's granulomatosis, sarcoidosis
  — Idiopathic

Erythema is a term which refers to the presence of red papules, macules or vesicles. In erythema multiforme, there is vasodilation and inflammation within the epidermal layer.

Q2 What is Stevens–Johnson syndrome?
- This is an immune-mediated hypersensitivity reaction, most commonly to drugs, which can be fatal.
- It is a more severe form of erythema multiforme, where it also called erythema multiforme major.
- It is thought Stevens–Johnson syndrome is clinically related to toxic epidermal necrolysis, simply differing in their expression.
- There are multiple eruptions of the bullae seen in erythema multiforme, leading to extensive denudation of skin, with an associated fever.
- Typically, there is oral, eye and genitalia involvement in initial presentation, progressing to significant involvement of the respiratory and GI systems leading to necrosis, significant fluid and electrolyte disturbances with associated increase in morbidity.
- Erythema multiforme is a cell-mediated hypersensitivity reaction to any of the above conditions (*see* Viva Q1). It is a self-limiting condition, unlike Stevens–Johnson syndrome, which is a medical emergency and requires admission to a dedicated burns unit. Treatment methods are controversial, but generally include intravenous fluids, antibiotics, corticosteroids, high-dose immunoglobulin, immunosuppressants such as azathioprine, ciclosporin and in select cases aciclovir.

Honours response

Case 7: Erythema ab igne

Instructions: Please examine this lesion.

Key features to look for

❏ there is a reticular erythematous rash
❏ usually on the abdomen, but can be lower legs and back

Complete the examination

❏ **Further examination**

- *'To complete my examination, I would like to evaluate the patient for possible hypothyroidism.'*

An important differential is livedo reticularis, which can be seen in SLE, occult malignancy and can be a normal feature in young women, particularly in cold temperatures.

❏ **Thank the patient**
❏ **Wash your hands**
❏ **Present your findings**

AUTHOR'S TOP TIP

This reticular rash if found on the abdomen is commonly seen in those who use hot-water bottles; however, you must always consider pancreatitis or any other abdominal malignancy as a possible cause. This is a commonly tested feature in the exam.

Viva questions

Q1 What is erythema ab igne?
- This reticular pigmented rash occurs due to repeated exposure to a localised heat source, most commonly a hot-water bottle for those who use this as a form of pain relief, thus commonly seen on the abdomen and back.
- It can be also be seen on the lower legs of patients who sit in front of fireplaces.

Case 8: Digital clubbing

Instructions: Please examine this lesion.

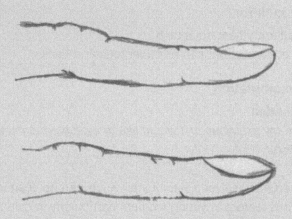

FIGURE 9.2 Clubbing

Key features to look for

❑ swelling of the terminal phalanx like a drumstick with increased curvature of the nail
❑ increased angle between nail and nail bed; demonstrated by diamond sign test
❑ increased fluctuance on palpation
❑ there may be nicotine staining

Complete the examination

❑ **Further examination**
 ■ *'To complete my exam, I would like to examine the feet for clubbing of the toes and palpate the wrists for tenderness.'*
 ■ *'I would also like to look for a cause of clubbing.'*

Try to quantify the phase of clubbing, if at all possible (*see* below).
❑ **Thank the patient**
❑ **Wash your hands**
❑ **Present your findings**

Viva questions

Q1 What are the causes of clubbing?
 'The causes of clubbing are idiopathic, lung cancer, inflammatory bowel disease and cystic fibrosis.'

Average response

'The most common cause of digital clubbing is idiopathic. However, there are many causes of clubbing, and they can be classified into:

TABLE 9.8 Causes of clubbing

Classification	Causes
Gastrointestinal causes	Inflammatory bowel disease
	Primary biliary cirrhosis, liver cirrhosis
	Coeliac disease, tropical sprue
	Lymphoma of the GI tract
Respiratory causes	Bronchogenic carcinoma
	Suppurative lung disease, e.g. bronchiectasis, cystic fibrosis, lung abscess, empyema
	Mesothelioma, fibrosing alveolitis
Cardiac causes	Congenital cyanotic heart disease
	Endocarditis, atrial myxoma
Other causes	Familial
	Idiopathic
	Graves' disease (thyroid acropachy)

Good response

This is a perfect example of how one can demonstrate their breadth and depth of knowledge using aetiological sieves. It is very easy to jump in with numerous random causes of clubbing; as previous finalists ourselves, we can understand that in the pressure of finals, being given a relatively easy question such as this can make some candidates rush their answer, with an almost comical sigh of relief at the end of their response that they've managed to mention so many causes. This is not the appropriate response to such a question. It is important to remain composed and not to read off lists as quickly as possible. The examiner will only get confused and this will not help you. It is far better to classify as described above and give a few examples of each. This gives you time to collect your thoughts and think of answers instead of memorising lists. Try to stand out from the crowd and give a well-thought-out structured response to a very common question!

EXAMINER'S ANECDOTE

He spoke so fast I barely understood a word he said. Classify, classify, classify!

If you come across unilateral digital clubbing and are asked for possible causes, consider aneurysm of the axillary artery or AV malformations of the brachial artery; these are rare.

Q2 Do you know of any stages of clubbing?

Honours question

TABLE 9.9 Grades of clubbing

Phase	Description
Grade 1: Terminal phalanx swelling	The soft tissue of the terminal phalanx swells, leading to a fluctuant nail bed. This increased fluctuance can be palpated on examination. Cyanosis and glossiness of the skin at the nail root is also seen.
Grade 2: Loss of angle between nail plate and fold	This is a permanent and defining feature of clubbing. The diamond sign test is useful in demonstrating this. The angle may also be increased > 180.
Grade 3: Increased nail curvature	Occurs due to soft tissue hypertrophy leading to the drumstick appearance.
Grade 4: Hypertrophic pulmonary osteoarthropathy (HPOA)	The most severe form. Patients complain of wrist and ankle joint tenderness, and occasionally the elbow and knees on palpation due to bony changes.

Digital clubbing will move through the above four phases consequentially, with HPOA representing the severest form. Rapid onset of HPOA should alert you to consider a diagnosis of bronchogenic carcinoma.

In our experience, many students demonstrate the diamond sign with their patient but don't actually know what it means. Most understand that by asking the patient to approximate with their fingers and noting the absence of the normal diamond-shaped window confirms the presence of clubbing. Although what most students don't know is that by demonstrating this sign, they are in fact proving that the clubbing is indeed in either Grade 2 or 3 of development, a fact which would impress any examiner as well as demonstrate your understanding of why you are doing certain clinical tests. (*See* companion text, *The Ultimate Guide to Passing Surgical Clinical Finals*, Figure 4.3.)

Q3   Do you know why clubbing occurs?

Honours question

- The pathophysiology of clubbing is ill understood.
- It may be related to increased growth hormone activity causing excessive tissue growth in the nail bed, tumour necrosis factor and even the vagus nerve has been implicated as vagotomy can reverse clubbing.
- Vasodilation of vessels in the nail due to an unknown vasodilator agent leading to increased blood flow to fingers. Defective inactivation of this unknown vasodilator is thought to be the mechanism.

The important thing to remember from a finals point of view is that there are numerous theories that have been put forward to explain the pathophysiology of clubbing. Simply being aware of one of the above will impress the examiner.

Q4   What other nail changes are associated with disease?

Difficult question

TABLE 9.10 Nail changes

Nail sign	Description
Mees' lines	Linear white discolouration seen in arsenic poisoning
Leukonychia	White discolouration seen in chronic liver disease, but can also be congenital or fungal in origin
Beau's lines	These are transverse depressions of the nail, which occur in severe disease states. Although a non-specific sign, it may represent altered growth rates, even temporary arrest in growth. Consequently this can help approximate length of disease state, as nails normally grow at 0.1mm daily, taking almost 4 months to grow out fully
Koilonychia	Nails look spoon-shaped, i.e. brittle and concave. Commonly seen in iron-deficiency anaemia, but is also a feature of thyrotoxicosis
Nail discolouration	**Blue:** a blue lunula is associated with Wilson's disease and antimalarial drugs
	Yellow: associated with rheumatoid arthritis, nephrotic syndrome, pleural effusions, tetracycline use, dystrophic nails
	Brown: a feature of chronic renal failure (CRF) and dystrophic nails; a distal transverse band of brown is seen in liver disease and heart failure but can also be a normal sign in the elderly (Terry's nails). 'Half and half' nails are seen in CRF and rheumatoid arthritis, whereby the distal half of the nail is brown-pink and the proximal end pale (Lindsay's nails)
	Green: *Pseudomonas* infection of nail
Nail pitting	Numerous depressions or 'pits' are seen in the nail. Associated with psoriasis, vitiligo, alopecia areata and dermatitis
Onycholysis	This is when the nail plate is separated from and literally lifted off the nail bed. This is seen in psoriasis and thyrotoxicosis as well as hypothyroidism and diabetes, where it is important if found to exclude an underlying fungal infection. Excessive exposure to detergents has also been implicated
Onychomycosis	Fungal infections leading to nail dystrophy. A fungal nail infection will lead to features of discolouration, nail thickening and onycholysis. Bacterial infections tend to be due to *Staphylococcus* species
Onychogryphosis	This is hypertrophy and thickening of the nail plate. Associated with chronic traumatic injury

9.2   MISCELLANEOUS SKIN CONDITIONS

The following are other possible cases that may come up in finals and that you would be expected to recognise.

TABLE 9.11A Miscellaneous skin changes

Condition	Description
Dermatomyositis	Polymyositis is an inflammatory skeletal muscle disorder of unknown aetiology. In the presence of skin lesions, it is termed dermatomyositis. Patients may complain of proximal muscle weakness, manifested as difficulty in climbing stairs or standing up from a chair. You should always consider possible malignancy, as dermatomyositis is associated with colorectal, breast, ovarian and lung cancers. Investigations include ANA, specifically anti-Jo-1, abnormal EMGs, elevated CK, AST and LDH.

(*continued*)

Condition	Description
Dermatomyositis (*cont.*)	**Morphology:** heliotrope (lilac coloured) rash around eyes, Gottron's papules (red scaly eruptions) on the MCP and IP joints of the hands. Knee and elbow erythema (Gottron's sign). Erythema of the nail folds, nail infarcts and telangiectasia. **Treatment:** management of underlying cancer if any, most patients are given steroids (prednisolone), for refractory cases, high-dose iv immunoglobulin or methotrexate and/or azathioprine. There is an 80% 5-year survival rate for those on treatment.
Ichthyosis	A skin disorder characterised by abnormal keratinisation and epidermal differentiation. It can be acquired or inherited in a number of ways (X-linked, autosomal dominant or recessive). Its presence may be seen as a cutaneous marker of malignancy, particularly Hodgkin's disease and multiple myeloma. **Morphology:** rough, dry, fish-scale-like skin. Scarring alopecia may be seen and hyperkeratotic palmar creases. **Treatment:** emollients and moisturisers containing urea.
Lichen planus	This relapsing remitting condition of unknown cause leads to thickening of the epidermis with excessive keratinisation. Patients complain of excessive pruritis. **Morphology:** well-demarcated shiny elevated plaques with purplish flat tops and intermittent fine white streaks (Wickham's striae). Scratch marks due to excessive itching. Distribution tends to be on flexor aspects of the wrist and ankles, but can be seen in the mouth, genitalia, nails and scalp. They may exhibit the Koebner phenomenon. Note that lichenification itself can be seen in many other skin disorders. **Treatment:** topical steroids, UV light
Impetigo	This is a skin infection typically affecting children; *Staphylococcus aureus* is the usual organism. **Morphology:** honeycomb-coloured well-defined crust-like lesions with an erythematous base. Distribution tends to be on nose and face. **Treatment:** oral antibiotics and topical fusidic acid.

TABLE 9.11B Miscellaneous skin changes

Condition	Description	
Pemphigus & pemphigoid	**Pemphigoid** This a benign relapsing remitting condition typically affecting the elderly. Occurs due to IgG autoantibodies to basement membrane. **Morphology:** tense blister-like lesions of a few mm to cm in size. Distribution tends to be on flexor surfaces and the trunk. Oral lesions are rare. Skin biopsy confirms diagnosis **Treatment:** steroids and immunosuppressants	**Pemphigus** This is a rare group of disorders causing widespread epidermal blisters. The commonest type, pemphigus vulgaris typically affects the mucous membranes of the mouth, progressing to widespread superficial blisters and bullae that break easily. Sloughing of the normal epidermis on rubbing contact (Nikolsky's sign) is a feature. Bacterial secondary infection is a risk. Morbidity is high. Affects young patients (< 40 years). Occurs due to IgG autoantibodies to desmosomal components. **Morphology:** flaccid blisters, which easily lead to bullous eruptions rendering red tender patches or widespread erosions. Lesions can be 1–2 cm. Oral lesions are common. Skin biopsy confirms diagnosis. **Treatment:** high-dose systemic steroids (prednisolone), azathioprine, MTX and ciclosporin. Patients also require iv fluids, antibiotics and barrier nursing.

(*continued*)

Condition	Description
Shin-related disorders	**Pretibial myxoedema**

Pretibial myxoedema

This rare sign is pathognomonic of Graves' disease. Its presence is a late manifestation and patients often exhibit thyroid eye disease as well by this stage.

Morphology: raised symmetrical lesions over the anterior aspect of lower legs, but can occur elsewhere. They are well-demarcated red/brown lesions with shiny overlying skin and a peau d'orange appearance. Lesions may be tender to palpation and can demonstrate non-pitting oedema in the advanced stage. **Treatment:** manage underlying cause, intralesional steroids, octreotide.

Erythema nodosum

Classically seen in sarcoidosis and tuberculosis, but can also be a feature of many other conditions: lymphoma, pregnancy, IBD, drug induced (sulphonamides, tetracyclines & OCP), infective causes such as *Salmonella*, *Campylobacter* and *Streptococcus* species.

Morphology: tender bilateral erythematous nodular lesions found over the anterior aspects of the leg. Nodules tend to flatten with healing as the lesion evolves over several weeks. They may be warm to touch and can be multiple and variable in size. Not limited to the legs. Diagnosis is made definitively by wedge biopsy. **Treatment:** manage underlying cause; hot/cold compresses, NSAIDs, steroids, salicylates.

Pyoderma gangrenosum

Classically found on the lower limbs, but can be seen on any body part, including the face. Associated with inflammatory bowel disease, especially ulcerative colitis, whereby its presence indicates active UC. It is also seen in rheumatic disease, hepatitis, diabetes, sarcoidosis, myeloproliferative disorders and can be idiopathic in over half of cases.

Morphology: painful necrotic ulcer, with irregular hypertrophic edges and surrounding purple erythematous plaques and pustules. **Treatment:** manage underlying cause, high-dose oral and intralesional steroids, immunosuppressants and/or antibiotics. A skin graft or muscle flap may even be required.

CHAPTER 10

Rheumatology

Rheumatology is much like endocrinology in that many of the cases involve pattern recognition of a syndrome or a cursory examination comprised mainly of inspection. This lends itself well to case pictures examination, such that in any one station you may be shown several photographs of patients' signs and asked to comment on these. As before, although you are not actually physically examining a patient, it is important to let the examiner know what other associated features you would look for or ask the patient about; this is how you will gain extra marks. If you were to examine a patient, the most common instruction would be to 'look at this patient's hands'. Other locomotor system examinations such as the elbow, knees, etc. are more surgically derived and are very rarely seen in medical finals. As with all the locomotor system examination routines, the Look, Feel, Move model is integral to its successful execution.

10.1 EXAMINATION OF THE HANDS

Most rheumatological disorders you will come across in finals will be presented to you as a case in which you are asked to examine the patient's hands. It is therefore important you have some sort of examination schema in your mind with which to follow. This must appear logical and meaningful, such that you can recognise the many rheumatological conditions that occur in everyday practice. However, luckily there is only a handful of cases that could possibly be seen in finals. Below we describe the more common ones.

Clinical examination

Introduction

As for any clinical encounter (*see* Chapter 1, Section 3); specifically for this case:
- ❏ **Explain purpose and gain consent:** Explain that you will be looking at, moving and feeling the joints of the hand and wrist. Ask if the patient is in any pain (this is especially important in a hand examination, where many patients will have painful joints with restricted movement); if not, ask them to let you know if you cause them any pain during the examination, so that you can adjust or stop what you are doing.
- ❏ **Expose patient adequately:** The patient usually has on a short-sleeved shirt; otherwise, ask them to roll up their sleeves to above their elbows.
- ❏ **Position patient appropriately:** Rest a pillow on the patient's lap and ask them to place both their hands on this pillow, palms facing up.

AUTHOR'S TOP TIP

A kind and thoughtful student will always be looked upon more favourably than an abrasive one, and remember, stress is no excuse for being abrupt with your patients, as this is a reflection on what your actual clinical practice will be like once qualified. Always keep the patient's well-being above your need to examine them. When it comes to borderline cases, those few extra marks gained from building a good rapport will come in very handy.

If there is no pillow, do not make an issue of it by looking for one. Simply lay their hands on the table or, perhaps easier, get them to lay their arms out onto their own lap.

EXAMINER'S ANECDOTE

I once heard a candidate say 'You can place your arms onto MY lap'. We both knew what he meant, but it could have been clearly interpreted in a whole different manner. Be careful with instructions given to patients; they will often follow them to the letter. Practise what you plan to say to patients beforehand with a colleague so that it sounds professional and isn't derogatory.

AUTHOR'S TOP TIP

In this specific situation, it may be advisable not to offer to shake the patient's hands on formal introductions. This is because the patient may have a painful arthropathy and shaking their hands may only make them feel pain.

Look
❑ **Check around the room for any aids or appliances**
  ▪ The patient may have a walking stick or have an arm splint; comment on these as they give an indication of the patient's functional level.
❑ **Observe the palmar and dorsal aspect of hands**
  ▪ Simultaneously examine both hands, inspecting the dorsal surface, and then ask the patient to turn their hands over to inspect the palmar surface.
  ▪ Whilst doing this, assess the ease with which they can achieve this. This will give you a crude indication of the ease of supination and pronation and whether this is inhibited by pain or deformity which may be obvious.
  ▪ **Scars:** from previous surgery may be seen, e.g. Z scar from Dupuytren's repair, carpal tunnel release – associated with RA.
❑ **Identify any swelling**
  ▪ **Soft tissue swelling:** marked involvement of the wrists, MCP and PIP joints with sparing of the DIP joints is classically seen in RA; this gives the appearance of spindling of the fingers.

❑ **Describe obvious deforming joint involvement**
  - **Distribution:** is this asymmetrical (psoriatic arthropathy) or symmetrical (as seen in RA)?
  - **Pattern recognition:** *see* table below

TABLE 10.1 Deformities seen in RA

Deformity	Description
Ulnar deviation	Ulnar deviation of the MCP joints due to subluxation
Swan neck	Hyperextension of PIP joints with flexion of MCP and DIP joints. Occurs as a result of tendon prolapse
Boutonniere	Flexion of PIP joint with extension of DIP and MCP joints. Occurs due to rupture of the central extensor tendon
Z thumb	A flexed MCP joint with an extended IP joint of the thumb

Note that these are all features of rheumatoid arthritis, the most likely deforming polyarthropathy you will see in finals.

❑ **Examine the nails**
  - **Nail infarcts:** this is a vasculitic process which is immune mediated
  - **Pitting of fingernails, onycholysis, and hyperkeratosis:** features of psoriatic arthropathy. If this is evident, then look for a red scaly psoriatic rash and any subcutaneous nodules (seen in RA) at the elbows and extensor surfaces of the arms and forearms
  - **Nail fold telangiectasia:** seen in scleroderma

❑ **Examine the skin**
  - **Palmar erythema:** associated with RA
  - **Scleroderma:** look for shiny and tight skin around the fingertips
  - **Finger lesions:** ischaemic lesions on digits seen in scleroderma
  - **Skin integrity:** bruising or thin skin suggests steroid treatment

❑ **Look for joint lesions**
  - **Heberden's nodes:** affecting the DIP joints; feature of OA
  - **Bouchard's nodes:** affecting the PIP joints; feature of OA

❑ **Assess for muscle wasting**
  - **Thenar eminence:** median nerve palsy
  - **Hypothenar eminence:** ulnar nerve palsy
  - **Small muscles of the hand:** wasting of the small muscles of the hand is usually secondary to disuse from pain or a particular nerve involvement

Feel

❑ **Systematically palpate all joints**
  - **Tenderness**
  - **Warmth:** warm MCP, IP and PIP joints, indicating active disease
  - **Swellings:** are these solid or fluctuant? Can you feel any nodules on the palmar surface of the fingers? These may contribute to the formation of a trigger finger
  - **Lesions:** you may be able to feel Herberden's or Bouchard's nodes, sometimes easier than seeing them; gouty tophi

It is probably easiest to palpate from distal to proximal, i.e. from the DIP joints to the wrist bilaterally.

AUTHOR'S TOP TIP

When feeling for warmth, you can assess both hands at the same time using the dorsal surface of your hands to assess the joint temperatures in tandem.

❏ **Palpate the palmar surface**
  ■ **Dupuytren's contracture:** a thickened palmar fascia

Move

Assess both active and passive movements and always let the patient try and complete any movements first before you move the joint.

❏ **Assess wrist extension/flexion**
  ■ Hold just above the patient's wrist to stabilise the joint and ask the patient to move the wrist up and down, eliciting palmar flexion and dorsiflexion. Ask them to move their hand around in a circle.

An alternative method is to ask the patient to demonstrate the 'prayer sign'. This involves extending the wrist to 90 degrees, by holding the two palmar surfaces together like during traditional prayer. Doing the opposite demonstrates dorsiflexion; also to 90 degrees normally.

❏ **Assess extensor tendons**
  ■ Ask the patient to spread their fingers apart; this should normally be easy for them to complete.

❏ **Assess fist formation**
  ■ Ask the patient to make a fist as tight as possible. Observe for any incomplete formation, as this may suggest joint deformities of the DIP, PIP or MCP joints.

❏ **Assess motor power**

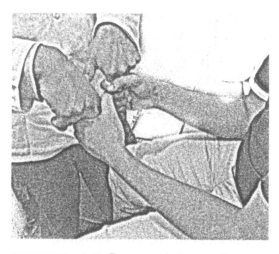
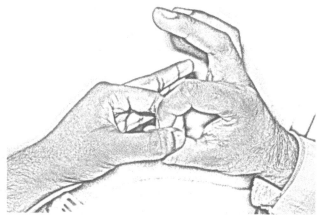

FIGURE 10.1A–B Power and pincer grip

- **Power grip:** ask patient to hold onto your two fingers (index and middle finger) in their fist whilst you pull your fingers away.
- **Pincer (precision) grip:** ask the patient to touch each of their finger pulps with their thumb. This can be demonstrated by asking the patient to pick up a coin.

AUTHOR'S TOP TIP

For the pincer grip, it is easier to demonstrate to the patient what you wish them to do.

❑ **Assess sensation**
- Assess for any deficit in sensation via light touch over the palmar aspect of the index finger (median nerve), little finger (ulnar nerve) and the anatomical snuffbox (radial nerve) (*see* companion surgical book for detailed assessments of each nerve).

Complete the examination
❑ **Thank the patient**
❑ **Wash your hands**
❑ **Further examination**
- *'To complete my exam, I would like to examine the joint above and below and request plain film radiographs of the joint.'*
- *'I would also like to look at the elbow and behind the ear for signs of rheumatoid nodules or psoriatic plaques.'*

It is good practice to also quickly look at the elbows and behind the ears in a short case, as you will more than likely find associated pathology.

AUTHOR'S TOP TIP

Remember, this is not surgical finals and you do not need to examine all the joints in the appropriate manner for an orthopaedic case. Simply saying what you see is probably more than enough in medical finals. These are almost always short cases, so time will not permit you to do so anyway. It is more your ability to recognise pathology as well as a basic understanding of the disease process which will help you pass the station.

Viva questions

Q1   What are Heberden's and Bouchard's nodes and when are they seen?
- Heberdens's and Bouchard's nodes are seen in osteoarthritis.
- They represent bony swellings of the DIP and PIP joints of the hands, respectively.
- These palpable lumps are calcification of the articular cartilage (osteophytes).

Q2   What is Caplan's syndrome?

Difficult question

- Caplan's syndrome is an immune reaction seen in rheumatoid patients which results in a massive fibrotic reaction with rheumatoid nodule formation (0.5–2 cm) in the lung.
- It was originally described in coal miners.
- The nodules may cavitate and resemble TB on a CXR.

Q3   What is Felty's syndrome?
- This is a triad of splenomegaly, RA and neutropenia.
- It occurs in patients with longstanding RA.
- It is associated with rheumatoid factor positive disease.
- The neutropenia can lead to serious infections, sepsis and even death.

Case 1: Rheumatoid arthritis

Case history: A 55-year-old woman presents with right hip pain progressively worsening, with a limp and pain which wakes her up at night. She is now walking with a stick, and her pain is most severe upon waking in the morning. She has no past history of damage to her knees. Please look at her hands.

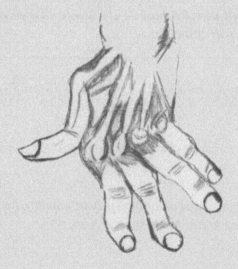

FIGURE 10.2 Rheumatoic

Key features to look for

Look
- ❑ **Symmetry:** symmetrical involvement (look at both hands)
- ❑ **Characteristic deforming features:** ulnar deviation, Z thumb, boutonniere and swan neck deformities
- ❑ **Swellings:** boggy swelling, particularly at the MCP and PIP joints; with characteristic sparing of the DIP joint; spindling of the fingers

❏ **Nails:** signs of psoriasis (pitting); vasculitic lesions
❏ **Muscle wasting:** of the dorsal interossei (particularly the first web space)
❏ **Elbows:** psoriatic plaques or rheumatoid nodules
❏ **Behind ears:** psoriatic plaques
❏ **Skin:** thin bruised skin with palmar erythema

Look for any joint incongruity, e.g. subluxation caused by cartilage deterioration in combination with degradation of the periarticular ligaments which allows forces exerted across the joints to deform them.

Feel
❏ Palpate over any swollen joints (e.g. MCP joint), checking for:
  ▪ **Temperature and tenderness:** seen in active RA
    — **Elbows:** palpate for subcutaneous nodules.

Move
❏ **Motor function assessment:** wrist flexion/extension, finger apposition and power grip
❏ **Sensation:** median nerve entrapment leading to carpal tunnel syndrome; ulnar nerve may be affected due to rheumatoid nodules at the elbow

---

AUTHOR'S TOP TIP

Don't forget that patients with RA have tender joints, so always ask the patient about pain before moving any part of their body.

Complete the exam
Present your findings.
  ▪ *'This patient appears to have signs suggestive of RA. Can I see the X-rays please?'*
                                                                    Average response

  ▪ *'This patient has a symmetrical deforming polyarthropathy. I would like to examine for extra-articular features of RA. May I see the X-rays?'*
                                                                    Good response

  ▪ *'This patient has a symmetrical deforming polyarthropathy. I would like to examine for extra-articular features of RA, assess the patient's functional status and check to see if the RA is active or quiescent. May I see the X-rays please?'*
                                                                    Honours response

❏ **Thank the patient**
❏ **Wash your hands**
❏ **Present your findings**

Rheumatoid arthritis is driven by an autoimmune process that leads to synovial hypertrophy and joint inflammation, leading to cartilage and bone destruction, in addition to possible systemic inflammation of many different organs. There is a strong genetic component with association to certain HLA groups: HLA-DR4/DR1. It typically affects females, with onset in 40- to 60-year-olds. It usually presents as a symmetrical polyarthropathy of the small joints of the hands and feet with morning stiffness.

It is important to always ask about the impact the disease has on a patient's day-to-day life, i.e. their functional status. The ability to get dressed, pick up items, turn a key in a lock are examples; bear in mind that despite marked deformity, some patients may retain reasonable function.

AUTHOR'S TOP TIP

Remember, management will involve an MDT approach with input from the OT, physiotherapists as well as the GP and rheumatologist for consideration of specialist disease modifying anti-rheumatic drugs (DMARDs).

The main differential diagnosis will be psoriatic arthropathy, which would be likely if there were signs of psoriasis and the articular changes were asymmetrical.

The diagnosis of RA is based on a combination of history, examination findings, serological tests and imaging. Diagnostic criteria do exist, as stated by the American College of Rheumatology; this is beyond the scope of this revision guide.

Viva questions

Q1   What is rheumatoid factor (RF)?
- Rheumatoid factor is an autoantibody against the Fc portion of the IgG antibody.
- These combine to form immune complexes which are involved in the underlying inflammatory process in rheumatoid disease.
- Up to 70% of patients with rheumatoid arthritis have a positive RF.

Q2   What features are associated with a worse prognosis in rheumatoid arthritis?
                                                                    Difficult question

- HLA-DR4
- raised ESR or CRP and RF positivity
- female
- severe disability or joint destruction at presentation
- extra-articular features
- multiple joint involvement

Q3 How would you investigate this patient?

- **Bloods:** rheumatoid factor and anti-citrullinated (CCP) antibodies, patients are often ANA positive. Raised ESR/CRP in flare-ups. Anaemia due to chronic disease among other causes (*see* Viva Q6)
- **Joint aspirate:** can be taken if there is an effusion. Usually cloudy in consistency due to raised WCC. Culture this if suspicion of septic joint exists, as this may be likely in those taking immunosuppression or who have coexisting diabetes
- **X-rays:** classically demonstrate
  — periarticular osteoporosis
  — loss of joint space
  — marginal erosions
  — absence of osteophytes

It is important to remember to look for atlantoaxial subluxation, which may be asymptomatic. As the RA progresses, erosion of bone occurs after cartilage destruction, which in the case of joints such as the hip can lead to perforation of the acetabulum.

Q4 How would you treat this patient?

TABLE 10.2 Treatment of RA

Classification	Description
Conservative	**Physiotherapy**
	Occupational aids: e.g. wrist supports for carpal tunnel syndrome
	Analgesia: NSAIDs are usually the mainstay of pain management; caution must be taken to monitor renal and cardiac function and to prescribe with gastro-protection to prevent gastric ulcers. Opioids may be prescribed if needed, and other analgesics such as amitryptilline and gabapentin have been tried
Medical	**Steroids:** can be used in acute flare-ups and are very effective at dampening down the inflammation; they do not modify disease progression. Steroids are not ideally used in the long term due to the side effects of osteoporosis, fragile skin, easy bruising and diabetes
	DMARDs: disease modifying anti-rheumatic drugs function by dampening the body's immune system to reduce the progression of and inflammation caused by RA. They delay disease progression and minimise disability. The patient cannot be on them if they have an active infection and must warned that they may become more unwell than normal if they do get an infection as a consequence of the medication. Examples include:
	Steroids: a form of immunosuppression or modulation but cannot be used long term as discussed above
	Methotrexate: needs regular monitoring of LFTs and FBC; can cause pulmonary fibrosis
	Sulfasalazine: causes rash and diarrhoea; can cause bone marrow suppression
	Gold: rarely used now; causes rashes and nephropathy, nephrotic syndrome
	Penicillamine: can cause loss of taste, bone marrow suppression, nephrotic syndrome, rashes, drug induced lupus
	Infliximab/etanercept/adalimumab: these are anti-TNF-alpha monoclonal antibodies. They usually have a better side-effect profile than traditional DMARDs. They can cause flu-like reactions. They are very costly and reserved for selected cases

(*continued*)

Classification	Description
Surgical	Once the cartilage and bone is destroyed, no medical treatment will halt the progressive destruction and deformity, so joint replacements are undertaken to improve the pain and mobility; other operative procedures include tendon repair, arthrodesis, osteotomy.
	Other operations may be required to treat nerve entrapment, e.g. carpal tunnel syndrome.

Treatment for RA has been revolutionised by the early introduction of DMARDs. Previously, the mainstay of treatment was analgesia, with DMARDs introduced later on in the disease process once joint destruction had already occurred. Now DMARDs are introduced earlier in the disease, as they can not only improve inflammatory markers but also minimise any future disability; they delay disease and radiological progression also.

AUTHOR'S TOP TIP

Note that a large number of patients suffer from depression and this should be managed appropriately.

Honours response

Q5 What are the causes of anaemia seen in rheumatoid arthritis?
- anaemia of chronic disease
- megaloblastic anaemia
- DMARD-induced bone marrow suppression
- NSAID-induced peptic ulceration
- splenomegaly in Felty's syndrome

AUTHOR'S TOP TIP

This is a question beloved by examiners; make sure you know this well.

Q6 What are the extra-articular manifestations of RA?

Honours question

Inflammation can occur in almost any area in the body in rheumatoid disease.

TABLE 10.3 Extra-articular features of rheumatic disease

Organ system	Features
Eyes	Episcleritis
	Scleritis progressing onto scleromalacia perforans
	Keratoconjunctivitis sicca
Skin	Rheumatoid nodules (common location is olecranon)
	Vasculitic lesions: purpura, digital infarcts
	Pyoderma gangrenosum, palmar erythema
	Tenosynovitis, muscle wasting
Neurological	Mono/polyneuropathy, carpal tunnel syndrome, cervical myelopathy
	Mononeuritis multiplex
Cardiac	Pericarditis, effusion, myocarditis
Respiratory	Pulmonary fibrosis, effusions, nodules
	(Remember methotrexate, a treatment for RA, can also cause pulmonary fibrosis)
	Caplan's syndrome
Haematological	Normocytic anaemia (anaemia of chronic disease), eosinophilia and thrombocytosis
Renal	Nephrotic syndrome due to amyloid accumulation in the kidneys
Abdominal	Splenomegaly (Felty's), hepatomegaly (amyloid)

Short Case 1: Osteoarthritis

Case history: A 67-year-old retired teacher complains of gradual-onset pain in her left hip on walking which is becoming more frequent and severe, limiting walking. Pain eases after rest. Taking simple analgesia controlled pain initially, but now this is not enough. Please look at her hands and describe what you see.

Key features to look for

❑ **Hands:** DIP joint swelling (Heberden's nodes); PIP swelling (Bouchard's nodes)
❑ **Hip:** the leg is externally rotated in adduction, with some muscle wasting. There is a fixed flexion deformity, with painless restriction of movement in all ranges. There is an obvious limp on walking and a positive Trendelenburg's test (*see* companion text for detailed examination sequence)

> **AUTHOR'S TOP TIP**
>
> *Some patients may have features of both RA and OA, i.e. a mixed picture, in which case examine as above for RA. OA of the hands is generally a non-deforming polyarthropathy compared to RA hands.*

Osteoarthritis is usually primary in form, but can also be secondary to other disease processes. It is more common in females and was previously thought of as a degenerative disease, but there has been increasing evidence of an inflammatory process leading to joint degeneration. There is loss of cartilage with narrowing of the joint spaces. The disease tends to affect weight-bearing joints as well as the hands, involvement of which is usually indicative of the primary form.

It usually presents as hip pain or groin pain radiating down to the knee and sometimes the back. The pain gradually worsens in severity, eventually leading to nocturnal pain which disturbs sleep. Rest initially eases the pain and later rest can cause stiffness. Pain in the hand joints results in reduction in function which may impact activities of daily living, an important feature to question in the history station. Diagnosis is a combination of clinical history and radiological findings.

Viva questions

Q1   What treatment options are available?
— *'The management of OA involves a **multidisciplinary team** approach with input from orthopaedic surgeons, the GP, physiotherapist and occupational therapist.'*
— *'But in general, it can be divided into conservative, medical and surgical measures.'*
- **Conservative measures involve**
   — lifestyle changes particularly functional aids to help with activities of daily living such as dressing
   — weight loss and regular physiotherapy
- **Medical treatments involve**
   — pain relief via adoption of the WHO analgesic ladder
   — particularly, the use of paracetamol as first-line, NSAIDs with prophylactic peptic ulcer medication
   — corticosteroid intra-articular injections, glucosamine and chondroitin supplementation, topical capsaicin
- **Surgical interventions**
   — arthroscopy with cartilage trimming
   — arthroplasty

Honours response

Short Case 2: Psoriatic arthropathy

Case history: A 40-year-old female presents to the clinic with worsening pain and swelling in her fingers, complaining specifically of a singular swollen 'sausage-shaped finger'; you note that she has a plaque-like disease on her elbows. Please examine this patient's hands.

Key features to look for

❑ **nails:** pitting, onycholysis, hyperkeratosis
❑ asymmetrical polyarthropathy involving DIP joints
❑ **psoriatic patches:** on extensor surfaces and scalp (*see* Chapter 9 for further details)

Viva questions

Q1 What other recognised clinical patterns of disease presentation are there?

Psoriatic arthropathy can follow or even predate psoriatic skin disease. There are many recognised clinical presentation patterns; peripheral joint involvement is by far the most common:

- **symmetrical polyarthritis:** commonest form, similar to RA
- **DIP joint involvement:** more common in men, can involve the nails
- **asymmetric oligoarthritis:** hands/feet affected first usually, dactylitis caused by synchronous inflammation of flexor tendons and synovium (sausage finger) often seen
- **spinal:** similar to ankylosing spondylitis and can include sacroiliitis
- **psoriatic mutilans:** severe deformity, telescoping of digits; 'pencil and cup' X-ray appearance

Q2 What are the radiographic findings of psoriatic arthropathy?

Honours question

- asymmetric destruction of small joints of hands and feet
- sclerosis of distal phalanx
- soft tissue swelling (sausage digit)
- erosive changes with 'pencil and cup' appearance in arthritis mutilans; usually affecting the DIP

Q3 What treatment options are available?

Difficult question

- topical treatments for psoriatic skin disease (*see* Chapter 9)
- **analgesia:** NSAIDs forms mainstay of treatment, also opioid analgesia
- **intra-articular steroid injections:** for symptomatic control, although disease progression remains unaffected
- **DMARDs:** e.g. methotrexate, sulfasalazine, anti-TNF therapies

Case 2: Ankylosing spondylitis

Instructions: This 23-year-old gentleman presents with lower back pain and stiffness, which is worst first thing in the morning, easing as he mobilises throughout the day. Please examine him.

Key features to look for

❑ **Spinal abnormalities:**
- there is **loss of the normal lumbar lordosis**
- increased forward curvature of thoracic spine (**increased and fixed kyphosis**)
- with a **compensatory cervical spine extension**; this prevents patients from looking down constantly and keeps the visual axis horizontal

- **Question-mark posture:** the above spinal abnormalities gives the classical stooped question-mark posture.
☐ **Others:**
  - reduced movement in all fields of spinal movement; patient will turn whole body as a block when asked to look to either side, due to rigidity and stiffness of spine
  - reduced chest expansion
  - prominent abdomen
  - positive Schober's test: this examines lumbar mobility, which will be reduced (*see* companion text for further details)
  - **wall test:** patient unable to place occiput of head against the wall when standing with feet against the wall.

AUTHOR'S TOP TIP

If you suspect ankylosing spondylitis, ask them to stand against a flat wall. In a normal individual, the heels, buttocks, scapula and occiput will be against the wall; however, due to the spinal changes in ankylosing spondylitis in the spine, this will not be possible. This is an easy-to-perform test in the exam.

Complete the examination

☐ **Further examination**
  - *'To complete my exam, I would like to assess for aortic regurgitation, examine the eyes and listen to the lungs.'*

The presence of severe aortic incompetence and pulmonary fibrosis are features of severe disease. Postural deformity makes tasks such as sitting on a chair or driving difficult. Indeed, the risk of cervical spine injury is increased in a road traffic accident. Patients with Achilles tendonitis may complain of heel pain.

☐ **Thank the patient**
☐ **Wash your hands**
☐ **Present your findings**

Ankylosing spondylitis is a form of spondyloarthropathy; the primary form. All spondyloar-thropathies share similar features, mainly being that their articular signs are asymmetrical, with arthritic involvement of major joints and associated sacroiliitis and spondylitis.

Ankylosing spondylitis is more common in males (M : F is 5 : 1) and white ethnic groups, with up to 95% of patients carrying the HLA-B27 genetic marker (white males). HLA-B27 is positive in up to 10% of the Caucasian population. It usually occurs in a young age group (15–35 years) and is associated with other HLA-B27 conditions, such as inflammatory bowel disease and Reiter's syndrome. There are several diagnostic criteria based on clinical and radiological features, referred to as the New York criteria; these are beyond the scope of this revision guide.

Viva questions

Q1   How does the patient classically present?
- Patients typically complain of lower back pain radiating to the buttocks with prolonged morning stiffness which is made worse after periods of prolonged immobility (e.g. sleep, sitting).
- The pain improves with exercise and movement.
- It is a disease of the axis – mainly affecting the spine (**spondylitis**), shoulders, knees, hips (i.e. **asymmetrical peripheral large joint monoarthritis**) and sacroiliac joints (**sacroiliitis**) with peripheral **enthesitis** (inflammation at insertion sites of a tendon).

Good response

Q2   How would you investigate this patient?
- **Bloods:** CRP/ESR may be raised in some but not all, even in active disease. ALP may also be raised
- **HLA-B27-positive**
- **X-rays of AP sacroiliac joints & lateral lumbar spine:**
  — loss of lumbar lordosis on lateral view
  — increased thoracic kyphosis and extension of C-spine on lateral view
  — **erosions and sclerosis of the sacroiliac joint**
  — **syndesmophytes** in the lumbar spine
  — **bamboo spine:** sign of severe disease.

The so called bamboo spine appearance on an AP view is due to calcification of the anterior and posterior spinal ligaments.

AUTHOR'S TOP TIP

A question beloved by examiners concerns the X-ray changes seen in ankylosing spondylitis, and although 'bamboo' appearance is commonly recited, these changes are not seen early in the disease process when symptoms may already be present. Imaging of choice in early disease is contrast-enhanced MRI, which is able to show the inflammatory areas of enthesitis at the corners of vertebral bodies (MR corner sign) and perivertebral joint inflammation and sacroiliac joints, which can later develop into the classic bony extensions seen on X-ray.

Q3   How would you treat this patient?

Difficult question

- **Conservative:** physiotherapy, exercise
- **Medical:** NSAIDs, e.g. indomethacin, DMARDs, e.g. sulfasalazine, anti-TNF therapy

- **Surgical:** osteotomy of the spine to partially correct the flexion deformity. In certain circumstances, joint replacements such as the hip may be undertaken

Previously, patients were treated with radiotherapy to the spine; unfortunately, patients were at increased risk of leukaemia many years after initial therapy.

Q4 What are the extra skeletal manifestations associated with ankylosing spondylitis?

Honours question

- <u>A</u>ortitis and <u>A</u>ortic regurgitation
- <u>A</u>pical pulmonary fibrosis
- Cardiac conduction defects (<u>A</u>trioventricular block)
- Secondary <u>A</u>myloidosis
- <u>A</u>nterior uveitis
- <u>A</u>chilles tendonitis

AUTHOR'S TOP TIP

A useful aide-mémoire is that they all begin with the letter 'A'.

Q5 What are the spondyloarthropathies?

Honours question

- These are conditions characterised by the absence of a positive rheumatoid factor.
- All are associated with HLA-B27.

There are four major spondyloarthropathies:
- ankylosing spondylitis
- psoriatic arthritis
- reactive arthritis
- enteropathic arthritis

There is normally a family history, and so HLA-B27 patients should be offered genetic counselling, as their children are likely to develop symptoms.

Case 3: Gout

Instructions: This 40-year-old obese gentleman presents with excruciating pain and swelling of his right big toe. Please examine him.

Key features to look for

❏ **Swelling of joint:** there may be erythema, hot and exquisitely tender joints, usually monoarticular but can be polyarticular. MTP of the large toe, ankle, knee and wrist are the most common sites

❏ **Chronic gouty tophi:** these are painless urate nodules found in the joints or soft tissues classically seen in the ear helixes, olecranon, achilles tendon and other tendinous sites
❏ **Asymmetrical joint involvement**

AUTHOR'S TOP TIP

Tophi tend to occur in areas exposed to cold, as the uric acid is less soluble in the cold temperature.

Complete the examination

❏ **Further examination**

- ■ *'To complete my exam, I would like to assess for and rule out septic arthritis.'*

If you haven't already done so, make sure you examine the ears, the elbow and feet or hands for the above signs, as these are typical areas of involvement.

❏ **Thank the patient**
❏ **Wash your hands**
❏ **Present your findings**

Gout is a metabolic disorder of purine metabolism and results in monosodium urate crystal deposition in the soft tissues and joints leading to acutely tender swollen joints, most commonly affecting the MTP joint of the big toe (podegra) but also other joints such as the knees and wrists. Gout is associated with hyperuricaemia, often with a recognised precipitant to acute attacks. It is more common in men.

Gout is one of the crystal arthropathies, of which an important differential diagnosis is pseudogout (*see* Viva Q6 below). You must also always consider septic arthritis as a cause for acute synovitis in a single joint in combination with fever.

Viva questions

Q1 How can gout present?
- ■ Gout can present acutely or in a chronic form
- ■ Signs and symptoms include:

TABLE 10.4 Presentation of gout

Presentation	Signs & symptoms
Acute synovitis	Red, hot, swollen joints which are extremely tender, usually monoarticular but can occur in a polyarticular form, worse at night
	MTP of the large toe, ankle, knee and wrist are the most common sites
	May have a pyrexia (difficult to differentiate from septic arthritis in the absence of other signs)

(*continued*)

Presentation	Signs & symptoms
Chronic hyperuricaemia	Gouty tophi seen in the ear pinna, achilles tendon and other tendon sites
	Degenerative arthritis
	Renal stones and nephropathy

Some patients may present with renal failure due to long-standing hyperuricaemia and hyperuricuria causing urate crystals.

Q2 What are the causes of gout?
- **Idiopathic:** most common cause
- **Increased purine intake:** dietary, alcohol excess
- **Drugs:** aspirin, diuretics, ciclosporin, nicotinic acid
- **Increased purine production:** chemotherapy, lymphoproliferative disorders
- **Decreased urate excretion:** renal failure, ketoacidosis, lactic acidosis

Q3 How would you investigate this patient?
- **Bloods:** raised WBC, serum urate levels may be normal in an acute attack and are generally unreliable even if raised
- **Joint aspirate:** the synovial fluid is examined for
  - **WCC:** this is often very high
  - **Polarised microscopy:** seen under polarised light, the fluid demonstrates needle-shaped, negatively birefringent crystals; this provides a definitive diagnosis of crystal arthropathy
  - **Culture:** the aspirate from joints should still be sent for culture to rule out an infection within the joint regardless of crystal findings
- **Joint X-ray:** in chronic disease, you may see lytic lesions, punched-out erosions (with sclerotic borders), joint destruction and sometimes calcified tophi.

AUTHOR'S TOP TIP

Hyperuricaemia does not prove a swollen joint is gout; it only makes the diagnosis more likely.

Q4 How would you treat this patient?
- Management can be divided up into treatment of acute attacks and prevention of attacks.

TABLE 10.5 Treatment for gout

Classification	Treatment
Acute flare-up (< 3 weeks)	**NSAID**, e.g. indomethacin
	Oral colchicine
	Occasionally intra-articular **steroid** injections in large joints

(continued)

Classification	Treatment
Prevention	The primary aim in chronic disease management is in reducing uric acid levels once the acute flare has settled
	Allopurinol (xanthine oxidase inhibitor) is the drug of choice
	If contraindicated to allopurinol, you can use uricosurics such as probenecid or sulphinpyrazone
	Uricase (used to prevent chemotherapy-related gout in bulky and high-turnover malignant disease)
	Lifestyle modification: dietary change will be required to avoid precipitants

Remember, allopurinol can also precipitate an acute attack; therefore, a careful history should be taken for onset of symptoms. This also highlights the importance of classifying treatment according to acute-attack management or prevention of future attacks.

AUTHOR'S TOP TIP

Remember to ask about a history of peptic ulcer disease, heart or renal failure, as this will influence the medications you will be able to offer the patient in an acute attack, e.g. NSAIDs.

Q5 Do you know of any precipitants of an acute gouty attack?

Difficult question

- **Dehydration:** lack of fluid intake, alcohol excess, diuretics
- **High intake of food rich in purines:** cheese, red meats, sardines, wine
- **Renal impairment:** acute or chronic
- **Medications:** allopurinol, bendroflumethiazide, other diuretics, ethambutol
- Chemo- or radiotherapy for large tumour bulk or disseminated malignancy
- Trauma, surgery and infection

Acute gout can occur whenever serum urate levels rapidly change (even a rapid fall); this is far more important than the actual absolute level in the serum. The above features are associated with such situations.

Q6 What is pseudogout?
- Pseudogout or calcium pyrophosphate arthropathy is caused by deposition of calcium pyrophosphate crystals in the bone and cartilage, classically in the knee, but can be polyarticular.
- It can be difficult to differentiate from gout on history alone.
- Differentiating features from gout include their positively birefringent crystals under polarised light; rhomboid-shaped crystals and joint predilection (usually the knee, shoulders and hip). It is more common in the elderly and usually has a slower onset; hours to days rather than in gout, which is hours.
- Treatment is the same as for an acute flare-up of gout, including hydroxychloroquine; unfortunately, however, there is no preventative treatment currently available.

Case 4: Systemic lupus erythematosis (SLE)

Instructions: This 45-year-old Afro-Caribbean woman presents with a rash across her face and painful non-swollen joints. Please examine her.

Key features to look for

Inspection

❑ **Malar rash:** the classical erythematous malar rash in a butterfly distribution across the nose and cheeks with nasolabial sparing.

❑ **Discoid lesions:** may have disc-like lesions in discoid lupus.

❑ **Photosensitive rash:** skin rashes may demonstrate photosensitivity; the rash is distributed in sun-exposed areas.

❑ **Mouth:** painless oral or nasopharyngeal ulcers are commonly seen.

❑ **Other:** there may be a patterned rash, such as livedo reticularis, purpura or alopecia.

Palpation

❑ **Arthritis:** commonly non erosive and affecting at least two joints

Complete the examination

❑ **Further examination**

■ *'To complete my exam, I would like to assess for other manifestations of SLE.'*

❑ **Thank the patient**

❑ **Wash your hands**

❑ **Present your findings**

SLE is a relapsing remitting autoimmune disease of unknown cause which is characterised by the production of autoantibodies leading to inflammation. It is typically seen in female patients (F : M ratio is 9 : 1) of African descent in countries such as the UK, but this is not replicated with high rates within African countries.

Viva questions

Q1   How else may this patient's disease manifest?

■ Constitutional features of SLE include: arthralgia (often with minimal joint swelling), myalgia, rash, fever and fatigue. There is an association with antiphospholipid syndrome.

■ May affect other organ systems, leading to:

TABLE 10.6 Manifestations of SLE

Organ system	SLE manifestation
Renal	Renal failure
	Different forms of glomerulonephritis
	Nephrotic syndrome
	Lupus nephritis
	Proteinuria
Cardiac	Pericarditis
	Myocarditis
	Libman–Sacks endocarditis (rare)
Pulmonary	Pleural effusion
	Pulmonary hypertension and embolism
	Pulmonary fibrosis
Neurological	Strokes, seizures and psychological changes (psychosis)
	Peripheral neuropathy, cranial nerve involvement
Haematological	Hypocomplimentaemia, leucopenia and lymphopenia
	Thrombocytopenia, raised APTT
	Autoimmune haemolytic anaemia
Other	Raynaud's phenomenon
	Scarring alopecia

The above signs on examination and associated medical history form several criteria as part of the American Rheumatism Council (ARC) criteria for diagnosing SLE; only four criteria are required. Although you would not be expected to know the ARC criteria in detail, they do point out the different manifestations and signs of SLE, which could be a viva question instead.

Q2   How would you investigate this patient?

Difficult question

- **Routine bloods:** high ESR but may have normal CRP, low WBC, renal function, thrombocytopenia, lymphopenia, anaemia
- **Immunological bloods:**
  — **ANA, anti-dsDNA (double stranded) and anti-Sm (Smith)** – positivity virtually diagnostic of SLE
  — **rheumatoid factor**
  — **complement:** low C3/4 (suggests lupus nephritis)
  — **anticardiolipin:** screening for antiphospholipid syndrome, a common association
  — **lupus anticoagulant**
  — **antihistone antibodies:** classically seen in drug-induced lupus

Note that a syphilis serology may also be falsely positive.
- **Urine:** protein/haematuria
- **X-ray of joints:** often little to be seen; there may be periarticular osteopenia and soft tissue swelling

- **CT chest:** used to assess pulmonary disease
- **MRI brain:** used for cerebral disease (infarctions) secondary to disease
- **Echo:** pericardial effusions, Libman–Sacks endocarditis

Serological evidence of ANA positivity with anti-dsDNA and anti-Sm are considered criteria for diagnosis under the ARC diagnostic criteria. ANA is a sensitive screening test for SLE and is positive in over 95% of cases. A negative ANA brings the diagnosis of SLE into doubt.

Note that drugs can induce SLE, classically procainamide, hydralazine, phenytoin, isoniazid and penicillamine, amongst many others. Therefore, a careful drug history is paramount in your investigations, as cessation of the offending drug often leads to resolution.

Q3   What treatment options are available?
- **Conservative:** sunblock, and avoid sun exposure and offending drugs
- **Medical**
  - NSAIDs and hydroxychloroquine are very effective for arthritis
  - steroids and immunosuppressants such as methotrexate, cyclophosphamide for lupus nephritis (often in pulses intravenously)

Good response

Mortality from SLE occurs from renal failure and infections. It is important to remind patients that there is no cure and management is focused around symptom control and disease manifestations.

Case 5: Polymyositis

Instructions: This 45-year-old woman presents with progressive difficulty in climbing stairs and a facial rash. Please examine her.

Key features to look for

Inspection

☐ **Heliotrope rash:** a lilac-coloured rash classically around the eyes but may be seen on the hands and face also

☐ **Macular rash:** the so called shawl sign, i.e. a rash over neck and shoulders

☐ **Gottron's papules:** red papules seen on the MCP and ICP joints of the hands, sometimes on the knees and elbows; this is pathognomonic

☐ **Polydermatomyositis:** erythema of the nail folds

☐ **Proximal muscle weakness:** there is a symmetrical weakness with muscle wasting of the pelvic and shoulder girdle muscles, i.e. patient is unable to climb stairs, stand from a chair or raise their arms over their head

☐ **Dysphonia:** if bulbar muscles are involved

AUTHOR'S TOP TIP

Bilateral symmetrical muscle weakness is suggestive of some form of myopathy. If however there is asymmetrical involvement, you should consider an alternative neurological diagnosis.

Palpation
- ❏ **Muscle tenderness:** suggestive of an inflammatory myopathy
- ❏ **Arthralgia**

Complete the examination
- ❏ **Further examination**
  - ■ *'To complete my exam, I would like to assess for evidence of malignancy associated with dermatomyositis.'*
- ❏ **Thank the patient**
- ❏ **Wash your hands**
- ❏ **Present your findings**

Polymyositis and dermatomyositis are the most common cause of striated muscle inflammatory myopathies. Both conditions are similar; with dermatomyositis having additional skin signs. Systemic symptoms include weight loss, fever and malaise.

Muscle weakness can lead to respiratory and swallowing difficulties, although an important exception is eye muscle involvement with very rarely any facial muscle involvement. There may be subcutaneous calcification and gastrointestinal ulcers. (For further details *see* Chapter 9)

An important differential diagnosis is polymyalgia rheumatica (PMR), which also presents with proximal muscle involvement. The key difference is that there is more pain and stiffness of the proximal muscles, not weakness, especially in the morning, and the ESR is very high.

Viva questions

Q1 How would you investigate this patient?

Difficult question

- ■ **Bloods:** anti-Jo-1, anti-Mi-2, raised CK, raised ESR
- ■ **EMG:** spontaneous fibrillation potentials, short duration complexes, polyphasic potentials
- ■ **Muscle biopsy:** inflammatory myositis, necrosis

Almost all patients are screened for an underlying malignancy, especially if dermatomyositis is present. In general, patients are managed with steroids. Occasionally, imunosuppressants such as cyclophosphamide or methotrexate are required.

Case 6: Systemic sclerosis

Instructions: This 45-year-old woman presents with restricted mouth opening. Look at her face and hands.

Key features to look for
Inspection

TABLE 10.7 Signs of scleroderma

Feature	Examination findings
Hands	**Sclerodactyly:** smooth shiny and tight skin over fingers, i.e. finely spindled digits
	Nails: nail fold infarcts, **telangiectasia** of the nail fold capillaries
	Fingers: pulp atrophy, digital ischaemia, ulcers; there may be amputations, **calcinosis** (subcutaneous calcium deposition)
Face	**Skin:** telangiectasia, shiny and tight skin
	Nose: beak-like appearance
	Mouth: restricted mouth opening with skin puckering around the mouth; microstomia

Complete the examination
❑ **Further examination**
  ■ *'To complete my exam, I would like to assess for signs of pulmonary hypertension.'*
❑ **Thank the patient**
❑ **Wash your hands**
❑ **Present your findings**

Scleroderma is a multisystem connective tissue disorder that leads to excessive organ fibrosis of unknown aetiology. Systemic sclerosis is a connective tissue disease consisting of scleroderma (skin thickening) in combination with varying levels of other organ involvement, including vasculitis. There is excessive collagen deposition and fibrosis within the skin and other organs. The cause is currently unknown, and there is no cure for the underlying disease process. Raynaud's phenomenon is present in nearly all cases and may precede other signs.

Viva questions

Q1 How do you classify systemic sclerosis?
There are two main disease patterns that exist:

TABLE 10.8 Sclerosis types

Classification	Description
Limited systemic sclerosis	**Also referred to as CREST syndrome, as this refers to several coexisting signs:**
	Calcinosis
	Raynauds
	o**E**sphageal dysmotility (also general gut dysmotility)
	Sclerodactyly
	Telangiectasia: seen on fingers and across face
	Skin involvement is limited to the arms distal to the elbow, legs distal to knees, neck and face. Pulmonary hypertension is more commonly seen in this form
	Investigations: anti-centromere antibodies, seen in > 50% of cases
Diffuse systemic sclerosis	Carries a worse prognosis than limited
	Scleroderma affecting whole skin surface, especially trunk and proximal limbs
	Organ involvement:
	• **Pulmonary:** fibrosis, less incidence of pulmonary hypertension than in limited disease
	• **Renal:** impaired renal function, may present with renal crisis (severe hypertension and rapid decline in renal function); onion-skin vasculature seen on biopsy
	• **Cardiac:** pericardial and myocardial fibrosis, conduction defects and heart failure
	• **Musculoskeletal:** arthralgia and erosive arthritis, myositis
	• **GI:** GORD with dysmotility and bacterial overgrowth, long-term risk of Barrett's oesophagus
	Investigations: Anti-topoisomerase-1 (Scl-70) or anti-nucleolar antibodies seen in > 50% cases

Investigations would also include the associated organ systems involved; this may include renal function tests to assess renal failure, pulmonary function tests in interstitial fibrosis and an echocardiograph to assess LV function, amongst others.

Honours response

AUTHOR'S TOP TIP

On examination of a patient with suspected systemic sclerosis, to help differentiate a limited type with a diffuse sclerosis pattern, pinch the skin gently, starting at the wrist and work your way up the arm. In a limited pattern, the skin tightness should return to normal as you ascend the arm; if the skin remains tight, this suggests a diffuse disease pattern.

Q2   What treatment options are available?

Difficult question

- Most treatments are for the organ systems involved and symptomatic relief; there is no curative treatment available for the underlying cause.
- **Physiotherapy:** to help prevent contractures.
- **NSAIDs:** for arthritic pain.
- **PPI:** for acid reflux; antibiotics for bacterial overgrowth.
- **ACEi/ARB:** in those with renal disease.
- **Prostacyclins/calcium channel blockers:** for Raynaud's and digital ischaemia.
- **Immunosuppressants and immune-modulating drugs:** such as cyclophosphamide to try to prevent organ and skin disease progression, especially interstitial lung disease. It has been noted, however, that steroids do not help improve skin disease.
- **Penicillamine D:** shown to slow skin disease progression.

10.2 HISTORIES IN RHEUMATOLOGY

By far the most likely case you will come across in finals will be joint pain. *See* Chapter 2 for the general history-taking schema described; here we focus on specific points related to rheumatology.

History Case 1: Joint pain

Instructions: This 47-year-old woman presents with joint pain. Please take a focused clinical history.

Key features to look for

❑ **History of presenting complaint**
- **Site of pain:** Where is the pain, especially if it is any particular joint? Upper limb or lower limb? If it is upper limb – which is their dominant hand? If lower limbs – does it affect their walking? Is just one joint affected? (monoarticular) or are many joints affected? (polyarticular) Are they symmetrically involved? (symmetrical polyarthropathy)

TABLE10.9 Commonly associated sites of pain

Condition	Site predilection
Osteoarthritis	Hands, hips, knees and spine
Rheumatoid arthritis	Small joints of hands and feet (proximal joints), i.e. MCP and PIP joints in hands and MTP in feet; progresses to involve other joints, including the ankles, wrist, elbows
Paget's disease	Can affect any bone, but has predilection for axial sites, i.e. skull, spine, sacrum, humerus and femur
	Hands and feet are rarely involved

(continued)

Condition	Site predilection
Polymyalgia rheumatica	Girdle joints, e.g. shoulders
Reactive arthritis	Often oligoarticular (progressive, i.e. moves from joint to another) involving large joints and asymmetrical pattern of polyarthropathy
Gout	Podagra (large toe; not pathognomic), ankle, knee and wrist
Pseudogout	Shoulder, wrist, knee
Ankylosing spondylitis	Spine with peripheral enthesitis; insertion of Achilles tendon, plantar fascia, patella, iliac crest

❑ **Onset:** Is the pain of sudden onset? Or does it come on gradually after use? Is it a chronic pain? Has it got progressively worse or maintained the same intensity? Gradual pain is suggestive of OA. After use or sudden onset may suggest fracture; sudden-onset back pain in an elderly osteoporotic woman would suggest a wedge fracture or a pathological fracture in a patient with known metastatic cancer. Sudden onset is also associated with infection; this may be septic arthritis or a flare up of previous OA/RA. RA and ankylosing spondylitis is associated with morning stiffness.

❑ **Character:** Describe the nature of the pain; it might help if you suggest some terms for them, e.g. 'sharp, stabbing, dull ache, etc.' How severe it is on a pain scale of 1–10, where one is no pain and 10 is the worst pain ever? Does the pain wake them up from sleep?

❑ **Radiation:** Remember, in joint pathology the pain can radiate to the joint above or below the joint affected. For example, in teenagers with Osgood–Schlatter's disease affecting the knee, they may present with hip pain. Conversely, an elderly lady with OA may present with back pain which was originating in the hip. This is due to the compensatory effort other joints must take when a diseased joint cannot support its normal full load.

AUTHOR'S TOP TIP

Always remember, in the examination of a joint where the patient is complaining of pain, you must examine the joint above and below. However, in the OSCE you will not normally have time to do this, but you must clearly state this when presenting your findings.

- **Alleviating factors/Exacerbating factors:** What makes the pain better? Is it analgesia? If so, which type? Or does rest improve the pain – suggesting OA. Or does activity ease the pain – suggesting RA and ankylosing spondylitis, which are both worse after waking, with the latter especially due to periods of immobility.
- **Timing:** Is the pain there every day? Any particular time? How long does it last?

❑ **Associated symptoms**
- **Associated symptoms:** Do they get swelling, stiffness, locking/giving way of the joint? Fever? Feeling generally unwell? Loss of sensation?
- **Functional limitation:** Important to ask about their functional status; what does the pain stop them from doing?
- **Systemic involvement:** Many conditions have systemic involvement. Enquire about any extra-articular involvement, especially eye and skin involvement.

TABLE 10.10 Extra-articular features

Condition	Extra-articular features
Gout	Tophaceous deposits (auricular cartilage, Achilles) Renal failure
Septic arthritis	Fever, sepsis, weight loss
Psoriatic arthritis	Psoriatic plaques, eye involvement, e.g. uveitis
SLE	Photosensitive rash, alopecia, Raynaud's phenomenon, stroke, depression and mood change

❑ **Past medical history**
- ■ **Medical:** gout, malignancy, osteoporosis, any other previously affected joints
- ■ **Prior investigations:** X-rays, DEXA, MRI
- ■ **Prior treatments:** any treatments in the past with, e.g. analgesia, immunomodulatory drugs such as infliximab; operations such as joint replacements, fusions

---

AUTHOR'S TOP TIP

Also keep in mind that joint pain/rheumatic complaints might be the presenting symptom of a systemic disorder.

❑ **Family history**
- ■ **HLA-B27 conditions:** ankylosing spondylitis, psoriatic arthropathy, reactive arthritis, seronegative arthropathies
- ■ **Genetic components:** RA has a large genetic component

❑ **Drug history**
- ■ **Diuretics:** those such as thiazides could predispose to gout
- ■ **Analgesia:** current requirements; whether pain controlled or not
- ■ **Specific agents:** use of allopurinol or probenicid; prophylactic treatment in patients with recurrent episodes of gout
- ■ **Immunomodulatory agents:** methotrexate, infliximab

❑ **Social history**
- ■ **Occupation/hobby:** This may cause joint damage leading to, for example, OA; this may be seen in runners, footballers, dancers and certain occupations involving predominantly outdoor work, e.g. builders or gardeners. Another important reason to ascertain occupation is if your patient is self-employed; the amount of time off work for a joint replacement may cost them more than another patient in receipt of sick leave
- ■ **Smoking:** Increased risk of osteoporosis

Completion

AUTHOR'S TOP TIP

Remember to start the history as you would for any pain history using SOCRATES.

> **AUTHOR'S TOP TIP**
>
> *Adapt the history so you know how to take a history for the three main symptoms of any rheumatologic condition – joint pain, swelling and stiffness – and think of the differential diagnosis related to each principal symptom.*

Viva questions

Q1 What are the causes of joint pain?
There are many causes, however in general:

TABLE 10.11 Aetiology of joint pain

Classification	Aetiology
Infections	Septic arthritis
Inflammation without joint degeneration	SLE
	Reactive arthritis
	Bursitis, enthesitis
Inflammation with joint degeneration	OA, RA, psoriatic arthropathy, ankylosing spondylitis
Crystal arthropathies	Gout
	Pseudogout
Vascular	Sickle cell, Raynaud's disease, thrombosis
Trauma	Damage to joint and surrounding bone, referred pain of a fracture
Neuropathic	Diabetes (remember, Charcot joints are painless), stroke

Q2 What organisms are linked to septic arthritis?
- *S. aureus* is the most common.
- Others include *Neisseria gonorrhoea*, group B *Streptococcus.*

Q3 Name some secondary causes of OA.

Difficult question

- **Underlying joint disease:** RA, avascular necrosis, gout, infection, Paget's disease
- **Localised disease:** chondrocalcinosis, neuropathies
- **Systemic diseases:** sickle cell, acromegaly, haemophilia, haemochromatosis
- **Mechanical:** hypermobility, trauma, SUFE, Perthe's

Q4 How would you distinguish OA from RA in a joint on plain film radiography?

TABLE 10.12 Radiological features of RA vs OA

Condition	Radiological features
Osteoarthritis	Loss of joint space
	Osteophytes
	Subarticular bone cysts
	Subarticular sclerosis
Rheumatoid arthritis	Loss of joint space
	Marginal bony erosions
	Periarticular osteoporosis
	Joint line thickening
	Soft tissue swelling
	Joint deformity

Q5 What are the common causes of acute joint swelling?

Difficult question

- **Flare underlying arthritic process:** RA/OA/psoriatic
- **Crystal arthropathy:** gout/pseudogout
- **Infection:** septic arthritis, osteomyelitis
- **Trauma:** fracture (intra/extraarticular)/penetrating injury/haemarthosis
- **Haemarthrosis:** collagen disorders, clotting abnormalities (haemophilia), trauma, medication (overtreatment with warfarin)
- **Others:** ruptured Baker's cyst

History Case 2: Vasculitis

Instructions: This patient is known to have a vasculitic process. Please ask her some questions; you may wish to focus on organ-specific questions.

Key features to look for

❑ **Constitutional symptoms:** fever, malaise, weight loss, myalgia, arthralgia
❑ **Organ-specific signs:**

TABLE 10.13 Organ-specific manifestations of vasculitis

Organ	Features
Neurological	Fits, stroke, mono- or polyneuropathies
Cardiac	MI, heart failure
Pulmonary	Haemoptysis
Eyes	Visual loss, episcleritis
GI	Bowel ischaemia
Renal	Renal failure, haematuria, proteinuria
Skin	Purpura, livedo reticularis, nail bed and finger pulp infarcts

Completion

Vasculitis refers to conditions characterised by blood vessel inflammation within the body. Patients usually present with constitutional symptoms in combination with any organ with vasculitic involvement. The inflammatory process may result in thickening of vessel walls, with endothelial cell injury, stenosis and eventually ischaemia of parts of the body caused by vascular occlusion.

Vasculitis can be classified according the size of vessel affected and whether they are ANCA positive or negative.

TABLE 10.14 Vasculitis classification

Classification	Description
Large vessel	**Aortitis associated with AS:** murmur may be present on auscultation
	Takayasu's arteritis: affects aorta and major branches. More common in females of Asian decent. Absent central and peripheral pulses with limb claudication; difference in blood pressure between left and right arms
	Vascular imaging shows narrowing of part or all of the aorta and its major branches
	Giant cell arteritis: temporal arteritis
Medium/ small-sized vessel	*Granulomatous*
	Churg–Strauss syndrome (pANCA +ve): initially features of asthma or rhinitis which are usually present for months. Subsequent development of eosinophilia with eosinophilic tissue infiltration, pneumonias, haemoptysis and eventually systemic vasculitis
	Wegener's granulomatosis (cANCA +ve): chronic sinusitis, epistaxis and rhinitis, saddle-nose development, pulmonary nodules and infiltrates; renal disease; focal proliferative glomerulonephritis (GN)
	Non-granulomatous
	Microscopic polyangiitis (p/c ANCA +ve): purpura (palpable), leucoclastic angiitis, glomerulonephritis, neuropathy, GI/pulmonary haemorrhage
	Vasculitis of conditions such as SLE: *see* Cases 1 and 4 above
	Polyarteritis nodosa: microaneurysm formation, typically at vessel bifurcations; can affect any system, but more commonly renal (leading to hypertension), skin, peripheral nerves, joints and gut. Associated with hepatitis B infection
	Sjögren's syndrome: *see* History Case 4 below
	Kawasaki disease*:* common in children under 5 years, especially of Japanese descent, fever, rash, strawberry tongue, red cracked lips, conjunctivitis, thrombocytosis. Patients can develop coronary aneurysms which need treatment with aspirin in the acute phase and are the most common cause of death
Small vessel	**Cryoglobulinaemia:** disease caused by immunoglobulins that when cold undergo reversible precipitation; associated with conditions such as haematological malignancy, Sjögren's, infections, e.g. hep C
	Henoch–Schönlein syndrome: haemorrhagic purpura commonly appearing on the buttocks and thighs with or without GN, arthritis and abdominal pain. Usually a precipitating infection or medication with prodromal viral-like infection, e.g. streptococcal infection, penicillins
	Drug induced vasculitis

Viva questions

Q1 What is ANCA, and what is the difference between pANCA and cANCA?

Honours question

- ANCA stands for antineutrophil cytoplasmic antibodies.
- Usually of the IgG subclass, it is recognised commonly in two forms depending on staining results when looking for autoantibodies:
  — **p-ANCA (perinuclear antineutrophil cytoplasmic antibodies)**: perinuclear staining pattern, commonly anti-MPO antibodies
  — **c-ANCA (cytoplasmic antineutrophil cytoplasmic antibodies)**: diffusely granular, cytoplasmic staining pattern; commonly anti-PR3 antibodies.
- A ratio will be given to indicate the level of positivity, e.g. 1 : 10 or 1 : 6400.
- This indicates how many times the solution can be diluted and still be positive (i.e. the bigger the number, the more positive the result).

History Case 3: Raynaud's phenomenon

Instructions: This 18-year-old woman presents with painful cold hands whenever she is out in the cold. Please take a history.

Key features to look for

❑ **Age:** young females
❑ **Occupation:** use of vibrating tools
❑ **Characteristic colour changes:** cold white hands which turn blue then red (and painful)
❑ **Pain & cold hands**
❑ **Exacerbating features:** worse in cold weather or precipitated by emotion
❑ **Alleviating feature:** improvement with heat
❑ **Social history:** smoker
❑ **Others:** dysphagia, arthralgias, butterfly rash

Completion

Episodic digital vasospasm results in the characteristic colour changes of **(remember mnemonic WBC):**

1. **White:** caused by arterial spasm
2. **Blue:** deoxygenated blood slowly seeps through dilated capillaries
3. **Crimson:** occurs as a result of reactive hyperaemia secondary to relaxation of arteries

Viva questions

Q1 What are the causes of Raynaud's?

Difficult question

- Primary Raynaud's also called Raynaud's **disease**; it is idiopathic.
- There are many causes of secondary Raynaud's, i.e. Raynaud's phenomenon.

TABLE 10.15 Causes of Raynaud's phenomenon

Classification	Aetiology
Autoimmune/vasculitis	Scleroderma, CREST syndrome, RA, SLE, mixed connective tissue disease
Trauma/environmental	Vibrating tool usage, immersion of hands repeatedly in cold water, working with refrigeration units, lead and arsenic exposure
Drugs	COCP, beta blockers, bromocriptine
Haematological/malignancy	Polycythaemia, cold agglutinins, lymphoma, myeloma
Endocrine	Diabetes, acromegaly, phaeochromocytoma
Infection	Hep B/C, mycoplasma

Q2 How would you investigate this patient?
- Try to identify a cause of secondary disease (*see* above table)
- **Bloods:** FBC, ESR, RF, autoantibodies, clotting, glucose, TFTs, cold agglutinins, GH, catecholamines
- **CXR:** to look for a cervical rib; a differential diagnosis of arterial impairment
- **Barium swallow:** if suspicious of CREST
- **Radiological contrast studies:** e.g. MRA or CTA if arterial disease suspected

Q3 What treatment options are available?

Honours question

If there is a secondary cause, treatment should focus on managing this first. In general, treatment can be:
- **Conservative:** smoking cessation, avoid exposure to the cold, wear gloves (special electrically heated versions are available)
- **Medical:** calcium channel blockers, e.g. nifedipine, prostacyclins, ACEi
- **Surgical:** cervical sympathectomy to inhibiting vasoconstriction

History Case 4: Sjögren's syndrome

Instructions: Take a history from this 60-year-old lady who has come in complaining of a gritty feeling in her eyes, which are now feeling constantly sore. She has also noted that she has been having an increasingly dry mouth with altered taste.

Key features to look for

TABLE 10.16 Features of Sjögren's

Feature	Description
Sicca syndrome	The most common symptoms are dry eyes and mouth. Patient may describe dry, gritty, sore eyes, with sticky eyelids. Oral symptoms of inability to eat dry food, altered taste, tongue sticking to palate, increased dental caries and requirement for fillings are common
Eye signs	Mainly these are due to lack of tears, e.g. keratoconjunctivitis sicca, dilated conjunctival vessels
Exocrine function	Loss of exocrine function leading to vaginitis, difficulty swallowing
Systemic	Arthritis, Raynaud's, rashes and purpura, neuropathies, pericarditis, pancreatitis, gastritis, lymphadenopathy and gland swelling, e.g parotid

Completion

Sjögren's is a connective tissue disease which is characterised by lymphocytic infiltration of exocrine glands and their subsequent lack of function in combination with other features such as arthritis. Sjögren's may be primary or secondary if another connective tissue/rheumatic disease process is observed. It is commonly seen in association with RA and SLE. Female patients are more commonly affected than males.

Viva questions

Q1   How would you investigate this patient?
- **Bloods:** ANA and RF are commonly positive, hypergammaglobinopathy caused by B-cell hyperreactivity (can lead to renal disease), anti-Ro and anti-La (primary Sjögren's), anaemia and leukopenia. Raised CRP/ESR can be used as activity markers
- **Schirmer test:** used to diagnose lack of tear production

Treatment is mainly symptomatic with artificial tears and saliva; skin creams for dry skin and vaginal lubricants. Analgesics for related arthritis, e.g. NSAIDs/hydroxychloroquine.

CHAPTER 11

Medical emergencies

11.1 PRINCIPLES OF EMERGENCY MANAGEMENT

Emergency management of the acutely unwell patient is a commonly tested feature in OSCEs. The examiner is trying to assess whether you will be a safe junior doctor. It is therefore essential that you call for help early, as this is likely to form part of the mark scheme. But be careful: candidates assume that calling for help absolves them of any other management responsibilities. This is not true, as very often in actual clinical practice your senior is either en route, which takes time, and/or busy with another sick patient and cannot come to your aid immediately. You therefore need to be able to resuscitate the patient whilst awaiting senior review. You need to be logical, calm and methodical in your approach to an emergency. All acutely unwell patients should therefore be initially assessed and simultaneously managed using the ABCDE algorithm regardless of the cause. This initial assessment is the cornerstone of medical emergency management and should be ingrained into your minds for the remainder of your careers.

The initial assessment allows you to simultaneously perform a focused clinical examination and treat any abnormalities before moving onto the next system. As the A, B, C model prioritises the recognition and treatment of illness in order of its relative threat to life, you cannot for example proceed from B to C unless you have managed or treated any problems you have found in B.

Initial assessment of an emergency

❏ **Recognition of emergency**
- Examiners want you to appreciate the urgency of the treatment, and want to see this in your answer. Call for help early; this is what would be expected of you as a junior doctor.
- We suggest you simply state: *'This is a medical emergency. I will resuscitate the patient by . . .'*

❏ **Assess the Airway (A)**
- **Give supplemental oxygen:** Always give the patient high-flow oxygen (this is appropriate in all but known type 2 respiratory failure COPD patients, in which case oxygen can be started off high flow and then titrated to effect with regular blood gas analysis).
- **Assess patency:** Ask the patient a question; if they respond by speaking, then they can maintain their airway. If not, then:

— **Assess for evidence of airway compromise:** Look in the oral cavity for anything blocking their airway, such as blood or vomitus, and suction this using a Yankauer suction. Listen for noisy breathing, which may give clues as to level of obstruction; stridor suggests impending airway compromise.

— **Establish a patent airway:** Do this using the following airway manoeuvres
  - **Simple manoeuvres:** Jaw thrust, chin lift; remove any foreign bodies, use suction if necessary to remove secretions.
  - **Airway adjuncts:** If the patient cannot maintain their airway, then use simple airway adjuncts such as an oropharyngeal airway (Guedel) or a nasopharyngeal airway.
  - **Secure/definitive airway:** If the patient's GCS is < 8 or you are worried they may lose their airway for any reason, you will need anaesthetic support to insert a definitive airway. This can be in the form of an orotracheal intubation, e.g. endotracheal tube or a surgical airway, e.g. cricothyroidotomy.

❏ **Check the Breathing (B)**
  - **Monitoring:** Attach a saturation probe to assess the level of oxygen saturation, although ideally you would perform an ABG to determine the actual oxygen saturation in the blood.
  - **Inspection:** Do they look cyanosed, suggesting imminent respiratory arrest? Assess their respiratory rate; an increased respiratory rate > 20 is a sensitive sign of disease. Look for equal chest wall expansion and/or any distended neck veins in case they have a pneumothorax; paradoxical chest wall movement suggests evidence of a flail chest.
  - **Palpation:** Assess for tracheal deviation; percuss the chest wall for hyperresonance in a pneumothorax or dullness in post-operative basal atelectasis or a haemothorax.
  - **Auscultate:** Listen to breath sounds for lung pathology, e.g. loss of air entry, crackles, increased or decreased vocal resonance.
  - **Treatment:** Chest drains or needle decompression may be needed acutely.
  — The purpose of assessing breathing is to ensure adequate ventilation.

❏ **Assess Circulation (C)**
  - **Assess level of shock:** Look for signs of poor peripheral perfusion – cool, clammy, pale extremities or collapsed veins. Check capillary refill time (CRT), normally < 2 seconds; patients with impaired circulation in septic shock could also have CRT < 2 seconds.
  - **Monitoring:** Attach to monitor and check vital signs, i.e. HR, BP, ECG monitoring for rhythm abnormalities. Assess the peripheral pulse, which could be faint if low BP; remember to check a central pulse for strength as well. Blood pressure monitoring: arterial vasodilation is seen in septic shock and anaphylaxis; patients therefore have low diastolic pressures; in cardiogenic shock or hypovolaemia, patients have arterial vasoconstriction leading to a narrowed pulse pressure.
  - **Obtain IV access:** Insert two large bore cannulae (grey or orange), one into each antecubital fossa. Take this opportunity to take bloods for further investigation, including cultures if clinically appropriate.
  - **Resuscitation fluids:** If the patient is haemodynamically unstable, start resuscitating using intravenous fluids, e.g. crystalloid, colloids or blood to improve those with low circulating volumes; replace cautiously in those with LVF.
  - **Additional monitoring:** Consider inserting a urinary catheter and/or central line to

help gauge fluid resuscitation and response. Continuous ECG monitoring may be required.

- **Treatment:** Reassess HR and BP regularly to check response to fluid boluses given; if well filled and still hypotensive, the inotropic support may be required to maintain BP; the inotrope used will vary depending on the cause of shock.

❑ **Assess Disability (D)**
- Assess the patient's neurological status, pupil size, and BM glucose levels.
- **Neurological status:** can be estimated using the GCS score; or the AVPU (Alert, Verbal response, response to Pain; Unresponsive).
- **Pupils:** are checked to detect cases of opiate overdose (bilateral pinpoint pupils), or for a blown pupil (unilaterally dilated pupil) in a space-occupying lesion.
- **BM glucose:** should be checked in case the neurological status is secondary to blood glucose derangement, which is easily amenable to treatment.

❑ **Assess Environment (E)**
- Expose the patient; this may help in your diagnosis.
- For example, the hypotensive patient may be actively bleeding and the lost blood is being hidden by the bed sheets. Another good reason to expose the patient is to check for rashes, as the patient may be hypotensive from anaphylaxis.

❑ **Assess response to initial measures**
- If something has changed, be it in breathing or circulation, always start from the beginning again and reassess the patient's ABCs.
- Likewise, if the patient is showing signs of improvement after treatment, reassess; there may have been a hidden pathology that can now be unmasked.

AUTHOR'S TOP TIP

If the examiner is probing you for an answer and you are unsure of what to do, the best reply in this situation is to say that you will go back and reassess the patient's ABCs to see if there is anything you have missed. This shows you are being systematic in your approach and will not miss out on any life-threatening injuries.

❑ **Emergency investigations**
- Investigations can be done to help aid your diagnosis, e.g. requesting an ECG in ACS
- These are divided into:
    — simple bedside tests – ECG, pregnancy test, BM glucose
    — blood tests – FBC, U&Es, etc.; ABG as appropriate (especially if critically ill)
    — imaging: portable bedside CXR; CT head
    — specialist investigations: these depend on your differentials.

❑ **Call for senior help and advice**
- Note that you are calling for senior help and advice once the patient is stabilised.

In actual clinical practice, once your seniors have arrived, they may refer the patient or ask you to refer to other specialties for advice, e.g. ITU. In the exam, it may be easier to state this at the beginning in case you forget to mention that you will call for help.

❏ **Definitive treatment**
- This can be either conservative, medical or surgical
- Depends on the cause; the acute upper GI bleed may need resuscitation followed by emergency endoscopic treatment

---

Case 1: Asthma exacerbation

Instructions: This 25-year-old woman, a known poorly controlled asthmatic, has presented to A&E resus with an acute exacerbation. How would you manage her?

Viva discussion

❏ **Recognise urgency**
❏ **Initial resuscitation:** Assess ABCs. Make an assessment of the severity of exacerbation; remember, this can change rapidly, so frequent reassessment is required including after all treatment is given
❏ **Call for help:** Remember to contact seniors early if patient not responding to treatment or deteriorating despite treatment
❏ **Additional monitoring/investigations:** saturations should be kept at 94%–98%; **PEFR:** useful to know their normal or best PEFR, however if not known you can use predicted value. **ABG** if deterioration or Sats < 92%. **CXR** only usually carried out acutely if suspicion of underlying driver for exacerbation, e.g. pneumonia, other pathology such as pneumothorax or those with a severe exacerbation not responding to medical therapy
❏ **Assess severity:** *see* Viva Q1
❏ **Definitive treatment**
- **Oxygen:** high flow, if required through non-rebreather bag to maintain Sats between 94% and 98%
- **Nebulised beta-2 agonist (salbutamol):** should be oxygen driven if available, can be given back to back if required
- **Intravenous salbulatmol:** can be given if severe or deteriorating asthma or patient unable to swallow
- **Nebulised antimuscarinic (iptratropium bromide):** used if severe asthma or poor response to beta agonist
- **Steroids:** oral prednisolone if mild or moderate, intravenous hydrocortisone if unable to swallow or very unwell
- **IV magnesium (1.2–2 g):** can be given as a bolus in those with severe asthma and those not responding to nebulisers
- **ITU referral:** criteria include those requiring ventilatory support or those with deteriorating severe asthma:
  - deteriorating PEFR despite treatment
  - refractory hypoxia
  - hypercapnoea
  - ABG analysis showing acidosis
  - patient tiring and unable to maintain adequate respiration
  - drowsiness, confusion, altered conscious state
  - respiratory arrest

Viva questions

Q1   How would you assess severity of acute asthma?

TABLE 11.1 Asthma severity

Severity	Description
Moderate	PEFR > 50%–75% best or predicted
	Increasing symptoms
Severe	PEFR 33%–50% best or predicted
	Respiratory rate ≥ 25/min
	Heart rate ≥ 110/min
	Inability to complete sentences in one breath
Life-threatening	PEFR < 33% best or predicted, SpO2 < 92%
	PaO2 < 8 kPa, normal $PaCO_2$ (4.6–6.0 kPa)
	Silent chest, cyanosis, poor respiratory effort
	Arrhythmia, bradycardia, hypotension
	Exhaustion, altered conscious level
	Near-fatal asthma: raised $PaCO_2$ and/or requiring mechanical ventilation with raised inflation pressures

Case 2: COPD exacerbation

Instructions: This 65-year-old woman, known COPD, attends A&E acutely breathless with a fever and productive cough. How would you manage her?

Viva discussion
- ❏ **Recognise urgency**
- ❏ **Initial resuscitation**
- ❏ **Call for help**
- ❏ **Additional monitoring/investigations:** oxygen saturations, ABG, temperature, **CXR** – to help to identify consolidation or signs of heart failure, **bloods** – FBC/U&E/CRP/LFTs
- ❏ **Definitive treatment**
  - **Oxygen:** if a known retainer of CO_2 – for 24%–28% controlled oxygen to reduce chance of CO_2 retention, aim for Sats of 88%–92%. If no evidence of CO_2 retention on ABG, can use higher percentage oxygen but must always be at a controlled percentage (venturi masks)
  - **Nebulisers:** salbutamol (beta-agonist) and ipratropium bromide (anti-muscarinic), salbutamol can be given repeatedly; ipratropium is a QDS nebuliser maximum dose
  - **Chest physiotherapy:** this is an underused resource in the hospital; there are on-call physiotherapists for this very reason
  - **Steroids:** oral or IV if very unwell and unable to swallow
  - **Antibiotic:** type will depend on local antibiotic guidelines, but usually a tetracycline or macrolide for infective exacerbation (i.e. pneumonia also present)
  - **IV aminophylline:** used if patients remain wheezy with poor response after

nebulisers. Need to take levels if on oral theophylline; patients require a loading dose followed by a maintenance infusion
- **ABG/ventilation:** taken regularly (up to every 15 minutes in acute treatment to assess response). If in decompensated type 2 respiratory failure despite optimal medical management, patient will need NIV or intubation as appropriate. You should be talking to a senior early if you see a pattern of deteriorating ABGs or a severely deranged ABG on initial testing. Early on, a ceiling of treatment needs to be decided to stop inappropriate escalation of care; this again should be done by the senior member of the team, which should also include a decision on resuscitation status
- **Doxapram:** can be given IV if NIV not available or not appropriate; acts centrally as a respiratory stimulant

Viva questions

Q1 What pertinent features in the history would you wish to know?
Patients with COPD may be presenting for the first time when you see them or have a long history of hospital admission with frequent exacerbations. It is useful to ask a few pertinent questions if able to quickly assess the severity of their COPD.
- Do they have home nebulisers?
- Do they have home O_2?
- How many exacerbations have they had in the last year that required hospital admission?
- Have they ever been intubated?

Case 3: Diabetic ketoacidosis

Instructions: You are called to review a 28-year-old woman, known type 1 diabetic, with high BMs. How would you manage her?

Viva discussion
- ❑ **Recognise urgency**
- ❑ **Initial resuscitation**
- ❑ **Call for help**
- ❑ **Additional monitoring/investigations: Bloods** – WBC/CRP, i.e. signs of precipitating infection; renal function, glucose. **Urine** – testing for urine and ketones. **ABG** – for pH to identify acidosis seen due to lack of insulin causing ketoacidosis. **CXR** – signs of infection
- ❑ **Definitive treatment**
  - IV fluid resuscitation with normal saline
  - IV insulin sliding scale
  - potassium replacement (intravenously)
  - early low molecular heparin, as patient will be intravascularly volume deplete and more likely to suffer with venous thrombosis

- not recommended to give bicarbonate to reverse acidosis, as this will not reverse tissue acidosis
- antibiotics if underlying sepsis
- once BM is 10–15 mmol/L, switch to dextrose-containing fluids
- will need regular pH, bicarb and BM monitoring to assess response to treatment

Type 1 diabetics are insulin deficient; therefore, if they do not take their regular insulin or increase their insulin sufficiently during illness, their body will switch to fat and protein metabolism, which in turn generates ketones and eventually an acidotic state.

Case 4: Alcohol withdrawal

Instructions: You are called to review a known alcoholic on the ward who appears to be acutely withdrawing. How would you manage him?

Viva discussion
❑ **Recognise urgency**
❑ **Initial resuscitation**
❑ **Call for help**
❑ **Definitive treatment**
- IV thiamine should in practice be given to all alcoholics on admission to emergency departments to help prevent Wernicke's encephalopathy. This can usually be switched to oral preparation after 5 days (e.g. vit B co strong and thiamine tablets), unless the patient is proved not to have Wernicke's. In practice, 48–72 hours is normally given.
- Oral benzodiazepines are used in a reducing regime to help the physical withdrawal (e.g. chlordiazepoxide); remember, quite high doses may be required initially for those with heavy alcohol intake.
- If a patient has a seizure, PR or IV benzodiazepines can be used; phenytoin is not recommended for the treatment of alcohol-withdrawal seizures.

Viva questions

Q1 How would you recognise acute withdrawal from alcohol?
Those who are withdrawing from alcohol often exhibit signs of sympathetic activation:
- tremor
- tachycardia
- sweating
- anxiety
- vomiting

If the physical withdrawal from alcohol is not treated, it can result in seizures which may cause further injury to the patient.

Case 5: Hyperkalaemia

Instructions: A known renal failure patient has been found to have a potassium of 7 mmol/L. How would you manage her?

Viva discussion

- ❏ **Recognise urgency**
- ❏ **Initial resuscitation**
- ❏ **Call for help**
- ❏ **Additional monitoring/investigations**
  - ■ **Bloods:** lab or near-patient testing of potassium levels, also need a full blood count to rule out pseudo-hyperkalaemia caused by high cell counts and subsequent lysis in blood tubes or lysis of normal samples; need urgent repeat to confirm level
  - ■ **ECG:** tall tented T waves, small or absent P waves, increased PR interval, eventually prolongation of QRS with sinusoidal pattern formation and eventually VF and cardiac arrest
- ❏ **Definitive treatment**
  - ■ stop medications associated with hyperkalaemia, e.g. spironolactone, ACE/ARB, NSAIDs
  - ■ 10 mL of 10% calcium gluconate IV given over 10 minutes – short-acting membrane stabiliser to stop VF. If the patient is on digoxin, you may need to give the infusion more slowly to prevent calcium-induced myocardial digoxin toxicity
  - ■ 10–15 units of fast-acting insulin (Actrapid) with 50 mL of 50% glucose IV. Remember 50% glucose is very irritating to veins and can cause phlebitis; ensure the cannula is well flushed. The glucose works by transporting potassium intracellularly. The effect lasts for about 4–6 hours and you can expect to see a drop in serum potassium of between 0.5 and 1 mmol/L
  - ■ salbutamol nebulisers can be used to reduce potassium levels in combination with insulin/glucose
  - ■ calcium resonium: resin which binds potassium in the gut and removes it from the body. Remember to give with water, not squash, as the electrolytes in squash bind to the resin and inactivate it
  - ■ dialysis: a rapid method of reducing potassium levels, may be needed if other measures fail, the patient is unstable or hyperkalaemia is due to renal failure
  - ■ stop foods containing high levels of potassium, e.g. fruit juices, chocolate

Case 6: Status epilepticus

Instructions: You are called to the ward, where a patient is found fitting. How would you manage this?

Viva discussion

- ❏ **Recognise urgency**
- ❏ **Initial resuscitation:** secure airway, apply oxygen
- ❏ **Call for help**

❑ **Additional monitoring/investigations**
  ■ **Bloods:** emergency BM, infection screen, electrolytes, renal and liver function, FBC
  ■ **CXR:** can be used to assess for aspiration when fitting
❑ **Definitive treatment**
  ■ IV thiamine (Pabrinex) if suggestion of alcohol abuse or nutritional deficiency
  ■ IV glucose if low BM or nutritionally compromised
  ■ Stages for seizure control
    — PR diazepam can be given initially before IV access is gained; 10–20 mg or 10 mg midazolam buccal
    — IV lorazepam 4 mg, repeated at 10 minutes
    — phenytoin infusion with loading dose IV
    — if seizure still not controlled, needs ITU referral for sedation with agents such as propofol

Viva questions

Q1 How do you define status epilepticus?
  ■ This is a generalised convulsion lasting 30 minutes or longer.
  ■ Or repeated tonic-clonic convulsions occurring over a 30-minute period without recovery of consciousness between each convulsion.

Case 7: Acute left ventricular failure

Instructions: You are called to the ward, where a patient with known heart failure is found acutely short of breath. How would you manage this?

Viva discussion
❑ **Recognise urgency**
❑ **Initial resuscitation:** high-flow oxygen; may need assisted ventilation, e.g. CPAP
❑ **Call for help**
❑ **Additional monitoring/investigations**
  ■ **ECG:** rate and rhythm, signs of ischaemia (ST-segment and T-wave changes, Q waves), evidence of hypertrophy, bundle branch block, abnormalities of QRS and QT
  ■ **Chest X-ray:** pulmonary oedema, cardiomegaly
  ■ **Arterial blood gas analysis:** note levels of oxygen, carbon dioxide and pH due to poor perfusion and tissue acidosis
  ■ **Bloods:** renal function, LFTs, FBC (anaemia may increase cardiac workload), electrolytes – low sodium and high creatinine levels are poor prognostic markers. Elevated troponin is associated with worse outcome. BNP is raised in heart failure
  ■ **Invasive monitoring:** central line (for central pressures), arterial line if patient very unstable

❑ **Definitive treatment**
  ▪ **Analgesia:** patient may be in pain due to an acute myocardial infarction precipitating pain; morphine as well as being analgesic reduces cardiac afterload
  ▪ **Offload the heart/reduce pulmonary congestion:** loop diuretics, e.g. furosemide, vasodilators, e.g. GTN
  ▪ **Coronary angioplasty:** if the driver is thought to be due to acute ischaemic change secondary to coronary insufficiency
  ▪ **Inotropes:** may be required if the heart is unable to maintain sufficient output, e.g. dobutamine, dopamine
  ▪ **Vasopressors:** not used first-line, but may be used in cardiogenic shock or when patient does not respond to inotropes and fluid resuscitation, e.g. noradrenaline

Acute heart failure (AHF) is defined as 'a rapid onset or change in the signs and symptoms of heart failure, resulting in the need for urgent therapy.'

Case 8: Acute coronary syndrome (ACS)

Instructions: You are called to A&E, where a patient with chest pain was found to have ACS. How would you manage this?

Viva discussion
❑ **Recognise urgency**
❑ **Initial resuscitation:** high-flow oxygen; may need assisted ventilation, e.g. CPAP
❑ **Call for help**
❑ **Additional monitoring/investigations**
❑ **Definitive treatment**

TABLE 11.2 Treatment of ACS

ST elevation MI (STEMI)	*Non-ST elevation MI (NSTEMI)*
Initial treatment:	**Initial treatment:** similar to STEMI, except there is no use of PCI or thrombolysis
1. Aspirin 300 mg & clopidogrel 300 mg	1. Aspirin 300 mg & clopidogrel 300 mg; then continue both at 75 mg OD
2. GTN	2. GTN
3. 1 mg/kg enoxaparin (low molecular weight heparin)	3. 1 mg/kg enoxaparin (low molecular weight heparin) if PCI not occurring within 24 hours, otherwise unfractionated heparin infusion
4. IV morphine	4. IV morphine
5. Beta blocker (cardioselective atenolol/ bisprolol) and statin	5. Beta blocker (cardioselective atenolol/ bisprolol) and statin
6. GP IIb/IIIa antagonist, e.g. tirofibran	6. GP IIb/IIIa antagonist, e.g. tirofibran; used if PCI planned within 96 hours of admission and patient has medium to high risk

(*continued*)

ST elevation MI (STEMI)	Non-ST elevation MI (NSTEMI)
Definitive treatment: primary coronary revascularisation or thrombolysis ± rescue PCI	**Coronary angiogram:** should instead take place within 96 hours of admission; sooner if clinically unstable or very high risk
Primary PCI: should be within 2 hours of first medical contact or earlier if patient presents early to hospital. Patients may need GP IIb/IIIa infusions if clot occlusion of coronary vessels noted	**Following on from this patient may be offered:** ● percutaneous coronary intervention (PCI) ● coronary artery bypass grafting (CABG) ● or conservative medical management if low risk or not appropriate for either of the above.
Subsequent to intervention: ● lifelong beta blockers/aspirin/statin ● 12 months clopidogrel ● ACEi if signs of heart failure in the early stage or they have LVEF < 40%.	

In all patients who you will treat under the ACS, their bleeding risk must be considered, as most of the agents will impair clotting and platelet aggregation and increase risk of bleeding. If there is an increased risk of bleeding, discussion with seniors or a cardiologist should be had to determine optimal anticoagulation on a case-by-case basis. Bleeding is more likely in: elderly, recent operation/trauma, renal or liver disease, cancer, varices and recent stroke.

Viva questions

Q1   What is ACS and the difference between STEMI and NSTEMI?
  ■ ACS covers the spectrum of cardiac conditions from STEMI to NSTEMI and unstable angina, which are differentiated by ECG and positive troponin results.
  ■ Treatment pathways have changed due to the increased availability of primary coronary intervention services, in most centres available as a 24-hour 7-day-a-week service, which has replaced thrombolysis as the treatment of choice in STEMI but also plays an important role in those with NSTEMI as well. Most centres have local policy as to how they will manage STEMI, so it best to check with your local hospital for their treatment pathway.

TABLE 11.3 ACS

	STEMI	NSTEMI	Unstable angina
ECG	ST elevation	No ST elevation	No ST elevation
Troponin	Positive	Positive	Negative

Q2   What are the indications for thrombolysis in STEMI?

Honours question

  ■ Chest pain and ECG findings of:
    — > 2 mm ST elevation in two or more chest leads
    — > 1 mm ST elevation in two or more limb leads

— ST depression of > 2 mm in V1–V3 chest leads (posterior infarction) with
  dominant R waves
— new left bundle branch block.

Q3 What risk factors are used to profile patients with NSTEMI/unstable angina into different treatment pathways?

Honours question

- history of cardiac sounding chest pain
- PMH – previous MI/PCI/CABG/diabetes/HTN
- smoking history
- haemodynamic instability – BP/HR
- ECG findings – ST depression/T-wave inversion, Q waves
- troponin results

CHAPTER 12

Radiology, clinical procedures & data interpretation

12.1 RADIOLOGY FOR FINALS

Undoubtedly, you will spend a great proportion of your house officer years in the radiology department, where your negotiation skills and ability to compromise are tested to their very limits. Having a basic knowledge of the various image modalities available and the key features you are looking for will not only give you good grounds to make your case for your patient but will place you highly in the mind of your friendly radiologist!

Our goal is not to teach you to review images like a radiologist; that is beyond the scope of this book and is certainly not required for finals. You must, however, bear in mind that a doctor encounters a wide variety of image modalities in their day-to-day clinical practice, and accurate interpretation of those images will in some cases decide on the treatment plans for the patients under your care. As a house officer, you will be the one asked to request these images and will probably be the first team member to review them.

AUTHOR'S TOP TIP

Depending on your hospital, plain film radiographs may not be immediately reported, and so it is important you have a good understanding of how to interpret them as well as be able to spot any gross pathology.

The most common image modality you will come across in the hospital setting is the plain film radiograph. It is highly likely therefore that you will be presented with a chest radiograph during your final clinical examinations. Here, we will discuss a common approach when addressing the plain radiograph presented to you during your exam in order to help you to achieve the maximum available marks. It has been noted that some medical schools have a separate OSCE station devoted entirely to this purpose. Increasingly, more technical image modalities are being assessed during finals, not so much to test your understanding of the radiological principles, but to assess your ability to detect obvious gross pathology, which in the exam can act as a starting point for further clinically orientated viva discussions.

In most cases, you are simply given an image and asked to comment on it with minimal if any history at all. We feel this makes the case unrealistic, as in clinical practise you would often have some form of history, even if it's just a brief handover from the ambulance crew. If you find yourself stuck, it is perfectly acceptable to ask for any further history that you feel may assist you in your diagnosis. However, in the exam it is likely that no additional history will be available and so the examiner will ask you to proceed. But do not be flustered by this; the diagnosis may only be one mark, so remain cool and carry on with your systematic examination; the examiners are looking for confident and competent individuals. Also be aware that you may be given a normal image. If you are struggling to find any pathology, then you are probably right. If so, then state in your summary that this image is normal. Medical finals also want to check that you can spot the normal patient, as the more normal films you see, the more likely you are to spot an abnormality, should it arise.

AUTHOR'S TOP TIP

Avoid the use of the word 'X-ray', as technically you cannot see X-rays but can see the resultant radiographic image. We advise using the word 'radiograph' instead.

General principles of image reporting

To begin describing any piece of imaging, always start with the basics first.

❑ **Image details**
  ▪ **Patient details:** Identify the patient's name, gender and age.
  ▪ **Image details:** The date the image was taken. You can also state whether it is a supine or erect film (this will normally be marked on the radiograph).

❑ **Assess the technical quality of the radiograph**
  ▪ **Projection:** Identify whether it is an AP (film behind the patient, X-ray machine in front of the patient), PA (film in front of the patient), lateral or oblique film.
  ▪ **Orientation:** Identify which are the left and right sides of the film; there will normally be a marker on the film with an 'R' on the right and 'L' on the left side of the film.
  ▪ **Rotation:** This depends on the film, e.g. in a chest X-ray (CXR) the medial ends of the clavicles should be equidistant from the spinous vertebral processes that fall between them.
  ▪ **Penetration:** If bone is too clearly visible, then the film is overpenetrated; if you cannot see the bony structures clearly then it is underpenetrated.
  ▪ **Degree of inspiration (for CXR interpretation):** There should be six anterior ribs or 10 posterior ribs visible to the level of the diaphragm. If a greater number are visible, then the lung fields are hyperinflated; if fewer, then there has been a less than normal inspiratory effort. A poor inspiratory effort can give the misleading appearance of cardiomegaly and basal shadowing when there is no actual pathology. This is commonly seen in patients who are unable to take a deep breath either due to pain or lung pathology such as pneumonia.

AUTHOR'S TOP TIP

Even if a film is poorly penetrated or if you find any other discrepancy with the image quality, try to avoid saying so, unless it is really difficult to interpret certain aspects of the radiograph. Radiographers do try really hard to get you a good image, and despite their best efforts, some patients can be unable or unwilling to allow this to happen! Remember also that a lot of these films will be the old films kept by consultants from the time before computerised images when light boxes were used to view films, and so handle them with care and treat them with respect. It may be their gem!

The basic densities which will be visible on a plain radiograph include:

TABLE 12.1 Image densities

Structure	Image density
Gas	Black
Fat	Dark grey
Soft tissue/fluid	Light grey
Bone/calcification	White
Metal	Intense white

Specific image evaluation

- Follow your systematic routine for evaluating each image modality.

Some candidates go for the most obvious pathology first; although this is acceptable, you must remember to go back and evaluate the whole radiograph systematically, as you do not want to miss out on more subtle abnormalities. This is particularly true of medical finals, where a systematic approach is far more important than the actual diagnosis. Remember, your ability to be methodical is what is being tested here and not your knowledge. However, for purposes of clarity and avoiding repetition, the cases in this chapter will be described using the former approach.

Completion

Once you have summarised your findings to the examiner, offer a differential diagnosis. We suggest you use this opportunity to start a viva discussion. In some cases, the topic for discussion will be obvious. For example, if you diagnose acute left ventricular failure, the examiner will most likely ask you how to manage this. In some medical schools, however, there are standardised set questions which every student is asked, and in many cases these are fairly predictable.

AUTHOR'S TOP TIP

Pre-empt the examiner and start the viva discussion yourself. This not only demonstrates your confidence, but you have the added advantage of directing the viva, allowing you to concentrate on your strong areas.

Reporting the plain film chest radiograph

❑ **General principles** (as above)
❑ **Examine the lung fields**
  ▪ Compare the size; will be reduced in collapse.
  ▪ Look for discrete opacities; compare one side to the other.
  ▪ Compare transradiancy; they should be the same colour. If one is whiter than the other, this suggests fluid as seen in a haemothorax or effusion. If one is more black, this may indicate a pneumothorax.
❑ **Check the hilum**
  ▪ Compare shape and density, remember the left will be higher than the right.
❑ **Assess the heart**
  ▪ The normal width should be less than half the transthoracic diameter. However, in an AP film you cannot comment on this, as the heart is falsely enlarged. Comment on shape as well as size.
  ▪ Identify the heart borders. Any blurring may suggest consolidation.
❑ **Look at the diaphragm**
  ▪ Normally, right is higher than the left, as it is pushed up by the liver. A very high position may suggest a diaphragmatic hernia.
  ▪ Look at the area under the diaphragm for a rim of air, which is seen in the perforation of a hollow viscus within the abdominal cavity.
❑ **Examine the costophrenic angles**
  ▪ These should be sharp and clear.
  ▪ May be blunted in the presence of an effusion, haemothorax, consolidation or collapse.
❑ **Identify the mediastinum**
  ▪ Should be centrally placed; it may be shifted in an effusion or pneumothorax.
❑ **Assess for tracheal deviation**
❑ **Look at the bones**
  ▪ Examine the vertebrae, ribs and scapulae for any decreased density or signs of fractures.
❑ **Look at the soft tissues**
  ▪ There may be pockets of air (surgical emphysema) or swelling.
  ▪ Particularly the presence of breast tissue, as there may be an absence of breast tissue on one side, indicating a previous mastectomy.
❑ **Comment on any invasive devices**
  ▪ There may be an endotracheal tube, central line, chest drain, metal heart valve, NG tube or even a permanent pacemaker in situ. You must mention these to the examiner, or they will assume incorrectly that you have not seen them.
  ▪ These are independent indicators that this patient is unwell, including the degree to which they are. Clearly, an endotracheal tube in situ indicates the patient is at the very least an ITU-bound patient.

AUTHOR'S TOP TIP

In finals, it is important that you state the obvious, even if you think it seems likely the examiner knows that you know. We can assure you that the examiner does not know that you know. You have to spell things out, because if you don't say it, you will not get the marks for it.

EXAMINER'S ANECDOTE

I remember having to point out to the candidate the PPM on the X-ray in front of him. To which he replied, 'Yes, I know.' I said, 'Well, I don't know that you saw that!' It is important that you clearly state what you see; we are not psychic!

Viva questions

Q1 You are the house officer on call and have been asked by the nursing staff to review a chest X-ray for a patient who has just had a feeding nasogastric tube inserted. Please review this film.

Difficult question

This is a surprisingly common request, and one which you will regularly come across when on call as a house officer. Unfortunately, it seems no one really tells you what it is you are actually looking for when reviewing these films. You must remember that the purpose of the NG is for feeding, and so it is imperative the tube is in the stomach and not the lungs, as missing this can lead to significant morbidity and mortality from an avoidable aspiration pneumonia.

- The NG tube will have its guide wire in place and so this should aid identification, as this is radiopaque.
- The tip of the NG should be below the level of the diaphragm. This suggests the tube must be in the stomach, as the pleura does not extend beyond the diaphragm.
- If the tip is proximal to the diaphragm, then this may mean the NG has passed through a pulmonary bronchus and into the lung, in which case you must remove the NG tube and resite, as well as repeat the X-ray.

You must thereafter clearly document in the notes that the NG is in situ and feeding can be started. In cases of doubt, it is best to remove and resite the NG tube, as this takes a matter of minutes. However, you can assess correct positioning clinically by aspirating the NG for stomach acid, which when applied to litmus paper will react accordingly. Other tests include auscultating over the stomach with your stethoscope for borborygmi, which is a noise heard on passing air through the entry port of the NG tube with a syringe full of air in through the stomach.

Q2 You have successfully inserted your first central venous catheter in the right internal jugular vein. The post-procedural CXR arrives and is awaiting your review. What are you looking for?

Difficult question

- **Assess position:** Right-sided necklines will be seen to go vertically down into the superior vena cava. If too far, they may enter into the right atrium, in which case they need to be pulled back; commonly, right-sided internal jugular lines are left in at 15 cm. Bear in mind that left-sided necklines will need to traverse further, and so will appear to kink around and into the super vena cava.
- **Look for complications:** Carefully look for a pneumothorax, which is a well-known complication of any neckline. Assess for signs of a haemothorax, as lacerations of the vena cava have been seen with disastrous consequences.

Another form this viva question may take is by simply stating you have inserted a central line; what would you do next? Surprisingly, many junior doctors do not know that a post-procedure chest X-ray is required after any necklines are inserted. However, of far more concern are those who follow rules blindly, as we have seen requests made for post-central line chest X-ray reviews in patients who have had femoral central lines inserted!

AUTHOR'S TOP TIP

If a patient complains of shortness of breath following a central line insertion, be wary of a missed pneumothorax, as initially the post-procedure review film may demonstrate a small pneumothorax which may have been missed, and your now breathless and cyanotic patient may have developed a much larger pneumothorax in the interim period. Clinical signs are far more important than radiological, and if in doubt, repeat the chest X-ray.

Sometimes, it is difficult to appreciate or clearly delineate a central line in the superior vena cava, as more often than not these patients are critically unwell, so chest X-rays may be poorly penetrated, rotated and in AP view. Therefore, of more importance is assessing for the complications mentioned above.

You may also mention in your answer that for completeness, you will take a brief focused history and examine the patient looking for the above signs and symptoms. In actual practice, however, this is rarely done.

Q3 This patient has returned to the cardiology ward after having had a permanent pacemaker inserted. The nursing staff have called you to review his CXR. What are you looking for?

Honours question

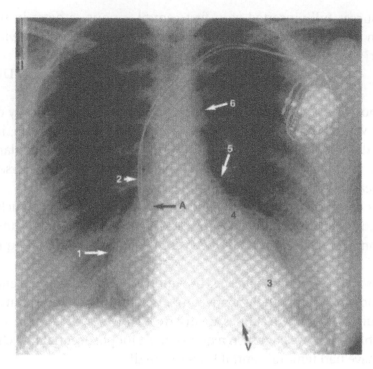

FIGURE 12.1 Pacing wires

- **Assess position:** The pacing wires should be seen to be positioned with the tip of the ventricular pacing wire in the ventricle and atrial wire in the right atrial appendage; the PPM is usually on the side of the non-dominant hand. Commonly this is on the left side, as most patients are right-handed.
- **Assess for complications:** Look for a haemothorax or pneumothorax.

Again, this is a common request in district general hospitals, requiring you to assess position and actively look for complications associated with this procedure, thereafter succinctly documenting your findings. A misplaced pacing wire will lead to non-functioning of the PPM, which is a possible complication, and you may be the first person reviewing the film to pick this up.

One of the authors remembers reviewing a chest X-ray in such a patient who had clinical signs of a pneumothorax, who was then shown radiologically to have a pneumothorax, requiring chest drain insertion. Therefore, do not underestimate the importance of making such checks.

You may also mention in your answer that for completeness, you will take a brief focused history and examine the patient, looking for the above signs and symptoms.

Case 1: Pneumonia

Instructions: This gentleman presented with productive cough and fever. Comment on his film.

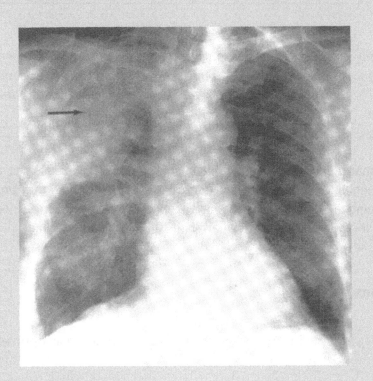

FIGURE 12.2 Lobar pneumonia

Key features to note

❏ *'This is a PA chest radiograph of patient x taken on x date.'*
❏ *'It is slightly rotated, but adequately penetrated with a good inspiratory effort.'*
❏ *'The most obvious abnormality is that of patchy shadowing in the right middle to upper zones.'*

Average response

❏ **The above plus:** *'This is most likely to be an area of consolidation in the right upper lobe due to pneumonia.'*
❏ *'There is an associated air bronchogram'* **(black arrow)**

Good response

AUTHOR'S TOP TIP

If you are unsure of which lobe is involved, then it is best to stick to zones. However, if you can work out which lobe is involved, then mention this in your answer. This will show you have a deeper understanding of the chest radiograph and will impress your examiners.

Completion

❏ *'This patient is likely to have lobar pneumonia. I would like to assess the severity of this using the CURB-65 scoring system, which will guide my management.'*

AUTHOR'S TOP TIP

By finishing your answer with this statement, you are likely to be asked about the management of pneumonia, as well as what the CURB-65 score is. This way, you are dictating the exam by convincing the examiners to ask you questions which you already know the answer to.

Remember that radiological signs of pneumonia lag behind clinical signs. So if your patient has signs suggestive of pneumonia with a clear chest X-ray, then they probably do indeed have a pneumonia. Occasionally, if your patient is severely dehydrated, consolidation may develop the following day after they have been given intravenous fluids.

Viva questions

Q1   How do you know this white shadowing is consolidation as opposed to anything else?

Difficult question

TABLE 12.1 Distinguishing features

Abnormality	Distinguishing features
Consolidation	**Whiteness:** non-uniform or patchy
	Borders: ill defined overall; however, can be well demarcated at lower edge (this is because fluid tends to fall with gravity)
	Others: presence of air bronchogram (air-filled small airways), transient nature of signs
Effusion	**Whiteness:** opaque whiteness or uniform shadowing
	Borders: well demarcated
	Others: presence of a meniscus
Fibrosis	**Others:** shadowing is more chronic, and so comparison of old X-rays will confirm its earlier presence
Collapse	**Whiteness:** opaque whiteness or uniform shadowing
	Borders: well demarcated

By far the easiest way to distinguish between the above is through a focused clinical history and examination. A productive cough with green sputum and fever is more likely to point towards consolidation than fibrosis. Ensure you state this in your answer also.

Q2   How can you identify which lobe is involved?

Honours question

Generally speaking, this is difficult to do and it is best to stick to zones when describing consolidation, as an appreciation of lobar anatomy is required for the former. However, certain patterns do make it more likely for one or more lobes to be involved.

- Blunting of the right heart border suggests right middle lobe involvement.
- A collapsed left lower lobe may lead to a 'sail' sign seen behind the heart on an AP film; classically, you will see deviation of the trachea and mediastinum to the left with rib crowding.
- The left heart border may be blunted when the left upper lobe collapses; occasionally in left upper lobe consolidation, there may be left shift of the trachea with consequent mediastinal displacement; there is a generalised increased density (veil-like shadowing) in the left upper zones.
- You may see a sharply demarcated horizontal border to the consolidation coinciding with the anatomical position of the horizontal fissure in a right upper lobe pneumonia; the horizontal fissure may also be pulled up.
- Collapse of lower lobes will lead to loss of the contour outlined by the hemidiaphragm, this is because lower lobes collapse posteriorly and inferiorly; in a right lower lobe collapse, the horizontal fissure may also be pulled down.

Patients with lobar pneumonia should be investigated further to assess whether there may be an underlying lung cancer or immunosuppression such as HIV. A more patchy distribution of shadowing throughout the whole lung suggests bronchopneumonia.

Although the terms pneumonia, consolidation and collapse tend to be used interchangeably, they actually have very specific meanings (*see* Viva Q3).

Q3 What is the difference between collapse and consolidation?

Difficult question

- Despite popular belief, these two words are not synonymous.
- Consolidation implies opacification as a result of fluid, blood or cells in the air spaces, and is therefore a component of collapse.
- Collapse occurs only when there is volume loss with the expected consequential displacement of anatomical landmarks.
- Collapse occurs due to a proximal obstruction from, e.g. foreign body, mucus plug or cancer.

AUTHOR'S TOP TIP

Collapse always has a cause, and this aetiology must be sought after.

Q4 What would you consider if the patient's pneumonia or shadowing on CXR is not resolving?
- Bronchogenic carcinoma

Average response

- Pulmonary fibrosis
- Empyema
- Pulmonary oedema

Good response

A repeat chest X-ray is often requested in patients who have had a radiological diagnosis of pneumonia 6 weeks after the initial film to look for an underlying bronchogenic carcinoma.

Q5 Do you know of any conditions that can cause a cavitating lesion on a chest radiograph?

Difficult question

- complications of pneumonia, i.e. cavitation around a pneumonia
- *Staphylococcus aureus*, tuberculosis and *Klebsiella* infections
- lung abscess, lung cancer and Wegener's granulomatosis
- Aspergilloma, rheumatoid nodules, lung infarction

Case 2: Pleural effusion

Instructions: This 84-year-old lifelong smoker presented with long-standing shortness of breath. Comment on his film.

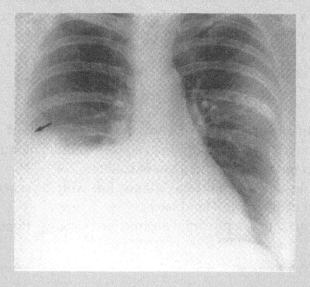

FIGURE 12.3 Pleural effusion

Key features to note
- ❏ *'This is a PA chest radiograph of 'patient x taken on x date.'*
- ❏ *'The most obvious abnormality is that of a pleural effusion'*

Average response

- ❏ *'The most obvious abnormality is that of a moderately large right-sided pleural effusion. There is mediastinal shift away from the effusion.'*

❑ *'The right lung field is white with a meniscal edge* [black arrow], *suggesting an effusion is the most likely diagnosis.'*

Good response

AUTHOR'S TOP TIP

Remember that you will need to be able to accurately describe such a film over the phone to a colleague who cannot view the films themselves. You must therefore be pedantic and use descriptors like right or left, estimating size whenever possible.

Completion

Although an effusion is the most likely cause, there are many other causes of such an appearance, e.g. consolidation, collapse or a raised hemidiaphragm and you should be able to distinguish between these. *See* Case 1, Viva Q1; Case 2, Viva Q1. For further details of pleural effusions, *see* Chapter 4, Case 3.

Viva questions

Q1   What features on any chest X-ray are suggestive of an effusion as opposed to any other differential diagnosis?

- **Whiteness:** Opaque whiteness or uniform shadowing in an effusion as opposed to heterogeneous or patchy shadowing in consolidation with an air bronchogram. The presence of an air bronchogram is typical of consolidation, not an effusion.
- **Mediastinal shift:** It is difficult to differentiate between collapse and an effusion, as in lung collapse the mediastinum shifts towards the affected side. It can be taken, therefore, that the absence of such a mediastinal shift is suggestive of an effusion. However, this is not always the case, as an effusion can occur with a collapse, and so this is an unreliable sign. With a moderate to large effusion, the mediastinum shifts away from the affected side. In the case of collapse due to, e.g. a proximal obstructing tumour with an associated ipsilateral pleural effusion, the loss of lung volume from the collapse may be greater than the increased volume of the hemithorax from the effusion, leading to an overall shift of the mediastinum to the right.
- **Meniscus:** In an erect film, there should be a visible fluid level and the presence of a meniscus, which is suggestive of fluid in the pleura; a lateral film allows the meniscus to appear more obviously. The upper outer border of the shadowing should therefore be concave in an effusion. Approximately 200 mL of fluid must be present for the normally sharp sulcus between the ribs and diaphragm to be effaced.

Remember to look at the chest X-ray for any obvious possible causes, such as cardiomegaly in heart failure, solid-mass lesions in the visible lung fields and particularly the apices for tuberculosis and lung cancer. The ribs and other bony structures may also shown signs suggestive of metastases.

Opacification of a hemithorax may also be due to complete lung collapse with mediastinal shift towards the affected side. A pneumonectomy can also lead to a complete white-out appearance on the ipsilateral side, due to fluid and fibrotic material accumulation occupying the now empty hemithorax.

Case 3: Cerebral infarction

Instructions: This 65-year-old diabetic and hypertensive gentleman presented with acute-onset left-sided weakness. His BP on arrival was 210/112 mmHg. He underwent CT scanning of his brain. Please comment on his film.

Difficult case

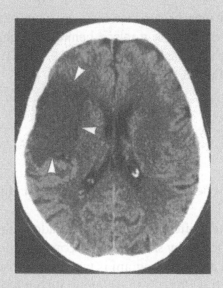

FIGURE 12.4 CT head of cerebral infarction

Key features to note

❑ *'This is a single slice of a CT brain of patient x taken on x date.'*
❑ *'The most obvious abnormality is that of an area of low attenuation in the right cerebral hemisphere in the temporoparietal region.'* [white arrows]
❑ *'There is some compression of the right lateral ventricle.'*
❑ *'In summary, these findings are consistent with an acute cerebral infarction in the territory of the right middle cerebral artery.'*

Honours response

Completion

This is a difficult case to comment on in finals, mainly because many students are unprepared for interpreting CT head scans. However, most examiners would have expected you to have at least identified that there is an abnormality in the scan fairly easily. From the brief history given in instructions alone, you should already be considering a CVA as your initial diagnosis, even before looking at the CT head.

Viva questions

Q1   How do you know this is an infarct versus a bleed?
- An acute bleed on an unenhanced (i.e. non-contrast) CT head will demonstrate an area of higher density than the surrounding brain, i.e. brighter/whiter.
- As the bleed becomes older, it becomes more isodense over a period of 1–2 weeks, thereafter eventually becoming hypodense (low attenuation) with respect to the surrounding brain parenchyma.
- The acute history is a key feature in helping distinguish this hypodensity as being an infarct.

Non-contrast CT head scanning is the investigation of choice in acutely unwell patients with focal neurological signs, due to its almost universal availability in UK hospitals, speed of testing and ability to exclude an acute bleed.

It must be remembered that within the first 6 hours of a cerebral artery infarction, the CT head may be normal. The purpose of scanning a patient within 24 hours of a suspected CVA is to exclude a bleed. An MRI head can then be performed in those with suspected infarction. Some specialist neurology centers offer hyperacute stroke services, whereby any patient with a suspected infarction undergoes early specialist goal-directed scanning and treatment, including thrombolysis, much like how acute ST elevation MI is managed in cardiac centres.

Case 4: Asbestos plaques

Instructions: This gentleman who worked his entire life in a naval dockyard had a chest radiograph as an inpatient when he presented with an upper GI bleed. Comment on his film.

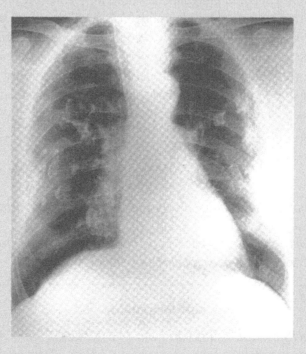

FIGURE 12.5 Asbestos plaques

Key features to note

❑ 'This is a PA chest radiograph of patient x taken on x date.'
❑ 'There are multiple lesions in the lung and a central line in situ.'

Average response

❑ 'This is a PA chest radiograph of patient x taken on x date.'
❑ 'It is well centred, with a good inspiratory effort; however, the film is poorly penetrated but adequate.'
❑ 'The most obvious abnormality is that of multiple calcified pleural plaques bilaterally.'

Good response

❑ **The above plus:** 'There is also a central venous catheter in the right internal jugular vein entering the SVC. I cannot see the distal tip, and hence its terminal location (due to poor penetration of film); however, it appears to be correctly positioned. There is no haemo- or pneumothorax on the ipsilateral side.'
❑ 'In summary, these lesions are most likely due to previous asbestos exposure.'

Honours response

AUTHOR'S TOP TIP

The difference between an average, good and honours response is clear. Although stating the same pathology, it is the level of detail and accuracy with which this is mentioned, e.g. the central line location not only being in the internal jugular vein but stating the important identifier of 'right side' does make a significant difference. Although to some, this may seem pedantic, even in postgraduate exams differentiating and stating whether left or right side, counts as marks and easy marks which are all too often forgotten or missed by good candidates. Some candidates believe to be awarded honours you need to talk about the latest scientific evidence or have a postgraduate level of knowledge, but this is simply not the case. Doing what you normally do but with accuracy and competence is more than enough to be awarded top marks. Evidence-based medicine and knowledge beyond the syllabus is more suited for gold-medal awards.

Completion

❑ 'In summary, this patient has bilateral pleural plaques, which is consistent with a diagnosis of asbestos exposure.'
❑ 'The patient also has a central venous catheter in situ, most probably related to his upper GI bleed, which is likely to be guiding fluid resuscitation.'

AUTHOR'S TOP TIP

Although not directly related to this particular OSCE station itself, you may be asked regarding the emergency management of an upper GI bleed. There are both medical and *surgical aspects to its treatment. However, it is important to remember to state that you would resuscitate the patient according to ABCs, which is essentially what the examiners are looking for. Note that the presence of a CVP line in this case highlights that the patient is likely to be unwell. A detailed overview of management of emergency upper GI bleeding is covered in our companion text,* The Ultimate Guide to Passing Surgical Clinical Finals.

Although you would not be expected to know much about asbestos exposure, this is an important case which highlights the need for being able to recognise esoteric signs on a chest X-ray, as sometimes, fair or not, these films do crop up in finals. However, it would have been enough to simply describe the lesions to pass the exam, but recognising that they are pleural plaques, and better yet, that this suggests asbestos exposure, means you are doing far better than the average response to this case.

Viva questions

Q1   What features make you think these are pleural plaques?

Honours question

- Pleural plaques are areas of pleural thickening due to asbestos fibres.
- Several features help differentiate them from other lung shadows.

TABLE 12.2 Features suggestive of pleural plaques

Feature	Description
Distribution	Typically axillary and midzones
	Sparing of upper zone and costophrenic angle
	Bilateral lesions
	Peripherally located
Shadowing	Patchy shadowing or calcification (map-like appearance)
	Well-demarcated margins
	Lesions along diaphragm tend to be calcified
Longevity	Lesions may be visible on previous X-rays

Asbestosis can cause cryptogenic fibrosing alveolitis, a form of pulmonary fibrosis. Asbestosis occurs from occupational exposure, classically a lifelong shipyard or factory worker. The effects take over 20 years to notice. Patients suffer from restrictive lung disease and are at an increased risk of developing lung cancer.

Such a diagnosis is important to document, as in the UK there are industrial injury benefits available for such patients. Asbestos exposure can also lead to mesothelioma.

Chest X-ray findings for asbestos include a honeycomb appearance in advanced disease to multiple irregular opacities in the lung fields. A pleural effusion, pleural plaque and pleural calcification will also be seen in asbestos-related benign pleural disease, whereby patients in general are asymptomatic and the features are coincidental findings on a routine chest X-ray done for another reason.

Case 5: Bronchogenic carcinoma

Instructions: This 78-year-old gentleman presents with haemoptysis and weight loss. Comment on his film.

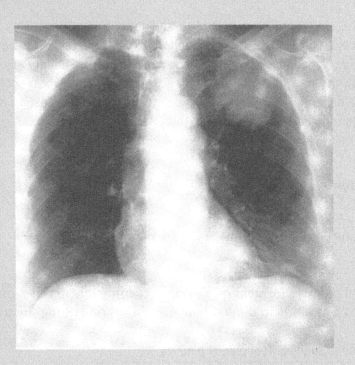

FIGURE 12.6 Coin lesion

Key features to note

❏ *'This is a PA chest radiograph of patient x taken on x date.'*
❏ *'It is well centred and adequately penetrated with a good inspiratory effort.'*
❏ *'The most obvious abnormality is that of a large well-demarcated irregular lesion in the left upper zone; it measures x cm by x cm.'*
❏ *'This is most likely due to a bronchogenic carcinoma; however, my differentials would include . . .'.*

Viva questions

Q1   What are your differential diagnoses for a coin lesion?
   ■ A metastatic deposit from an unknown primary cancer.
   ■ This could be an area of consolidation, e.g. a left upper lobar pneumonia, if based on this particular CXR.

- This could be tuberculosis, or a tuberculous abscess. These lesions tend to be seen in the upper zones; a corroborating clinical history would help guide you towards this diagnosis.
- A lung abscess due to, e.g. *Staphylococcus* species, *Klebsiella*, etc.
- A benign hamartoma, rheumatoid nodule.
- An infarction.

A coin lesion is a term used to describe any well-demarcated discrete opacification within a lung field. Although there are many possibilities, it is important to get across to the examiner that your primary consideration would be to exclude a lung cancer, in which case most patients would go on to have a CT chest and specialist referral to a respiratory physician. Remember, if you are asked how you would manage this patient, always begin by saying you would take a clinical history, asking specifically about night sweats, weight loss and haemoptysis, amongst many other symptoms, as well as performing a clinical examination of the chest and investigate methodically.

Q2 How would you distinguish a malignancy from any other cause of shadowing on a chest X-ray?

Difficult question

TABLE 12.3 Malignant versus benign opacification

Feature	Description
Cavitation	If there is a central darkness within this lesion suggestive of a cavitating lesion, then consider other causes of cavitating lung disease
Calcification	The presence of areas of calcification within the lesion (i.e. more densely white, e.g. like bone) is rarely found in malignancy
Lesion edge	Irregular, spiculated and/or a lobulated lesion suggests malignancy
Plurality	If there is more than one lesion, this is highly suggestive of metastatic disease, e.g. cannonball metastases are classically due to renal cell carcinoma
Comparison with previous films	If a previous film demonstrates the presence of this lesion and no change in size, particularly if there has been a long gap such as a period of years, then it is highly unlikely to be cancer
	If the lesion has increased in size or was not present earlier, you should consider cancer
Others	**Air bronchogram:** if present, this suggests an area of consolidation
	Lymphadenopathy: mediastinal lymphadenopathy suggests malignant tumours
	Bony metastases: suggests malignancy

AUTHOR'S TOP TIP

A commonly asked question in finals is what the differentials are when presented a patient with a widened mediastinum. Aside from aneurysms, you should mention bronchogenic carcinoma, lymphoma, thymoma and even thyroid goitres are possible causes.

Case 6: Left ventricular failure

Instructions: This lady was admitted to the ward yesterday with an acute myocardial infarction. You have been called to review her, as she has become increasingly short of breath. Comment on her film.

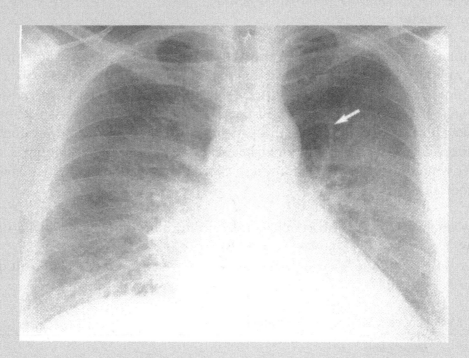

FIGURE 12.7 Acute left ventricular failure

Key features to note

❏ *'This is a PA chest radiograph of 'patient x taken on x date.'*
❏ *'The most obvious abnormality is that of cardiomegaly with Kerley B lines (horizontal septal lines) at the peripheries.'*
❏ *'The upper lobe blood vessels are dilated and prominent.'* [white arrow]
❏ *'There is a small pleural effusion.'*
❏ *'There is "bat's wings"-type hilar shadowing consistent with pulmonary oedema.'*
❏ *'In summary, my findings are consistent with a diagnosis of left ventricular failure.'*

Good response

AUTHOR'S TOP TIP

If it is obvious to you that the film demonstrates acute pulmonary oedema and you know the classical signs of LVF on chest radiography, then mention each of these terms in your description, as this not only shows to the examiner that you know the signs but that you are also actively looking for them. This is particularly true of Kerley B lines, which if you didn't specifically look for, you probably wouldn't have noticed otherwise.

Completion

A common point of discussion would be the management of acute left ventricular failure (*see* Chapter 11).

Viva questions

Q1 What are the CXR features of left ventricular failure?
- **Alveolar shadowing:** Bat's wings appearance is suggestive of pulmonary oedema.
- **Kerley <u>B</u> lines:** These are horizontal, non-branching white lines found peripherally, superior to the costophrenic angle. They occur due to oedema of the interlobular septa.
- **Cardiomegaly:** This suggests heart failure. The heart diameter normally should not be more than 0.5 of the cardiothoracic ratio. In acute LVF, the heart may not be enlarged.
- **Upper lobe blood <u>D</u>ilation:** Normally, the upper lobe blood vessels are narrower than the lower lobes. If wider, then this is the first sign of heart failure on an erect film.
- **Pleural <u>E</u>ffusion**

Non-cardiogenic pulmonary oedema may lead to a very similar-looking CXR; however, the heart size is likely to be normal.

Case 7: Pericardial effusion

Instructions: This 67-year-old gentleman was booked for an elective inguinal hernia repair. As part of his preoperative evaluation, a routine chest X-ray was performed. Comment on his film.

Difficult case

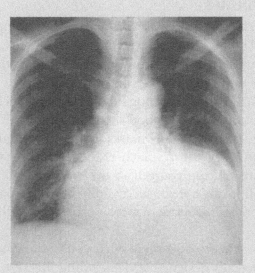

FIGURE 12.8 Pericardial effusion

Key features to note

❑ *'This is a PA chest radiograph of patient x taken on x date.'*
❑ *'The most obvious abnormality is that of cardiomegaly, which is globular in shape covering both hila.'*
❑ *'This is most likely to be due to a pericardial effusion.'*

Completion

Normally, there is 15–50 mL of fluid in the pericardial space acting as a natural lubricant for the visceral and parietal layers of the pericardium. A pericardial effusion is the presence of an abnormal amount and character of fluid in the pericardial space, of which there are many causes. They can be acute or chronic, and this determines the clinical symptomatology with which they present. Rapidly accumulating effusions will have more acute symptomatology in comparison to slowly progressing effusions, even in those up to 2 L in volume, which can be asymptomatic. ECG will demonstrate low-voltage complexes, and an echo is diagnostic.

Viva questions

Q1   What are the causes of a pericardial effusion?
- idiopathic
- infectious: TB, HIV, viral (Coxsackie virus, hepatitis), fungal, protozoal
- neoplastic: malignant effusions, e.g. lung, breast, lymphoma
- iatrogenic: post-cardiac surgery
- others: trauma, acute MI with free wall rupture, aortic dissection, rheumatoid arthritis, rheumatic fever, SLE, drug associated, e.g. phenytoin

This list is not exhaustive.

12.2   CLINICAL PROCEDURES

Performing practical procedures in OSCEs for finals is becoming more and more popular. Indeed, venepuncture and taking blood cultures are featured even in postgraduate membership exams. Therefore, do not underestimate the importance of doing these procedures confidently and competently. Despite what you may see on the wards, which may or may not be what is required to pass in an OSCE setting, learning how to perform such tasks properly early on in your career will enable you to maintain good such habits in the future. Much like the history and examination stations, there are many marks to be awarded just by your approach to the case and remembering some key features, such as always washing your hands before and after the clinical encounter, introducing yourself to the 'patient' and demonstrating good communication skills. After all, being able to successfully bleed the patient is only but one mark.

Below, we describe some of the more common procedural skills you may be asked to perform in medical finals.

It is important to remember to document what you've done in the clinical notes. Indeed, some NHS trusts have specially designed stickers aiding this very task, whilst enabling audit traceability. Also, for the more invasive procedures such as central lines, the lot number of the catheter used is an important identifier to document so that this can be easily traced in case there are equipment problems in the future. It also acts as a medicolegal statement of what you have performed in case of future complications.

AUTHOR'S TOP TIP

Always mention in the OSCE that you will document what you have done. It is a commonly forgotten but easy mark to gain in the exam.

Procedure Case 1: Venepuncture

Instructions: This 24-year-old woman is being seen in the clinic for chronic anaemia. This is her blood request form. It says she needs a full blood count (FBC). Please take blood.

Introduction

As for any clinical encounter (*see* Chapter 1, Section 3); specifically for this case:

❑ **Gain consent:** Explain what you are proposing to do and ensure that the patient is happy for you to take blood from them.

❑ **Identify patient:** Check that you are taking blood from the correct patient, as errors can happen and misinterpreting the wrong blood results taken from the wrong patient can have disastrous consequences for your patient.

AUTHOR'S TOP TIP

At the bedside before you take blood, ensure you have the correct blood request form and always remember to countercheck the patient details with the patient's wristband. Do not prelabel blood bottles; this should be done at the bedside, after you have taken the blood.

❑ **Wash your hands**

❑ **Maintain aseptic technique:** Remember, this procedure needs to be done under aseptic conditions, as you have the potential to introduce infection, so ensure you wear gloves and clean the area with alcohol wipes.

❑ **Expose patient adequately:** Try to take blood from the non-dominant hand; in the exam, you are likely to have a dummy prosthetic hand only, and so this limits your options.

❑ **Prepare your equipment**

  ▪ **Sharps bin:** this is commonly forgotten and is a very important piece of equipment when taking blood, as sharps injuries can occur.

  ▪ **Ensure you have:** tourniquet, alcohol wipe, vacutainer, swabs, gauze bandage/plaster, gloves, tape, blood request form.

  ▪ **Blood bottles:** correctly identify and use the blood bottles for the test you require. The FBC will be a purple bottle (*see* Viva Q below).

With the ever-increasing exposure of infection-control protocols, there has been a move towards preprepared venepuncture packs, with disposable single-use tourniquets and swabs. This is, however, unlikely to be the case in the OSCE. More commonly, there may be a trolley with a lot of different equipment available and you need to select and place everything on a tray, which is to be taken to the patient's bedside.

In the OSCE, it is best to use the vacutainers, as they are fairly easy to assemble and in most cases being able to get blood back from the patient will be fairly easy on the prosthetic arms, without the need for seeing a 'flashback'. In actual clinical practice, however, there are varying methods for taking blood; some like to use butterfly needles or a basic needle and syringe. Do note that the needle-and-syringe method is not recommended in the OSCE, as the risk of a sharps injury is much higher.

❑ **Position patient appropriately:** lay the arm on a pillow

Procedure

❑ **Don gloves & apply tourniquet**
❑ **Identify vein**
- Examine the arm for palpable or distended veins.
- They are most easily located in the antecubital fossa, forearm or on the dorsum of the hand.

AUTHOR'S TOP TIP

Some find it easier to palpate for veins without gloves on. Do whatever feels easiest for you. However, don't forget to put both your gloves back on when taking blood, as not doing so will not be looked upon favourably by the examiner and in some marking schemes results in an automatic fail.

AUTHOR'S TOP TIP

Being able to 'feel' the vein is far more important than 'seeing' the vein. This is particularly true in patients whose arms are hairy.

❑ **Clean the area**
- Using an alcohol swab or ChloraPrep, swab the skin over the anticipated puncture site.
- Leave this to air-dry; do not blow or hand-dry.
❑ **Use the vacutainer**
- Assemble the vacutainer, if not already done.
- Hold skin taught and insert needle at a 30-degree angle, advancing until a 'give' is felt; this implies you are in the vein.
- Attach the appropriate blood bottles for investigation to the vacutainer and remove each bottle in turn when the bottle has filled up to the required volume; this is denoted by a black mark on the side of the bottle.

❑ **Remove tourniquet**
❑ **Withdraw needle**
- Use gauze to apply pressure over the puncture site whilst simultaneously removing the needle.

❑ **Dispose of needle in sharps bin**
- Do this immediately upon withdrawing the needle.
- The sharps bin should be ideally positioned close to you to enable this process to be swift and safe.

❑ **Apply bandage**
- Apply a bandage over the puncture site, or apply gauze and tape to stop the blood from oozing.

❑ **Label blood bottles**
- At the bedside, hand-label the bottles.
- A minimum of date, time, patient name, hospital number and date of birth is normally required.
- Countersign the request form that you have taken the blood, along with your bleep number.
- Tip the blood collection bottles upside down several times to enable mixing.
- Place them into biohazard transparent transfer bags and either place them in a collection box, ready to be transported to the pathology lab, or place them in the transfer chute in a pod. In the OSCE exam, the former is more likely.

Some hospitals will have computer printout stickers designed specifically for the blood bottle and so do not require separate request forms or handwritten details. In general, however, most hospitals do not have this facility. Also, do not be tempted to use the patient labels meant for clinical notes. Some bottles require handwritten details whatever the case; specifically group and save bottles.

If a patient is known to be HIV-positive or has any other infection risk such as hepatitis C, then there is a 'high risk' tick box on the request form that should ideally be filled in, so as to warn lab technicians to be extra-vigilant when handling the samples.

Completion

❑ **Thank the patient**
❑ **Wash your hands**
❑ **Document the procedure**

Although perhaps the most basic of clinical procedures you will perform as a doctor, it is undoubtedly the most commonly performed, particularly as a house officer, and will remain so for the remainder of your careers. It is therefore good to learn to be proficient to take blood in your final year at medical school just before you start your foundation year training.

There are many tricks of the trade when dealing with patients who have difficult veins for taking bloods. In some cases, simply trying a different site such as the other hand or feet, or using smaller needles such as blue butterflys solves the dilemma. Patients with difficult veins would in general be difficult to take blood from using a vacutainer; it is easier to identify that you are in a vessel with a flashback method, and this is only really possible with a needle/

syringe or butterfly. If despite all of this, it is very difficult and the examiner is still probing to see what you would do, say that you would always seek senior help and advice, but that a femoral vein stab is a possibility, but only as a last resort. And if this is not possible, then seek expert advice from an anaesthetic colleague.

Renal patients in particular should be approached with caution. Never take blood from their AV fistula; it may seem tempting, but we assure you, you will regret this! This is their lifeline or may be in the future, so do not compromise its integrity or future use by using a vein which could be later utilised for fistula creation. Always speak to the renal team before taking bloods from their patients; they will gladly give you strict guidelines on what can be used.

IV drug users frequently have terrible veins as a consequence of their drug use. If you ever need to take blood from an IV drug user and you cannot identify a vein, ask the patient, as often they will know the best veins to use.

AUTHOR'S TOP TIP

When on your clinical placements always take the initiative and ask to be supervised doing this procedure as junior doctors would be more than happy to delegate this task to you; this is the best way to learn.

Viva questions

Q1   Which blood bottles are for which commonly ordered tests?
- **Purple:** haematology, e.g. FBC
- **Pink:** G&S
- **Yellow:** biochemistry, e.g. U&Es, LFTs, troponin
- **Blue:** coagulation studies, e.g. clotting screen, INR

Of note, there are some variations between hospitals, but in general these coloured tubes correspond to the above tests. If in doubt, call the respective labs and ask, e.g. call the biochemistry lab regarding troponin sample bottles.

If you use a vacutainer, fill plain blood bottles first, as the anticoagulant from the blue coagulation screen bottle if used first can contaminate and cause errors in subsequent samples. Also, do not take blood from the same arm that has an intravenous infusion running through it, as this will cause spurious results.

Procedure Case 2: Peripheral vein cannulation

Instructions: This 42-year-old woman has been admitted with severe dehydration. She requires a cannula for intravenous fluids. Please place a drip in her arm.

Introduction

As for any clinical encounter (*see* Chapter 1, Section 3); specifically for this case:

❑ **Gain consent:** Explain what you are proposing to do and ensure that the patient is happy for you to cannulate them.

❑ **Identify patient:** Check that you are placing a cannula in the correct patient by verbally checking the patient's details when introducing yourself and reading the patient's wristband before performing the procedure.

❑ **Wash your hands**

❑ **Maintain aseptic technique:** Remember, this procedure needs to be done under aseptic conditions, as you have the potential to introduce infection, so ensure you wear gloves and clean the area with alcohol wipes.

❑ **Expose patient adequately:** Try to place the cannula in the non-dominant hand; in the exam, you are likely to have a dummy prosthetic hand only, and so this limits your options.

❑ **Prepare your equipment**

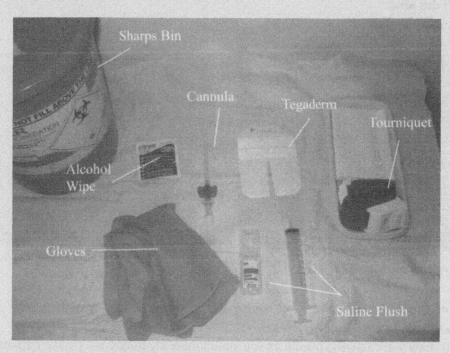

FIGURE 12.9 Cannulation equipment

- **Sharps bin**
- **Ensure you have:** tourniquet, alcohol wipe, swabs, gauze bandage/plaster, gloves, tape, tegaderm dressing, saline flush.
- **Cannula:** there are many different sizes, and used for different purposes. In the exam, we suggest you select pink, which is the most commonly used size.

With the ever-increasing exposure of infection-control protocols and minimising MRSA infections, there has been a move towards preprepared cannulation packs with disposable single-use tourniquets and swabs. This is however unlikely to be the case in the OSCE. More commonly, there may be a trolley with a lot of different equipment available, and you need to select and place everything on a tray, which is to be taken to the patient's bedside.

AUTHOR'S TOP TIP

The dressing will have a sticky label meant for dating the insertion time. This is for infection-control purposes, as peripheral cannulae should be removed and resited after being in situ for a maximum of 3 days. This is likely to have been incorporated into current OSCE marking schemes, so remember to date your cannulas.

❑ **Position patient appropriately:** lay the arm on a pillow

Procedure
❑ **Don gloves & apply tourniquet**
❑ **Identify vein**
❑ **Clean the area**
❑ **Cannula insertion**

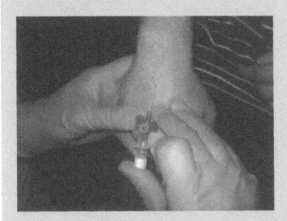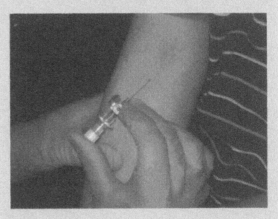

FIGURE 12.10A-B Using a cannula

- Hold the skin taught and insert needle at a 30-degree angle, advancing until a 'flashback' is seen.
- Carefully withdraw the needle as you simultaneously thread the plastic catheter over this needle into the vein.
- Release the tourniquet, as blood will rush out of the cannula otherwise.
- Remove the needle entirely whilst placing swabs underneath the cannula so that any blood is soaked up while you attach the cap.
- Ensure you place the needle directly into the sharps bin immediately.

AUTHOR'S TOP TIP

Some like to compress the tip of the catheter when removing the stylet and screwing on the stopper cap, so that blood doesn't spill over onto the patient. In the exam, it would be difficult to compress the veins in the prosthetic arm, so we advise you to avoid this technique and use swabs instead.

❑ **Check patency**

- Flush the cannula with 10 mL of normal saline.

Ensure you tell the patient they will feel a cold rush of water, but that if it hurts to let you know, as this may indicate the cannula is incorrectly sited or has tissued.

❑ **Secure cannula**

- Apply a tegaderm to fix the cannula in place.

❑ **Documentation**

- Date the cannula insertion; place sticker over dressing.
- Preprepared stickers are now available in hospitals as part of infection-control policy.
- Otherwise, state to the examiner that you would document in the notes what you have done, noting the size of cannula, date of insertion and site.

Completion

❑ **Thank the patient**

❑ **Wash your hands**

This is a procedure which with practice you will become very skilled at performing. Some patients will be very difficult to cannulate, and there are various methods available to make their veins more prominent. This ranges from using GTN spray to placing their arms in a hot-water bowl. Sometimes, the simplest solution is the best; patience in allowing the vein to become prominent with the hand dependent is all that is needed in most cases. Lightly tapping the vein or area may make veins appear more prominent.

Viva questions

Q1   What would you do if you could not cannulate this patient?
In the OSCE, the examiner is likely to ask you what you would do if you found it difficult to cannulate and your patient needed intravenous access urgently. If after attempting the opposite arm or feet, state that you would seek senior help and advice, which may even include speaking to anaesthetics or ITU for help, particularly if your patient is in extremis or periarrest, as their venous access experience will be invaluable. Although central venous access is ideal, with femoral venous cannulation relatively quick, it is seldom performed quickly enough to gain access in cases of extremis. However, the examiner is looking for you to say that in such extreme situations, a venous cut-down of the long saphenous vein is a possibility and that in children, the intraosseous route is an option.

TABLE 12.4 Examples of cannulae

Cannula	Details
Blue	22G; low flow rates (25 mL/min), ideal for children or patients with difficult veins
Pink	20G; standard for routine use, most intravenous infusions, including blood transfusion
Green	18G; faster flow rates (90 mL/min), ideal for blood transfusion, giving fluids quickly
Grey/orange	16G & 14G, respectively; high flow rates up to 250 mL/min. Standard for use in obstetrics or emergency/trauma cases where patients are shocked or bleeding profusely and need massive fluid resuscitation

See our companion text, *The Ultimate Guide to Passing Surgical Clinical Finals*, for more on intravenous cannulae.

Procedure Case 3: Arterial blood gas sampling

Instructions: This known COPD patient has been admitted to the ward acutely short of breath. You call the medical registrar on call, who asks you to do an ABG on this patient and inform him of the results. Please perform an arterial blood gas.

Introduction

As for any clinical encounter (*see* Chapter 1, Section 3); specifically for this case:

❏ **Gain consent**
❏ **Identify patient**
❏ **Wash your hands**
❏ **Maintain aseptic technique**
❏ **Expose patient adequately:** if taking a femoral artery approach, you will need to expose the groin.
❏ **Prepare your equipment**
  ▪ Ensure you have a tray containing local anaesthetic with needle and syringe, 22G needle, swabs, tape, alcohol wipe, sharps bin, ABG syringe (*see* below).
  ▪ **ABG syringe:** Usually, this is a self-filling 1.5- to 2-mL syringe, containing electrolyte-balanced heparin (60–80 IU); this is not for injection. Some come with a 22G needle, others do not, and are therefore not self-filling, so will require a needle to be attached and aspiration applied when using.

Procedure

❏ **Palpate artery**
  ▪ **Radial artery:** With two fingers, palpate the radial aspect of the wrist where the artery lies fairly superficial and proximal. It lies medial to the radial styloid and lateral to the flexor carpi radialis tendon, 2 cm proximal to the wrist crease.
  ▪ **Femoral artery:** This is at the mid inguinal point, which is a point halfway along the inguinal ligament running from the ASIS to the pubic tubercle. This is fairly deep, so will require a longer needle and firm pressure to palpate.

The radial artery is commonly used, as it is easily accessible and can have local pressure applied post-procedure. The femoral artery tends to be used in emergencies for easy access, e.g. cardiac arrest. Brachial and dorsalis pedis arteries can also be used.

❏ **Perform modified Allen's test**
- With the patient's arm raised straight up, apply firm pressure over the radial and ulnar arteries to cause occlusion.
- The patient is to clench their fist several times until the palmar skin blanches.
- Pressure over the ulnar artery is released whilst maintaining radial artery occlusion.
- Take note of the time for the arm to reperfuse.
- Repeat the test, only this time release pressure over the radial artery whilst maintaining occlusion of the ulnar artery and note time to reperfusion.

This is to confirm sufficient ulnar collateral blood supply to the ipsilateral hand.

AUTHOR'S TOP TIP

This is a commonly forgotten test and will definitely be looked upon favourably by examiners if mentioned. It is however unreliable and has a poor positive predictive value for limb ischaemia.

❏ **Don gloves:** preferably sterile, but can be non-sterile gloves.
❏ **Clean the area:** use ChloraPrep solution or alcohol wipes and allow to air-dry.
❏ **Drape the area**
❏ **Apply local anaesthetic**
- Palpate the artery again and either just lateral to or superficial to this area where you will insert your needle, infiltrate with local anaesthetic with an orange needle.

Having an arterial blood gas taken is a painful procedure and is rarely appreciated by patients who have them regularly, such as frequent attenders with exacerbations of their COPD. The authors have met many such patients who will absolutely refuse an ABG even when acutely unwell; therefore, LA is a very sensible solution to this dilemma and your patients will be grateful. You will see in actual clinical practice that many patients have an ABG without LA. This may be acceptable if the patient has an easily palpable artery and you are certain you will hit the artery in the first pass cleanly. In the exam, however, we advise you at the very least to offer LA to the patient or demonstrate that this would be your usual practice.

❏ **Direct arterial puncture**
- Stabilise the artery with your fingers.
- Hold the syringe like a pen and insert distal to your applied finger at a 30- to 45-degree angle.
- Advance slowly until you see flashback, after which if you are in the vessel the self-filling syringe should fill in a pulsatile manner; if it does not, then withdraw or advance further until this occurs.

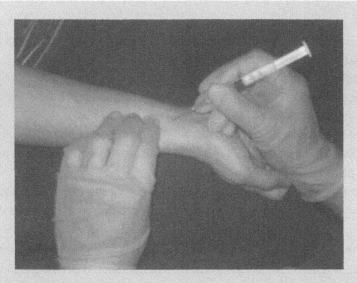

FIGURE 12.11 ABG sampling technique

- ■ Withdraw the needle entirely when a sufficient volume of blood is obtained. Most ABG machines required at least 0.5 mL of blood for analysis; most syringes are 1–2 mL.
- ■ Apply firm pressure over the puncture site with gauze for 3–5 minutes, after which you should tightly tape the gauze to the puncture site (remember to return after ABG analysis and release this pressurised tape).
- ■ Dispose of sharps in sharps bin.
- ❏ **Remove air bubbles**
  - ■ Attach the cap to the syringe and ensure any air bubbles are removed, as this will falsely raise the pO_2 during analysis.
- ❏ **Send for analysis**
  - ■ Tip the syringe upside down several times before analysis.
  - ■ You will either need to take the sample to the ABG machine for immediate testing or place in ice if you will test later.
  - ■ Take note of the fraction of inspired oxygen the patient was breathing, i.e. if the patient was on any supplemental oxygen or breathing room air.

Completion
- ❏ **Thank the patient**
- ❏ **Wash your hands**
- ❏ **Document the procedure**

If an artery is difficult to locate, then USS guidance should be considered. Sometimes it is difficult to tell whether a sample is venous as opposed to arterial. Blood colour is not as helpful as you may think. Darker samples may also be found in hypoxic patients. The oxygen saturations on the ABG result will be a helpful indicator, as a low saturation of 60% is more likely to be venous.

Viva questions

Q1 What are the indications for arterial blood gas sampling?
- monitoring of acid-base status in, e.g. diabetic ketoacidosis
- identification of any respiratory, metabolic or mixed acid-base disorders
- measuring arterial pO_2 and pCO_2 to assess adequacy of ventilation and oxygenation

The above is not exhaustive, but certainly represents the more common reasons, as there are many. There are some contraindications to ABG sampling, which include relative contraindications, such as coagulopathy or anticoagulant therapy, excluding aspirin use. Absolute contraindications include patient refusal, an abnormal Allen's test, severe peripheral vascular disease, an AV fistula or local site infection.

Q2 What are the possible complications of arterial blood gas sampling?
- haematoma
- local site tenderness
- LA anaphylaxis (if using local anaesthetic)
- infection at puncture site
- air embolism, arterial vasospasm
- vasovagal response
- arterial thrombus and subsequent embolisation or limb ischaemia
- median nerve damage from a brachial artery approach

Most patients have an adequate collateral arterial circulation to their hand, however this is variable and should arterial thrombosis occur and an Allen's test was positive, the limb is likely to become ischaemic.

Procedure Case 4: Prescribe antibiotics

Instructions: You have been asked by your consultant to prescribe intravenous Augmentin 1.2 g three times a day for the next 2 days for this patient with a urine infection. Please prescribe using this drug chart.

Introduction

❑ **Identify correct patient**
- The drug card should have at least three patient identifiers, usually the name, date of birth and hospital number.

❑ **Assess allergy status**
- There is normally an area on the drug chart in red notifying healthcare providers regarding the patient's allergy status.
- Check this first, but always confirm with the patient verbally if they have any allergies.
- Document any new allergies and the specific reaction, e.g. rash, anaphylaxis.
- If there are none known, then document no known drug allergies (NKDA).

Remember that Augmentin is co-amoxiclav, which contains penicillin. It is not unknown for

OSCE stations to have penicillin allergy documented on the drug chart, only for students to prescribe Augmentin. The station may simply be testing your ability to be a safe doctor and for you to recognise this oversight by your senior. The follow-up to this would be that you would seek an alternative antibiotic after discussing with your senior colleague or the microbiologist.

❑ **Prescribe drug**

REGULAR PRESCRIPTIONS			Month			Year		
			Date					
		Time						
Drug (Approved Name)		02						
CO-AMOXICLAV		[06]	Signed Staff Nurse					
Dose	Route	Frequency	08					
1.2 g	**iv**	**TDS**	12					
Additonal Information/Indication		[14]						
UTI; switch to oral in 2/7		18						
Signature/Print Name	Date	Pharm.	[20]					
FY1 DOCTOR	**8/8/11**		24					

FIGURE 12.12 Drug chart

- **Correct section:** this is a regular drug for the next few days and should be written in the regular prescription section of the drug chart
- **Generic names:** avoid use of trade names whenever possible
- **Date started:** the date prescription is to start; if you anticipate an end date, then mark this out as well; this is particularly relevant to antibiotics when you know the course is for x number of days
- **Dose:** legibly write out the dose and units, taking care not to confuse micrograms (mcg) with milligram (mg); it is better to write out 'micrograms'; it is better to write out the word 'units' as opposed to documenting 'U'
- **Route:** in this case, intravenous (IV); abbreviations are commonly used
- **Frequency:** this is three times a day (tds); ensure you circle the times the drug is to be given
- **Specific instructions:** whether the drug needs to be taken with food, or any other instructions you wish to give, such as withhold drug if systolic BP < 90 mmHg
- **Signature:** if it is not signed, the drug will not be given by nursing staff; at the very least, your surname, signature and a contact bleep number is required

---

AUTHOR'S TOP TIP

Write legibly or in capitals and use black ink.

TABLE 12.5 Commonly used abbreviations

Feature	Abbreviations
Routes of administration	po: by mouth
	iv: intravenously
	pr: rectally
	sc: subcutaneously
	im: intramuscularly
	neb: nebulised
	inh: inhalational
Dosage	iu: international units
	g: grams
	mg: milligrams
	T: one tablet or one puff
	TT: two tablets or two puffs
Frequency	stat: immediately
	prn: as required
	od: once a day
	bd: twice a day
	tds: three times a day
	qds: four times a day
	mane/om: in the morning
	nocte/on: at night

Completion

There are many reasons for prescription errors, but an easily rectifiable one is in taking care when writing dosages and avoiding any ambiguity. If in doubt, write it out! There is no harm in writing out in words any prescription instructions if you feel there may be confusion. This is especially true when it comes to insulin prescriptions, as it is very easy to confuse 4U (4 units) with 40 units.

Drug charts normally have various sections for the different urgency and frequency of drugs; some drugs even have their own specific dedicated sections, such as warfarin for anticoagulation; also, the 'regular prescription' section for usual drugs taken daily, e.g. anti-hypertensives or antibiotics over a period of a few days or longer; the 'as needed' or PRN section normally located at the back page containing drugs to be given whenever the patient needs them, e.g. analgesia such as morphine. There is a 'stat prescription' section for drugs that are to be given immediately, usually emergency drugs or a single one-off drug. Fluid prescriptions are occasionally part of the drug chart as well, although some hospitals have separate fluid prescription charts.

However, the most commonly prescribed drug in clinical practice, oxygen, is often forgotten, even though there is, again, a dedicated section on the drug chart for supplemental oxygen prescription.

This station could easily have had an empty drug chart on top of the instructions already given to you, and you would have to complete the allergy status and write the patient details in the chart as well as prescribe antibiotics. Prescribing fluids, warfarin or insulin sliding scales have been known to come up in finals.

Verbal prescriptions over the phone are a necessary part of hospital medicine, as of course you cannot be in more than one place at one time. This is acceptable for some common prescriptions, such as paracetamol or intravenous fluids, but you must sign for it as soon as possible and not make a habit of it, as drug errors are more likely to occur.

Procedure Case 5: Blood pressure measurement

Instructions: This known hypertensive attends the GP clinic for routine measurement of his blood pressure. Please take a manual blood pressure recording.

Introduction

As for any clinical encounter (*see* Chapter 1, Section 3); specifically for this case:

❑ **Maintain rapport**
- Inform the patient that the cuff when inflated may cause some discomfort, but that this will be short-lived.

❑ **Position patient**
- The patient's arm should be at heart level; this is easiest achievable by placing their arm on the desk or holding their arm in your arm at heart level if there is no desk to lean on.

❑ **Locate brachial artery**
- Palpate over the medial aspect of the arm, 2 cm superior to the antecubital fossa.
- The artery lies between the medial epicondyle of the humerus and the biceps brachii tendon, located in the antecubital fossa.
- It can be felt higher in between the groove of biceps and triceps tendon.

❑ **Prepare equipment**
- Manual blood pressure machine.
- Appropriately sized cuff; too small or too big for the patient's arm will cause an inaccurately high or too low a reading.
- The cuff markings will help orientate you as to how to apply the cuff around the patient's arm, including which side is to the patient, and that the bladder of the cuff should be over the artery.
- Stethoscope.

❑ **Palpate approximate systolic BP**
- Palpate either the brachial or radial artery, and inflate the cuff to the point where you can no longer feel the arterial pulsation.
- This is an estimate of the systolic pressure.

❑ **Take blood pressure**
- Repeat as above, with the estimated systolic pressure in mind, and inflate the cuff to 20 mmHg above this point.
- Release the pressure by 2 mmHg every second until you can hear the first Korotkoff sound.
- The first sound indicates the systolic blood pressure.

- When the sound disappears or becomes muffled, this indicates the diastolic pressure.
- Record readings to the nearest 2 mmHg.

Completion
☐ **Thank the patient**
☐ **Wash your hands**

You may wish to offer to measure the blood pressure with the patient standing up or in the opposite arm. There are some classical associations with blood pressure measurements (*see* table below)

TABLE 12.6 Blood pressure readings

Conditions	Blood pressure
Aortic stenosis	Narrow blood pressure e.g. 140/120
Aortic regurgitation	Wide blood pressure e.g.160/40
Aortic dissection	Difference on either arm, e.g. L arm (160/100) R arm (100/60)

Procedure Case 6: Death certification

Instructions: You are called by the bereavement office to complete the death certificate for this 84-year-old gentleman who died from a chest infection; his past medical history includes diabetes and high cholesterol. His notes are available for your perusal.

Key features to mention
☐ **Ability to complete form**
- You have seen the patient within 14 days of their death.
- Patient was > 18 years old.
- Patient was seen after death by you or another medical practitioner.
- Are there grounds for referring to coroner? If so, you cannot fill in the certificate and must discuss with the coroner on duty.

AUTHOR'S TOP TIP

Remember, you can only fill in a death certificate for a patient whom you have seen in the previous 14 days before their death.

- **Fill in the certificate**
  - name of deceased

- date of death and patients age
- place of death: the hospital name
- last seen alive by you
- time interval between onset of condition and death: normally the duration of hospital stay
- **Cause of death:** fill in to the best of your knowledge
  - **I(a) Disease or condition directly leading to death:** bronchopneumonia
  - **I(b) Other disease or condition if any leading to (a)**
  - **I(c) Other disease or condition if any leading to (b)**
  - **II. Other significant condition contributing to the death but not related to the disease or condition causing it:** diabetes mellitus

Completion

This type of scenario lends itself well to a short case procedural assessment. After completion of any death certificate and documentation to that effect in the notes, you need to go and see the patient in the morgue to identify them and confirm absence of a pacemaker, if the patient is to be cremated.

Do not use abbreviations, use question marks or include diagnoses in I(a) that include the word 'failure' in general. Section I(a) is where the disease that actually caused death should be documented, not the mode of death, e.g. heart failure or in this case respiratory failure. The subsections I(b) and I(c) should read in a logical sequence of events, i.e. I(c) led to I(b), which caused I(a), which led to death. For example, I(c) Osteoporosis, which led to I(b) Fractured neck of femur, which led to I(a) Pulmonary embolism.

Old age can be used as a cause of death but only in those > 70 years old and after you have discussed with the consultant in charge.

Do not feel obliged to fill in all subsections and look hard through the patient notes to find suitable diagnoses to document; I(a) is all that is required at the very least.

There are many grounds for referring a death to the coroner. These include, but are not limited to, death within 24 hours of admission to hospital, unknown cause of death, violent or suspicious death, death intraoperatively, death in police custody, or when death may be due to an industrial disease, abortion, suicide or an accident, and when the patient has not been seen by the certifying doctor within 14 days before their death or after their death.

The coroner is also a very useful resource to you if you are not sure what to document for the cause of death and have already spoken to your seniors. By going through the case history with the coroner and discussing what you think may be the cause of death, and assuming you do not think there are grounds for referral to a coroner for investigation, the coroner will then, in collaboration with yourself, offer you what to document on the certificate. The bereavement officers are also an invaluable resource, as they have seen countless doctors filling in certificates and can tell you straight away if your certificate will be rejected; therefore, always get them to read over what you plan on documenting before you write on the certificate.

Q1   How do you certify or confirm death?

- **Response to verbal or painful stimulus:** Patient does not respond to your commands and does not react to a painful stimulus, e.g. sternal rub.
- **Absent arterial pulse:** Palpate the carotid artery for 1 minute.
- **Auscultate for absence of heart sounds:** Listen for 3 minutes over the precordium.
- **Assess for absence of breath sounds:** Listen for 3 minutes over the anterior chest wall bilaterally and in the axilla.
- **Assess for presence of pacemaker:** Palpate the chest wall bilaterally for the presence of a pacemaker and make a note of this in the patient record.
- **Assess pupils:** Look for dilated and non-reactive pupils to light.
- **Documentation:** State that you would clearly document your findings, including the time you certified the patient deceased, as this will be taken as the legal time of death.

Some physicians document what they think the cause of death is and/or give suggestions as to what should be written on the death certificate. This is not advisable unless you know this patient and are part of the team taking care of them. The reason for this is the doctor filling in the certificate is usually someone other than the one who initially certified the patient deceased, and if when presented with the notes sees this, they may feel tempted to copy it verbatim, the caveat being that it could be inaccurate and require an amendment later, further delaying the burial/cremation process and adding undue stress upon the deceased's family.

Do not be tempted to write any personal or religious views on death or the deceased in the notes when reviewing a patient for death certification. We have come across actual notes whereby doctors certifying death have written with the best intentions in mind – 'Rest in Peace' or 'RIP' – and this has been criticised by family members. There is no need for such comments in the notes; you must remain impartial, no matter what your thoughts on death are. Your well-intentioned actions may well be seen in a completely different light.

12.3   DATA INTERPRETATION

Increasingly test results are being incorporated into clinical finals. The OSCE format helps make this achievable particularly after performing a clinical procedure as part of an overall clinical encounter. This can take the form of a short viva question after performing venepuncture whereby the candidate is presented with a sheet containing blood results and asked to interpret them. Below we describe several possible investigation results that you may come across in finals.

Blood Test Case 1: Urea and electrolytes

Instructions: The following are U&E results for several patients, please interpret.

TABLE 12.7 Urea and electrolyte readings

Normal value	A	B	C
Na			
(135–145 mmol/l)	149	148	129
K			
(3.5–5 mmol/l)	6.6	4.7	2.9
Urea			
(2.5–6.7 mmol/l)	15.7	37	11.1
Creatinine			
(70–150 μmol/l)	309	165	72

Interpretation

A. **Raised urea, creatinine and potassium:** renal failure

B. **Disproportionately raised urea to creatinine:** consider gastrointestinal (GI) bleed, dehydration or steroid use

C. **Raised urea, low sodium and potassium:** dehydration possibly due to vomiting or lack of oral intake

Complete the examination

AUTHORS TOP TIP

You would not be expected to memorise normal ranges for most of the blood results you will be asked to interpret, as the ranges will almost certainly be provided. However, having a general idea of what is grossly abnormal is always helpful.

It is important to remember that with any abnormal results, especially if unexpected, to take a repeat sample. However if the result is clearly dangerous, you should err on the side of caution and treat as required. Whilst a potassium of 7 mmol/l would require emergency treatment, in a previously well patient with a prior normal potassium and no obvious medical cause, a repeat sample is worthwhile sending, as haemolysis or any other cause of a spuriously high potassium could well be the reason for this unexpected artefact result.

The pattern of any previous results is also just as important as this will give you a clue to the underlying pathology. A chronically high creatinine over a period of weeks and months will alter your differential diagnosis in a patient who you may have previously thought had acute renal failure, but is more likely to have chronic kidney disease (CKD).

The weight and relative size of the patient is important when interpreting the creatinine as a creatinine of 120 μmol/l may be significant in an elderly patient who weighs under 50 kgs.

Blood Test Case 2: Full blood count

Instructions: The following are FBC results for several patients, please interpret.

TABLE 12.8 Full blood count results

Normal value	A	B	C
Haemoglobin (Hb)			
(13–18 g/dl Male; 11–16 g/dl Female)	13.5	9.5	8.9
MCV (76–96 fl)	89	92	70
White Cell Count (WCC) (4–11 × 10⁹/l)			
	18	11	10.6
Platelets			
(150–400 × 10⁹/l)	267	507	297

Interpretation

A. Raised WCC: infection, inflammation, steroid therapy or stress response; it is important to look at the differential, a neutrophilia suggests bacterial infection, lymphocytosis suggests viral infection and eosinophilia suggest parasitic infection

B. Low Hb, raised platelets: active bleeding, probable GI in origin (reviewing the patients U&Es would help aid in this diagnosis)

C. Low Hb, low MCV: microcytic anaemia most commonly due to iron deficiency, but can be anaemia of chronic disease; check ferritin, iron and transferrin levels; haemoglobin electrophoresis if suspicious for thalassaemia

ECG Case 1: Myocardial infarction

Instructions: This 56 year old male presented with central crushing chest pain. Please interpret his ECG.

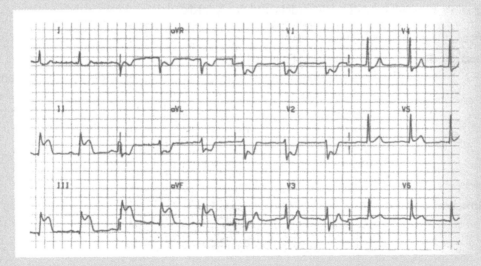

FIGURE 12.13 Inferior MI on ECG

Interpretation:

TABLE 12.9 ECG findings

Feature	Findings
Rate	66 bpm
Rhythm	Sinus; P waves are present
Axis	Normal
Durations	**PR Interval:** prolonged – 1st degree heart block
Morphology	**ST Changes:** ST elevation in leads II, III and aVF (inferior leads) and ST depression in leads V1–V2 (anterior leads)

'In summary these findings are consistent with an acute inferior myocardial infarction with lateral wall ischaemia.'

Completion

The leads of the ECG can help delineate where the infarction has occurred. This is because they represent areas supplied by the coronary arteries.

TABLE 12.10 ECG lead territories

Leads	Territories
II, III and aVF	Inferior leads; right coronary artery lesions
V1 and V2	Anterior leads; left main stem or left anterior descending artery lesions
V5 and V6	Lateral leads; left circumflex lesions

Occasionally, you may be asked about rhythm abnormalities you may see on any ECG no matter what else the pathology may be. It is useful to have an idea of what the common causes of a bradycardia and tachycardia are.

TABLE 12.11 Aetiology of tachycardias and bradycardia

Heart Rhythm	Common Causes
Bradycardia	**Physiological:** athletes (sinus bradycardia)
	Pharmacological: rate limiting drugs, e.g. betablockers, calcium channel blockers, digoxin
	Pathological: cardiac conduction, i.e. 1st, 2nd and 3rd degree heart block (this has many causes including: IHD, electrolyte imbalances, MI, cardiac fibrosis, amongst others)
	Other: sick sinus syndrome, hypothyroidism, hypothermia
Tachycardia	Atrial fibrillation or flutter
(Irregular rhythm)	Atrial and ventricular ectopic beats
	Endocrine: hyperthyroidism, phaeochromocytoma (can cause either regular or irregular)

(continued)

Heart Rhythm	Common Causes
Tachycardia **(Regular rhythm)**	**Sinus tachycardia:** following recent exertion, e.g. exercise
	Cardiac: supraventricular tachycardia (SVT), fast atrial fibrillation with 2:1 or 3:1 conduction block, ventricular tachycardia
	Abnormal conduction pathways: e.g. Wolff-Parkinson-White
	Pharmacological: caffeine, alcohol
	Metabolic: sepsis, dehydration, shock
	Endocrine: hyperthyroidism, phaeochromocytoma

ECG Case 2: Pulmonary embolism

Instructions: This patient presented acutely short of breath. Please interpret the following ECG.

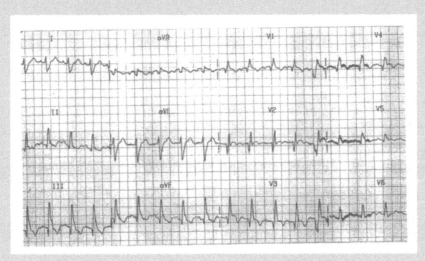

FIGURE 12.14 PE on ECG

Interpretation

TABLE 12.12 ECG findings

Feature	Findings
Rate	120 bpm
Rhythm	Sinus; P waves are present
Axis	Right axis deviation
Durations	**PR Interval:** Prolonged – 1st degree heart block
Morphology	**QRS complexes:** Right bundle branch block (RBBB), deep S wave in V1, Q wave in III
	T wave: T wave inversion in lead III

There is a classical but rarely seen S1, Q3, T3 pattern, suggestive of pulmonary embolism. However remember that the most common ECG finding in PE is in fact sinus tachycardia.

ECG Case 3: Left bundle branch block

Difficult Case

Instructions: This gentleman with an extensive cardiac history presents with cardiac chest pain. This is his ECG, please interpret.

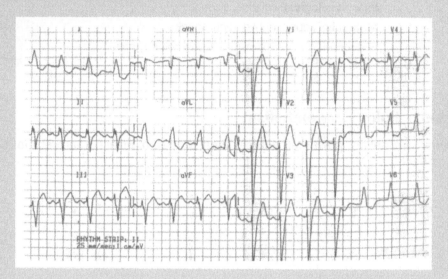

FIGURE 12.15 LBBB

Interpretation:

TABLE 12.13 ECG findings

Feature	Findings
Rate	100 bpm
Rhythm	Sinus; P waves are present
Axis	Left axis deviation
Durations	**QRS Interval:** >120ms
Morphology	S wave in V1
	R wave in V6 and lead I

'In summary, these findings are consistent with left bundle branch block (LBBB).'

Completion

A useful but simplified way of remembering the difference between left and right bundle branch blocks in the exam is that for RBBB, there is an M and W pattern on gross morphology, whereas for LBBB it is W and M.

RBBB: M a **RR** o **W**

LBBB: W i **LL** ia **M**

ABG Case 1: COPD

Instructions: The following are ABG results for several COPD patients, please interpret.

TABLE 12.14 ABG results COPD

Normal values	A	B	C	D
pH (7.35–7.45)	7.29	7.38	7.40	7.20
pO$_2$ (9.3–13.3 kPa)	7.8	7.5	7.2	7.0
pCO$_2$ (4.7–6.0 kPa)	7.4	5.8	6.6	7.5
Base excess (−2 to +2)	4	2	10	−5
HCO$_3$ (21–27 mmol/l)	28	26	36	15

Interpretation:

A. **Type 2 respiratory failure:** uncompensated respiratory acidosis – typical of an acute exacerbation of COPD that is admitted to hospital. Is a candidate for non-invasive ventilation (e.g. BiPaP) if this gas was obtained after medical optimisation, e.g. nebs/steroids

B. **Type 1 respiratory failure:** can be seen in mild COPD exacerbations, needs controlled oxygen therapy (24–28%)

C. **Type 2 respiratory failure:** compensated respiratory acidosis with metabolic alkalosis – can be seen in long standing COPD, often as a baseline blood gas

D. **Type 2 respiratory failure:** mixed respiratory and metabolic acidosis – can be seen in acute exacerbation of COPD, where underlying infection or hypoxia precipitates metabolic acid production, e.g. lactic acid

ABG Case 2: Asthma

Instructions: The following are ABG results for several asthmatic patients, please interpret.

TABLE 12.15 Asthma ABGs

Normal values	A	B	C
pH (7.35–7.45)	7.48	7.40	7.32
pO$_2$ (9.3–13.3 kPa)	10.0	9.5	8.7
pCO$_2$ (4.7–6.0 kPa)	3.5	5.8	6.6
Base excess (−2 to +2)	0	0	−2
HCO$_3$ (21–27 mmol/l)	25	25	24

Interpretation:

A. **Respiratory alkalosis:** due to an acute increase in respiratory rate, the patient 'blows off' extra CO_2 whilst trying to maintain oxygen saturations

B. **Special case:** don't be fooled by a relatively normal looking gas if the patient looks clinically unwell. The patient is probably tiring as seen by the normal/high CO_2 levels. This patient needs urgent senior review and repeat ABGs

C. **Type 2 Respiratory failure:** patient is no longer able to maintain ventilation (through a combination of non-compliant airways and fatigue; they need to be transferred to HDU/ITU for intubation and ventilation

Index